ROUTLEDGE HANDBOOK ON THE GLOBAL HISTORY OF NURSING

The *Routledge Handbook on the Global History of Nursing* brings together leading scholars and scholarship to capture the state of the art and science of nursing history, as a generation of researchers turn to the history of nursing with new paradigms and methodological tools.

Inviting readers to consider new understandings of the historical work and worth of nursing in a larger global context, this ground-breaking volume illuminates how research into the history of nursing moves us away from a reductionist focus on diseases and treatments and towards more inclusive ideas about the experiences of illnesses on individuals, families, communities, voluntary organizations, and states at the bedside and across the globe. An extended introduction by the editors provides an overview and analyzes the key themes involved in the transmission of ideas about the care of the sick. Organized into four parts, and addressing nursing around the globe, it covers:

- new directions in the history of nursing;
- new methodological approaches;
- the politics of nursing knowledge;
- nursing and its relationship to social practice.

Exploring themes of people, practice, politics, and places, this cutting-edge volume brings together the best of nursing history scholarship, and is a vital reference for all researchers in the field, and is also relevant to those studying on nursing history and health policy courses.

Patricia D'Antonio is the Killebrew-Centis Endowed Term Chair in Undergraduate Nursing Education, and Chair at the Department of Family and Community Health at the University of Pennsylvania, USA. She is the editor of the *Nursing History Review*, official journal of the American Association for the History of Nursing.

Julie A. Fairman is the Nightingale Professor of Nursing and Director of the Barbara Bates Center for the Study of the History of Nursing at the University of Pennsylvania, USA.

Jean C. Whelan is Adjunct Associate Professor of Nursing and the Assistant Director of the Barbara Bates Center for the Study of the History of Nursing at the University of Pennsylvania, USA.

ROUTLEDGE HANDBOOK ON THE GLOBAL HISTORY OF NURSING

Edited by Patricia D'Antonio, Julie A. Fairman
and Jean C. Whelan

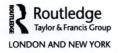

Routledge
Taylor & Francis Group

LONDON AND NEW YORK

First published 2013
by Routledge
2 Park Square, Milton Park, Abingdon, Oxon, OX14 4RN

Simultaneously published in the USA and Canada
by Routledge
711 Third Avenue, New York, NY 10017

Routledge is an imprint of the Taylor & Francis Group, an informa business

British Library Cataloguing in Publication Data
A catalogue record for this book is available from the British Library

Library of Congress Cataloging in Publication Data
Routledge handbook on the global history of nursing / edited by Patricia D'Antonio, Julie A.
Fairman, and Jean C. Whelan.
pages cm
1. Nursing–History–20th century. I. D'Antonio, Patricia, 1955– editor of compilation.
II. Fairman, Julie, editor of compilation. III. Whelan, Jean C. (Jean Catherine) editor of
compilation. IV. Title: Handbook on the global history of nursing.
RT31.R68 2013
610.7309–dc23
2012047333

ISBN: 978-0-415-59427-1 (hbk)
ISBN: 978-0-203-48851-5 (ebk)

Typeset in Bembo
by Keystroke, Station Road, Codsall, Wolverhampton

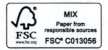

Printed and bound in Great Britain by
TJ International Ltd, Padstow, Cornwall

CONTENTS

CONTRIBUTORS

Katherine Abbott is a Research Scientist at the Polisher Research Institute and visiting Scholar at the University of Pennsylvania. As a Social Gerontologist, her research focuses on the social networks and health of older adults receiving long-term services and supports. She is now working on new methods for measuring social integration among cognitively impaired older adults residing in nursing homes, assisted living facilities, and dementia special care units.

Geertje Boschma is Associate Professor in Nursing at the University of British Columbia. Her research focuses on the history of nursing and mental health care. Current projects include the transition to community mental health services and the emergence of general hospital psychiatry in the latter half of the 20th century. She explores the ways in which nurses, other health professionals, clients, and families have experienced these changes and contributed to them. Her recent publications include refereed articles in *Histoire Social/Social History* (Volume 44, 2011) and *Nursing History Review* (Volume 20, 2012).

J. Margo Brooks Carthon is an Assistant Professor at the University of Pennsylvania School of Nursing. Her research focuses on early 20th-century racial health disparities and community health organizing. She is currently working on examining the socio-historical determinants of health inequities and understanding how nursing resources may be optimized to provide improved health outcomes for vulnerable populations.

Jonathan Cole is a PhD candidate at the University of California at Berkeley. His research focuses on the history of health and medicine in 20th-century Senegal. He is currently finishing his dissertation, "Planning the Family: The Politics of Reproduction in Twentieth Century Senegal," which explores how maternal and infant welfare policies have contributed to the construction of gender in 20th-century Senegal.

Winifred Connerton is an Assistant Professor of Nursing at the Lienhard School of Nursing, College of Health Professions at Pace University. Her research focuses on American-trained nurses' work in US-occupied territories and colonies in the early 20th century. Her current project is a book exploring the intersection of nursing and American imperialism. Dr Connerton is also a practicing nurse-midwife working with underserved populations.

Patricia D'Antonio is the Killebrew-Censtis Endowed Term Chair in Undergraduate Nursing Education, and Chair of the Department of Family and Community Health at the University of Pennsylvania, USA. She is the author of *Founding Friends: Patients, Families and Staff at an Early Nineteenth Century Insane Asylum* (2006), *American Nursing: A History of Knowledge, Authority, and the Meaning of Work* (2010), three edited books, and currently works on the history of early twentieth century health demonstration projects. She is also the editor of the *Nursing History Review*, the official journal of the American Association for the History of Nursing.

Dianne Dodd, PhD, a historian at Parks Canada, specializes in the commemoration of women's history in Canada. Past work includes a study relating to the designation of five nurses' residences, a summary of which appeared in *Nursing History Review*. In 2005, she co-edited (with Tina Bates and Nicole Rousseau) *On All Frontiers: Four Centuries of Canadian Nursing*, a bilingual volume of essays that accompanied a national exhibit on nursing at the Canadian Museum of Civilization. Her current research interests include a study of how Canadian military nurses who died in the First World War have been commemorated, nationally and regionally.

Julie A. Fairman is the Nightingale Professor of Nursing and the Director of the Barbara Bates Center for the Study of the History of Nursing at the University of Pennsylvania, USA. She is the author of *Critical Care Nursing: A History* (1998) and *Making Room at the Clinic: Nurse Practitioners and the Evolution of Modern Health Care* (2008), and currently works on the intersection of health policy and nurse practitioners in the US from 1980 to the present.

Jonathan Hagood is an Assistant Professor of History at Hope College in Holland, Michigan, where he teaches Latin American history as well as courses in the history of science and medicine. His research has focused on the history of social medicine and public health in mid-20th century Argentina. He is currently working on the history of international nursing in the early 20th century.

Christine E. Hallett is Professor of Nursing History and Director of the UK Centre for the History of Nursing and Midwifery at the University of Manchester, UK. She is Chair of the UK Association for the History of Nursing, and was founding Chair of the European Association for the History of Nursing. Her research interests encompass the history of wartime nursing, with particular focus on the First World War, the history of nursing education, and the history of nursing practice. Her most recent publications include *Containing Trauma: Nursing Work in the First World War* (University of Manchester Press, 2009) and "Nursing, 1830–1920: Forging a Profession," in Borsay, A. and Hunter, B. (eds) *Nursing and Midwifery in Britain since 1700* (Palgrave Macmillan, 2012).

Susanne Kreutzer is Professor of Nursing Ethics at Münster University of Applied Sciences, Germany, and Adjunct Professor at the University of Ottawa School of Nursing, Canada. Her research focuses on the history of religious and secular nursing in the 20th century. She has published on the reform of nursing in West Germany: *Vom „Liebesdienst" zum modernen Frauenberuf. Die Reform der Krankenpflege nach 1945*. She is now working on a research project: "Rationalization of Nursing in West Germany and the United States. A Comparative History of the Exchanges of Ideas and Practices, 1945 to 1975."

Thomas Lawrence Long, associate professor-in-residence at the University of Connecticut, has a dual appointment in the Department of English and in the School of Nursing, where he provides writing support services to faculty and doctoral students and teaches writing-intensive undergraduate courses. He is the author of *AIDS and American Apocalypticism: The Cultural Semiotics of an Epidemic* and co-editor with Zhenyi Li of *The Meaning Management Challenge: Making Sense of Health, Illness and Disease*. He is currently working a book-length study of AIDS and the rhetoric of dissent.

Karen Nolte is assistant professor at the Institute for the History of Medicine, University of Wuerzburg, Germany. Her research focuses on 19th- and early 20th-century history of nursing and social history of medicine in Germany. Her most recent publications deal with the history of caring for terminally ill patients from the perspective of physicians and Protestant nurses in the first half of the 19th century. She is also working on the social history of the early outpatient clinics in Germany in the first half of the 19th century.

Steven Palmer is Canada Research Chair in the History of International Health at the University of Windsor. His recent publications, *Launching Global Health: The Caribbean Odyssey of the Rockefeller Foundation* (University of Michigan Press, 2010) and "Toward Responsibility in International Health: Death Following Treatment in Rockefeller Hookworm Campaigns, 1914–1934," *Medical History* (2010), explore the way that actors on the periphery shaped the evolution of a global health system in the 20th century. He is currently researching the politics of medical research in late colonial and early republican Cuba.

Anne Marie Rafferty CBE is Professor of Nursing Policy and Director of Academic Outreach for King's College London, having completed her term as Dean of the Florence Nightingale School of Nursing and Midwifery in 2011. Her research interests combine health services research on workforce, health policy, and the history of colonial nursing. Her doctoral thesis, *The Politics of Nursing Knowledge*, was published as a book by Routledge in 1996.

Helen Sweet is Research Associate at the Wellcome Unit for the History of Medicine, Oxford University and Associate Lecturer with the Open University. Her research has focused on the history of primary health care, firstly in the UK and for the past 14 years in South Africa. The monograph from her PhD thesis, *Community Nursing and Primary Healthcare in Twentieth-Century Britain*, has recently been reprinted in paperback by Routledge. In 2009 she co-edited with Mark Harrison and Margaret Jones *From Western Medicine to Global Medicine: The Hospital Beyond the West* and she is currently researching the history of social medicine at the Valley Trust, KwaZulu Natal (c.1948–2008) while completing a monograph on the mission hospitals in the Province.

Kara Dixon Vuic is an associate professor of history at High Point University. Her research focuses on the connections between gender, war, and militarization in the 20th-century United States. Her first book, *Officer, Nurse, Woman: The Army Nurse Corps in the Vietnam War* (Johns Hopkins University Press, 2010), links the history of army nurses to larger political and cultural debates about gender norms, wartime roles for women and men, obligations of citizenship, and public memory of wars. Her current book project traces the military's utilization of women as entertainment for American soldiers from World War I through contemporary wars in the Middle East.

Rosemary Wall is a Lecturer in Global History at the University of Hull. She has previously worked at Imperial College London as a Lecturer in the History of Medicine, and has held post-doctoral research positions at the University of Oxford and King's College London. Wall's work focuses on the history of colonial nursing and on the social history of bacteriology in Britain. Her publications include "Using bacteriology in elite hospital practice: London and Cambridge, 1880–1920," *Social History of Medicine* (2011). Her forthcoming book, *Bacteria in Britain, 1880–1939*, explores the use of bacteriological resources and knowledge in the hospital, the workplace, and the community.

Jean C. Whelan is Adjunct Associate Professor of Nursing and the Assistant Director of the Barbara Bates Center for the Study of the History of Nursing at the University of Pennsylvania, USA. Her research focuses on the conventions and development of nurses' work, demographic characteristics of American nurses and their distribution to the public, and policy implications involved in maintaining adequate nurse services. Dr Whelan is President of the American Association for the History of Nursing, 2012–2014.

INTRODUCTION

Patrica D'Antonio, Julie A. Fairman and Jean C. Whelan

Almost a generation ago, both Ellen Lagemann and Celia Davis, in their respective introductions to edited collections of new essays on the history of nursing in the United States and Great Britain, captured the excitement that existed in this field of scholarship. New scholars with different backgrounds and experiences had come to the history of nursing with different methodological tools from women's history, labor history, and sociology. They also sought answers to innovative questions and mined new sources of evidence for insights that brought the history of nursing out of narrow disciplinary perspectives of institutions and people and into a broader historical world that placed their actors within the context of social and political imperatives.[1]

The succeeding years have seen an impressive range of work that builds upon this tradition. Recently, a new generation of scholars with, again, different backgrounds and experiences have been turning to the history of nursing with new paradigms and methodologies that bring new analytic tools and theoretical perspectives to traditional sources. Some of these scholars have also moved the history of nursing beyond a traditional nation-state analysis that structured Lagemann and Davis' collected essays and have used nurses to historically track the global flow of ideas and practices. Other scholars have turned to new actors in the history of nursing and have used such men and women to chart different forms of activism and ways of using power. Still others use nurses and nursing as a concept of analysis and, in doing so, tell a more nuanced and gendered history of hospitals and health care. And some are moving beyond the structure and function of a professionalization paradigm, focusing instead on the intersectionality of race, class, gender, and place on professional identity formation. The field of nursing history, to paraphrase Ellen Lagemann, is once again in ferment and its scholars, to paraphrase Celia Davis, see themselves working on the cutting edge of history, policy, and practice.

The *Routledge Handbook on the Global History of Nursing* brings these scholars and scholarship together in a way that captures the state of the science and invites readers to consider new understandings of the historical work and worth of nursing in a larger global context. The history of nurses and nursing is now mined for insights that help explain or illustrate the global circulation ideas about the care of the sick; about gender and the valuation of care work; about the intersections of lay and professional care; and about the definitions and valuations of vulnerable populations. This handbook is necessarily about the history of nursing; but the history of nursing also moves us away from reductionist foci on diseases and treatments and towards more inclusive ideas about the experiences of illnesses on individuals, families, communities, voluntary organizations, and states at the bedside and across the globe. It moves us away from amorphous definitions of care and towards clearer understandings of how those involved in care – both as caregivers and as patients – more fully operationalized their work. It allows new approaches to a construct about a fundamental human need that nonetheless finds different expressions in particular kinds of social, political, and religious contexts.

The genesis of this book reaches long back to our own discussions about the nature of care in general, and nursing care in particular, across time, place, and cultures. Our own position as clinicians as well as historians led us to wonder – who are the sick? Who has responsibility for them? How does the work of the individual, the family, the strangers – be they individuals, formal philanthropies, the community and the state – intersect with these responsibilities? We found, however, that we were not alone in posing and pondering these questions. A new generation of scholars – steeped in global studies – were looking outside their own nation states to examine the inevitable tensions that existed as the self-proclaimed "new ideas" associated with modernity confronted local assumptions about and traditions of care for the sick both in homes and in hospitals. Historians of medicine of the British Empire and of United States imperialism have long focused on disease eradication as central to colonial projects; they have pointed to the role of the state in forming the structures of power and policy that native communities might resist, accommodate, or incorporate into indigenous healing practices.

But when one turns one's focus to the history of nursing, quite different perspectives become more visible. Most concretely, the role of religion – notably Catholic and Protestant congregants whose orders did not neatly conform to nation-state boundaries – in developing systems of care appears more pronounced. But one also sees how the development of such systems was never hegemonic. As Ryan Johnson and Amna Khalid argue, what they term intermediaries and subordinates – those actually working in villages and towns – in the practice of public health in the British Empire influenced the implementation of national public health practices and, in some instances, changed the direction of policies of the Empire.[2] But where do trained nurses lie? With whom are they aligned? For what purpose? And how does this change over time and across place?

The history of nursing also complicates understanding of what is meant by the term "global." Certainly, the iconic figure of the nineteenth century, Florence Nightingale nursing the British troops in Scutari, fighting for health reforms for the British army, and capturing the public's imagination with the possibilities inherent in the training of women to care for strangers, represents the globalization of an idea that had a profound impact in Western Europe and in North America. From the beginning, this particular form of nursing was tightly linked to the development of later nineteenth and early twentieth century medicine – a form of practice rooted in rational science, the laboratory, and gendered practices. Yet the idea of care has its roots in very intimate and private processes built on deeply held assumption and long traditions of attention to details that escape a Western gaze. How, then, to trace the circulation of ideas about the care of the sick in ways that do not flatten the complexities of local customs? How do bio-medicine, on one hand, and local customs, on the other, shape or constrain circulation of ideas about the care of the sick? Or the challenges of a diaspora?

It is also important to note that the primary actors in these chapters are trained nurses. They are primarily (although not necessarily) women who received specialized training in Western knowledge about health and illness care, engaged in skilled practice, and identified as a professional member of any hospitals or clinics in which they worked. To be sure, their training could be very different, ranging from three year hospital-based diploma programs to shorter and more focused ones that dealt with the care of mothers and infants. The reciprocal recognition of their status also varied enormously. It ranged from the complete devaluation of the work and worth of black nurses in Helen Sweet's apartheid South Africa to nurses' recognition by the state, physicians, and patients in Jonathan Hagood's Peronist Argentina. But implicit in their identity was also a sense of authority. Karen Nolte's deaconesses' sense of themselves as facilitators of faith strengthened their positions with respect to ministers and physicians. And in Jonathan Cole's colonial Senegal formal training allowed women to challenge traditional roles as wives and mothers by providing them with new and significant opportunities. Indeed, issues involving knowledge, both nursing and gendered authority, practice and identity run through all the essays in this book. But we have decided to group the essays in ways that highlight the most significant contributions to new formulations of the global history of nursing. We recognize that our particular themes are an editorial decision that may not meet the needs of readers. We encourage you to reassemble the essays in ways that are most relevant to the questions you wish to ask.

Part 1: New directions in the global history of nursing

This part captures the two most significant perspectives that have emerged from a new generation of scholarship: that of situating nurses within a colonial (or post-colonial) agenda on a more global scale, and that of participation in war as a means of achieving full citizenship within one's own nation. Winifred Connerton shows the power of positioning nurses at the intersection of the interchange between the colonizers and colonized, as they at times mediate the exchange, and other times simply participate on behalf of the colonial power. Her essay on US nurses in the Philippines is emblematic of the ways in which looking at the history of nursing complicates dichotomies. Her nurses are not a monolithic group: they alternately or sequentially serve as civil service employees of the US government; as officers in the US Army; as missionaries; or as volunteers through the Red Cross, a non-governmental agency with its own global reach and perspective. Nor can their motives be generally characterized as benevolent or coercive, although they might be either at any point in time. Their work lies in an "in-between" state: in between benevolent or coercive practices, in between the structures that framed the delivery of care and, as importantly, in between national policy and practices at a patient's bedside. The power of the history of nursing lies in seeking to understand multi-determined ideas, motives, and actions.

Similarly, Kara Dixon Vuic complicates conventional understanding of the role of nurses in their nation's military forces by grounding their experiences in the context of changing gender roles, assumed and ascribed power, and the changing meanings of military service for both these women and their nation. Like Connerton, she acknowledges the humanitarian motives of service to country. But Vuic also explores how nurses not only waged war but also waged power. For much of the twentieth century women could only serve their country as nurses; and nurses' service slowly paved the way for an expanded role for women in the public sphere and, now, in the military itself.

Part 2: New methodological approaches in the history of nursing

This part moves to new methical approaches that can take the history of nursing in even more innovative directions. Thomas Lawrence Long urges us to consider the meaning of cultural representations of nursing to confront the US (if not the global conundrum) of nursing's place as the most trusted health profession while simultaneously struggling with issues of visibility and autonomy. Dianne Dodd shows the power of using the literature on historic memory to mine the meaning of representation of nurse categories. Her place is Canada, but her methods can be applied more globally to explore the ways in which memories and memorials might serve simultaneously as propaganda, tribute, and ambivalence about women's military roles. J. Margo Brooks Carthon and Katherine Abbott ask us to consider Social Network Analysis (SNA) as a valid tool in historical research. Their approach uncovers important – and often invisible – relationships among individuals, communities, and institutions that move beyond the traditional triumvirate of race, class, and gender.

Part 3: The politics of nursing knowledge

As we mentioned earlier, Parts 3 and 4 represent our intent to strive for a certain coherency among themes presented in the essays of our contributors. We make no claims to comprehensiveness: regrettably, histories of nursing in the Indian subcontinent and South America have not been captured. But we also believe that the essays included in these chapters highlight one of the most exciting developments in the history of nursing: exploring the fluid nature of nursing knowledge and practice. Part 3 focuses on the politics of nursing knowledge – a focus that allows one to see a much more subtle interplay of knowledge and context. As Christine E. Hallett indicates, this quest for what would be nursing knowledge began as a messy and inchoate process during the late nineteenth and early twentieth centuries. Her essay examines the efforts of a small group of leading British nurses to exploit the specific knowledge needed for wound healing demanded by World War I to advance an agenda of nursing knowledge as scientific, rather than innate, knowledge. Still the nursing–knowledge–science triad remained highly problematic.

But where nurses in Great Britain turned to their own internal professionalizing agenda, those in Jonathan Cole's Senegal had the power of the French empire behind them. To remake the African family in their own image in Senegal, the French had to expand educational opportunities so that women might serve as nurses and midwives. Granted, the work of nurses and midwives was to have been limited to the private sphere of home and household. But as women moved into these roles, they not only undermined the Senegalese traditional roles of wives and mothers, but also used their specialized knowledge in ways that created empowering opportunities. Still, as Steven Palmer argues, such specialized knowledge remains entangled with the politics of place. Palmer looks at the 1949 "sex scandal" of Windsor's Metropolitan Hospital School of Nursing, an imaginative and experimental school run by the Canadian Nurses Association. Although neither the nursing school students nor their faculty were implicated, the storm of negative publicity surrounding the discovery of the city's mayor and hospital administrator's entertainment of four hospital staff nurses at Detroit's glamorous Book-Cadillac Hotel undercut the political and social support the School needed to sustain its educational independence.

But if Palmer looks closely at the relationship between knowledge and context in one localized case study, Susanne Kreutzer widens the focus to encompass the state in the immediate aftermath of World War II. German nursing had been dominated for generations by the Catholic sisters and the Protestant deaconesses for whom the work of nursing was defined as a religious vocation. But, as Kreutzer points out, Christian and scientific concepts were not inherently incompatible: the denominational sisterhoods also believed in the value of theoretical and mid-twentieth-century scientific knowledge. But the sweeping changes of post-World War II German reconstruction reshaped all sectors of German society, and what counted as authoritative knowledge changed as well. New, more depersonalized forms of nursing knowledge emerged that fit better with the state and public ideas about the value of liberalization, individualization, and secularization of German society.

Part 4: Nursing and the "practice turn"

This part takes its title from Karen Nolte's exploration of Pierre Bourdieu's concept of social practice, a concept that asks us to focus on nursing's practices, discourses, and structures. An earlier generation of scholars focused on the meaning of nursing practice – to hospitals who needed students to care for patients; to families, physicians, and public health agencies who would employ them to care for the sick at home; and to the nurses themselves seeking respected and respectable work. More recent work, however, has focused on what nurses actually did and, while continuing an emphasis on nursing's work with families and communities as well as hospitals and health care agencies, it has found substantively broader sources of nursing authority and activism. This work has brought a new sense of agency to those who nursed, and creates a more powerful paradigm to understand the discipline's work and worth to both the public it serves and in the global context of the exchange of ideas.

Nolte's essay stands as a case in point. As we mentioned earlier, her mid-nineteenth-century deaconesses assumed an authoritative role in their spiritual care of the sick; but their working and reworking of the motherhouse's rules of service also suggest how they appropriated and influenced the framework for how they lived their lives and cared for their patients. However, as Jonathan Hagood argues in his essay on Perón's Argentina, changes in scope and authority in practice also come from the complicated historical interplay of the needs of the state for more intensive public health systems, the professionalization of a discipline seeking independent practice opportunities, and a willingness of the part of some physicians to see nurses as members of a health care team.

Like Hagood, Helen Sweet argues that the rural and underserved countryside offered some limited opportunities for black women whom the missionaries trained as nurses. But unlike Hagood's nurses, those in apartheid South Africa practiced in the face of stiff government sanctions, raising important questions about the pernicious influences of race as well as gender in decisions on who can access what kinds of nursing knowledge under what kinds of circumstances. And, as we bring this volume to a close, Rosemary Wall and Anne Marie Rafferty's essay about the critical support of British nurses in the post-WWII "hearts and minds" campaign of the Malayan Emergency challenges our traditional assumptions about the function of nursing practices, noting the complexity of practice entangled with political actions and the demands of colonized nations. Finally, Geertje Boschma's study of the intersections of nursing and consumer identities in post-World War II Canada highlights the complex transformations that occur when place and perspectives intersect and, often, collide. We come back full circle to the essay that begins this collection: what happens when new ideas and ideologies confront local assumptions about and traditions of care for the sick? How do we account for the values nurses bring with them when they provide public health care outreach? And can nurses truly be self-interested "culture-brokers"?

The essays in the *Handbook on the Global History of Nursing* raise more questions than they definitively answer. But perhaps, in the end, this is the overarching message in this perspective. A global history of nursing demonstrates the multi-dimensional encounters of nurses with patients, families, and communities. This multi-dimensionality also uncovers the many ways in which nurses reinvented, renegotiated, and reinterpreted the meanings of nationalism, imperialism, and their place within these ideologies and practices. The nurses did not construct simple narratives; rather, they created multiple ones brimming with self-awareness, hubris, political insights, and quests for social, cultural, and professional authority. And this multi-dimensionality may be more emblematic of all encounters of people, professions, and cultures across the globe.

Notes

1 Lagemann, E. *Nursing History: New Perspectives, New Possibilities.* New York: Teachers' College Press, 1983; Davis, C. *Rewriting Nursing History.* London: Croom Helm, 1980.
2 Johnson, R. and A. Khalid, eds. *Public Health in the British Empire: Intermediaries, Subordinates, and the Practice of Public Health, 1850–1960.* New York: Routledge, 2012.

PART 1

New directions in the global history of nursing

1

AMERICAN NURSES IN COLONIAL SETTINGS

Imperial power at the bedside

Winifred Connerton, PhD, CNM

Nurses are essential to studies of American imperialism of the early twentieth century because nursing as a profession embodied the "benevolent" approach of American colonialism; as individuals, trained nurses were the personal face of America in their contact with patients at the bedside and in the clinic.[1] Yet nurses are absent from nearly all studies of American imperialism, and conversely imperialism is absent from the few studies of nursing in the US colonial occupations. However, it is not easy to overlook the presence of nurses at every stage of operation: nurses worked with state agencies, with voluntary organizations such as Protestant missions, and with philanthropic foundations. New approaches to the US imperial era, which began with the Spanish–American War of 1898, include a wide set of historical actors and consider the power of cultural influence as an aspect of imperialism not constrained by the boundaries of colonial occupation. This chapter argues that including trained nursing in histories of the US imperial experiment of the early twentieth century offers an important perspective on imperialism and American influence in the world.

I begin with basic background to the 1898 transformation of the US into a colonial power. I then explore traditional historical interpretations of that transition, and new approaches to that history. Finally I explore the multiple approaches to historical analysis of the US imperial efforts of the early twentieth century that create opportunities to include nursing within the analytical field.

Background

The Spanish–American War began on April 23, 1898, after months of reports about Spain's brutal suppression of the Cuban revolutionary movement, and the destruction of the USS *Maine* in Havana harbor that killed 266 men in suspicious circumstances. The war was intended to be a war of liberation for the Cubans, not a war of acquisition. In fact, the declaration of war by Congress in April 1898 was only approved after

Congress added the Teller Amendment stating that the United States had no intention to annex or colonize Cuba. Although the Spanish–American War was focused on Cuba, the rest of Spain's colonies also became military targets and other Spanish territories of the Philippines, Guam, and Puerto Rico were taken by US forces.

The fighting was over by August 14, 1898, and the parties signed the Treaty of Paris on December 10, 1898. With the settlement the United States acquired the territory of Guam, Puerto Rico, and Cuba and paid Spain $20,000,000 for the Philippines. With the ratification of the treaty the United States formally became a colonial power for the first time in its history. Until this point the United States absorbed new territory with the intention of settling that terrain and eventually granting membership in the country.

The path of the US as an imperial power was not particularly clear, and the colonial occupations faced opposition from all points on the political spectrum. The Teller Amendment prevented any colonial ambition over Cuba, but did not specifically restrict colonial ambitions in any of the other territories taken in the war. Colonial proponents argued that the United States had a special destiny or duty to help reform other nations along an American model and to protect and guide them during the formative stages of this Americanization. Anti-imperialists, on the other hand, argued that there was no constitutional basis for a democratic country to have any colonial possession, that the native populations would not be intellectually capable of participating in democracy at the level necessary to maintain a civil society, and that the colonial populations would create an influx of cheap labor from the colonies. The national interest in colonialism waned after 1912, and by 1917 there were formal plans for each colony to move toward autonomy. This discomfort with the US imperial agenda has influenced how the meaning of American imperialism has been understood by historians.

American imperialism – oxymoron, historical anomaly, or natural progression?

Traditionally the US imperial period has been considered relatively short – beginning with the Spanish–American War, and ending with Philippine Independence in 1946 and Hawaii's statehood in 1959. The temporal boundaries of the US colonial period can be contested, however. For example, historians such as Thomas Hietala argue that the American imperial era began with the continental expansion of the 1840s, not the colonies of 1898.[2] Similarly, Julian Go argues that the US was experienced with territorial expansion by 1898 and that the only difference in the US occupation of the Philippines from that of the western territories was that the Philippines was not intended to be permanently settled by Americans or to join the Union, and thus had to be administered as a colonial territory rather than as a future state.[3]

The study of US imperialism has been complicated by disagreements over fundamental ideas, from those as basic as when the imperial process began to whether the US colonial possessions even constituted an empire at all. Historian Joseph Fry has noted that when the existence of an American empire has not been denied altogether, it has frequently been portrayed as a deviation from the American model of existence, and also as "more benign and more transitory than its European counterparts."[4] Similarly, Virginia Bouvier notes that there are many different explanations for the US imperialism of the early twentieth century, including accidental war and possession, premeditated expansion, inevitable progress, and unnecessary imperialism.[5]

There are two main groups of analysis for these years of explicit colonial possession: as either a historical anomaly or part of the natural progression of the nation. Those that subscribe to the "accidental imperialist" idea argue that the US did not enter the Spanish–American War with the intention of imperial occupation, but once in a responsible position over the colonies the US had a duty to protect and guide them. For example, Richard Hofstadter's analysis of the ideology behind the US occupation of Cuba and the Philippines explains the occupations as an aberration in American history, brought on by the closing of the American frontier to the west, a national sense of duty and a need for markets for American-produced goods.[6] Not all historians have explained the imperialist urge as an anomaly, however; some have described it as part of a natural progression – that once the United States had reached the western edge of the continent, it was natural to progress further into the Pacific.

These two versions are different in practice, but they share fundamental assumptions about the United States at the end of the nineteenth century. Both suggest that the US was naïve to imperialism prior to taking colonies itself. They portray a country surprised by the burden of colonial occupation, but willing and able to take responsibility to help other, weaker countries become independent nations. Both perspectives also represent the US occupation as a uniformly beneficial, if not always welcome, force for improvement in the colonial settings. Finally, they both also propose that US occupation was uniquely different (read: better) than other empires' colonial management, particularly the British. These perspectives underlie many historical assessments of the US imperial push, even those that otherwise present a unique perspective on American colonial occupation. For example, Kenton Clymer in his study of Protestant missionaries in the US-occupied Philippines expands the field of who could be considered imperialists, but ends his book with an exploration of how the Protestant ideals that the missionaries introduced into the Philippines also inculcated ideas of democracy that spurred resistance to Ferdinand Marcos.[7] Clymer does explore the negative aspects of the missionaries' evangelism in the islands, but his conclusion about the overall positive result of colonial occupation falls solidly within the traditional approach to American imperialism.

Amy Kaplan has argued that when historians fail to examine the imperial nature of American influence in the world, they inevitably fall into the trap of American exceptionalism. Kaplan suggests that excluding the US from discussion of empire creates the impression that there was no imperialism inherent in the spreading American influence in the twentieth century, and simultaneously that whatever imperialism the US engendered was somehow different (and better) than any other sort of imperialism present in the world.[8] Since the terrorist attacks of September, 2001 there has been a renewed interest in US internationalism and a discussion of empire, with some proponents embracing the idea of empire as a necessary policy for US foreign relations.[9]

This presents a new twist of the American exceptionalism that Kaplan addresses. When, in 2003, Donald Rumsfeld responded to a question in an interview on al-Jazeera with "We don't seek empires . . . we're not imperialistic. We never have been," he was denying the historical role the US took in the early twentieth century in the Pacific and Caribbean.[10] Similarly, Jeremi Suri has recently argued that the term "empire" is not large enough to encompass the benevolent aspects of American internationalism, suggesting that any negative aspects of US expansion are outweighed by the US-led reform and democratization projects.[11]

Histories of nurses abroad can easily fall into a similar exceptionalist approach by overlooking nurses' connection to the national political agenda. Nurses were part of the American administrative and social presence, and as a group are useful for examining the United States' imperial agenda. As individual women they offer the perspective of individual actors who chose to participate in the national mission for personal reasons, and, as a profession, they reflect the prevailing understanding of what it meant to be "American." Nurses as individuals may not have had overtly political interests in going abroad, as they may have been seeking adventure or simply new job opportunities, but they were operating within a political context that informed their work. Thus, nursing is a useful lens for examining colonial occupation because nurses were important to the functional work of the colony through public health programs, as well as promoters of the American ideology through their enforcing sanitary rules and teaching in nursing training programs.

Despite the recent resurgence of an exceptionalist rhetoric around US international expansion of the early twentieth century, Kaplan's challenge has been taken up by many historians who offer a wide variety of interpretations and approaches to this colonial period. These approaches also offer avenues for examining nursing within the US imperial expansion after 1898.

More inclusive approaches to American imperialism

In contrast to the "accidental imperialist" approaches to US imperialism, recent collections organized around the study of American imperial work offer useful examples of the trends in historiography of US international engagement. These new approaches make a comprehensive assessment of colonial locales and highlight the participation of non-state agents within the colonial apparatus. Others widen the focus and consider the US colonial occupations in the context of US history and world history – particularly focusing on the US as an empire in relation with other empires. Thomas Bender has long argued that it is impossible to isolate US history from worldwide developments.[12] Recently Jane Burbank and Frederick Cooper have included the US in a complex study of the intersection and interaction of empires.[13] Julian Go has taken up this inclusive approach in his examination of the similarities and differences between the colonial management of Puerto Rico and the Philippines.[14] These approaches to US empire may not directly include nursing, but their expansive approach to the subject also encourages historians to shift their focus, thereby deepening the analysis of the imperial experience.

The contributors and editors of *Colonial Crucible: Empire in the Making of the Modern American State* challenge "post-imperial denial" and include examinations of race, education, public health, and environmental management along with studies of the politics and military aspects of colonial occupation.[15] In *Competing Kingdoms: Women, Mission, Nation, and the American Protestant Empire* the collective editors and authors suggest that expanding the study of American empire to include not only colonial or territorial possessions, but also the power of international organizations to spread American influence, broadens the possibilities of understanding American history and of empire itself.[16] This collection notably includes women as central agents of cultural and national influence within their roles as Protestant missionaries, and although it does not include missionary nurses among its subjects, it gives several examples of how non-state actors participate in the spread of national interests. For example, Ian Tyrrell argues that the American version of empire was not built on overt territorial possession of colonies, but rather was embodied in the organizations that espoused a uniquely American cultural perspective, and through their projects spread the American influence all around the world.[17] Tyrrell's approach is particularly useful when considering US-trained nurses in American-held territories at the beginning of the twentieth century, because nurses influenced society both through their work and by their very presence in colonial settings. These collections are examples of alternate approaches to the US's colonizing era through their inclusion of many different colonial actors, and their recognition that colonial encounters took place on different fields, and were mediated by cultural and social context.[18] Histories that specifically use a social frame include those that examine gender and/or race within the colonial setting.

Historians of empire have examined women's roles from the perspective of those that were part of the colonized population, and women who were among the colonizers, with the understanding that all women in colonial settings were symbolically important for many reasons. Colonized women were the targets of reform in the areas of infant feeding, birth, and childrearing practices. Their needs – which were established by the colonizers – justified the need for colonial oversight.[19] No colonial occupation occurred in a vacuum, however, and Eileen Findlay has explored how Puerto Rican women successfully used the US colonial agenda to their own purposes.[20] Findlay notes that the US interest in creating a social structure similar to that of the "mainland" included introducing civil marriage and divorce, where religious marriage and annulment existed before. Puerto Rican women took advantage of the opportunity to seek divorce in large numbers, an unexpected consequence of the colonial administration's social policy.

Colonizing women, too, were important to supporting the colonial process. Nancy Rose Hunt explains that Belgian women in the colonies served as models for African women as well as a stabilizing center for the European family structure and maintaining the moral compass for Belgian men.[21] Antoinette Burton has argued that European women themselves identified their role in colonial settings as one of savior in which they offered an uplifting message to native women. Colonial women's efforts at reform could be used by both the women and the imperial government as evidence of the beneficial and benign nature of imperial expansion.[22] Catherine Choy has examined the long-term effects of the introduction of American-style trained nursing to the Philippines.[23] In her study Choy notes that the social patterns of nursing conflicted with traditional behaviors for Filipino women, from the expected uniform to caring for strangers of both sexes, working outside the home and family, and seeking advanced education.

The US expanded into Caribbean and Pacific islands that were already populated with ethnically and racially diverse peoples. Rudyard Kipling highlighted race as fundamental to the US management of its new colonial possessions in his 1899 poem "The White Man's Burden."[24] Historian Eric T. Love counters the idea that the colonial populations were being prepared for "benevolent assimilation" because in the racially charged atmosphere of lynchings of African-Americans in the US South, anti-Chinese legislation, and the disenfranchisement of Native Americans, no "pragmatic politician" would have supported any policy that aimed at improving the lot of "non-whites."[25] Rather, Love suggests, proponents of imperialism argued in terms of national gains and political duty rather than uplift.

Historian Paul A. Kramer also focuses on the role of race in the colonial acquisition of the Philippines, particularly in the way that race was part of the "hierarchies of difference" essential to imperialism, but also how the concept of race in a colonial setting is a "dynamic, contextual, contested and contingent field of power."[26] Warwick Anderson has chronicled how race played into the US colonial government's efforts at hygiene reform in the Philippines.[27] The Bureau of Health campaigns created an image of the unclean and inherently unwell native in contrast with the healthy, hygienic American colonizer.

There is little analysis of the intersection of race and gender for any of the US colonial workers, and this is a case where the absence of nursing from the analysis is glaring. The US nurses recruited to work in these new territorial possessions were white. They worked closely with native populations as caregivers and as instructors in nursing training programs.

American women participated in colonial work on a different scale than men – they did not run government agencies, nor did they set the agenda for colonial projects. Rather they worked in close contact with native people as teachers, nurses, and missionaries. They were busy representing the US and interpreting Americanization plans, while at the same time negotiating their own roles within the US and as colonial workers. Women's colonial work, then, requires a broader perspective – one that accounts for the intersection across groups, such as the interaction between the native and colonial peoples, as well as considering women's colonial roles in contrast or concert with those roles in mainland society.

Carol Chin suggests that women missionaries in China were "beneficent imperialists" because they understood their efforts to reform the Chinese culture in terms of unalloyed good, rather than as a hostile take-over.[28] Barbara Reeves-Ellington, Kathryn Kish Sklar, and Connie A. Shemo argue that as American women missionaries spread American influence around the world they crossed barriers of race and culture to make their work truly "transnational." Specifically they argue that these women were not "a homogenous group of cultural imperialists" but were rather "people who reinvented the meanings of American nationalism and imperialism as they negotiated competing nationalism and imperialisms in varying colonial settings."[29]

American nurses served in the American-held territories in a wide variety of roles and they negotiated their competing professional, national and personal agendas in all of their work. Some US nurses went abroad as missionaries, but even those without a religious mission had a secular mission, one that was sometimes obscured by the nature of their helping work.

Public health in colonial context

Public health was part of colonial administration and the area where nurses figured most prominently. Public health projects in the colonial territories served multiple constituencies, sometimes to the benefit of one group over another. Mariola Espinosa has documented how yellow fever eradication programs instituted by the US in Cuba served the US population more than the Cubans, though the Cubans bore most of the burden from the program. Yellow fever was not actually a threat to the Cuban population, who were generally immune to the disease from childhood exposure, but it was a threat to Americans living in Cuba, and the Southeastern US colonial health policy that focused exclusively on yellow fever in occupied Cuba benefited US nationals to the detriment of the Cubans, who suffered instead from tuberculosis, malaria, and enteritis, which were not identified as public health issues under the US.[30]

The beneficial results of colonial health programs have made them somewhat immune to critical examination. Anne Perez Hattori notes the accounts of the health programs organized by the US Navy in its occupation of Guam, which included sanitary inspections of homes and leper colonies, and the suppression of traditional *Chamorro* healers and midwives, are used by some Guamanian historians as examples of the "blessings of naval colonialism."[31] Similarly, historian Raymond Ileto has noted that even staunchly nationalist Filipino historians recount the US public health campaigns in the Philippines without any critique whatsoever, and that the cholera campaign, with its concentration camps that served the military's goals during the Philippine–American War, has been "assimilated into the universal history of medical progress, torn from its original moorings in a colonial war and pacification campaign."[32] Espinosa takes a slightly different perspective on the same critique when she points out that "public health efforts also sought to convince subjugated peoples of their own inferiority and, therefore, the desirability of continued colonial rule."[33] Thus successful public health campaigns that reduced disease also reinforced the colonial rule. Each of these authors takes other historians to task for not more critically examining the nature of public health programs in colonial context. Certainly some gains were made – maternal and infant mortality rates dropped, for instance – but these authors ask: what was the overall cost of those gains?

Nursing can be examined in the same light as other colonial programs. The colonial governments believed in their mission of uplift and improvement. The beneficent tutelage, however, coincided with the need to control an armed insurgency in the Philippines, and the goal to reform societal norms in all colonies. Health and hygiene programs fit within this structure of uplift and reform as colonial administrators aimed to improve the public health, and nursing was an essential part of that service. Nursing represented a particular, culturally bound, understanding of illness and of a scientific approach to treatment. American nurses in the colonies were what Sharon Nestel, in reference to European colonial nursing in Africa, has called "capillary power" – an extension of colonial power out to the extremities of its reach, because nurses participated in medical policies and performed regulatory tasks that were at heart coercive or intended to maintain the colonial power.[34] Charles McGraw identified this same pattern in the US nurses who went to Cuba prior to the Spanish–American War, where they were examples of what he calls "friendly power" – power exerted under the cover of aid.[35]

Americanization campaigns took place in public spheres as well as the intimate places in people's lives. Health was identified early as an avenue for inculcating American values in native populations, and nurses were a part of that campaign as caregivers in the public hospitals and as instructors in the government-run training school for nurses. Public health campaigns in each of the colonies were part of what were intended to be beneficial services, but those services had coercive aspects, as in the Philippines and Guam, or simply did not have the native population as the target audience, as in Cuba. Whether or not nurses were present during the most brutal parts of colonial occupation, they were associated with the colonial power and were part of the colonial apparatus, and consequently their participation deserves focused attention.

Conclusion

Although America's period of seeking colonial territories ended soon after the 1898 acquisition of the Philippines, Cuba, Puerto Rico, and Guam as a settlement from the Spanish–American War, historians who have begun to stretch the boundaries of the definition of empire have opened a new avenue for exploring nurses' roles in empire. American nurses were part of a system of colonial management. They supported the colonial presence by caring for the American workers in the islands, and they put a face on American policies as they taught in training schools or worked on public health campaigns. In fact, American nurses had a unique position within the colonial health program because their work brought them into direct contact with native peoples as patients, students, and colleagues. Nurses offer a glimpse of the negotiations between the colonial parties as the administration modified programs in response to the native people's participation and resistance.

As members of the American population in US-occupied territories, it is impossible to isolate the truly beneficial services trained nurses provided from the climate of coercion and sometimes violent suppression in which they were working. Even nurses somewhat removed from the colonial government itself, missionary nurses for example, were members of a colonizing population, and in the aggregate were representatives of the colonial mission. As individuals these nurses had stronger or weaker affiliation with their national mission. More research into the personal reflections of American nurses in the US territories will give context and depth to nurses' participation in the colonial project, and the reciprocal stories of the native nurses they trained would add an important counterpoint. As an almost exclusively female group of workers, nurses offer a vision of what it meant for women to participate in colonial activities. Did they protest maltreatment but were overruled, or did they subvert programs and policies they personally found unpalatable? How did they understand their work within the context of "Americanization" campaigns? Was there a hierarchy of ideologic identification, and if so how did nurses rank nation, religion, profession, race, and gender in their colonial work? Without those explanations we are left to wonder at nurses' motivations, but even without those personal recollections we must not fail to place nurses within the colonial context – including the context of coercive and punitive policies. To do so only creates an odd variant of American exceptionalism, a nursing exceptionalism that robs nursing of its cultural import and power at the crossroads of colonial contact.

Notes

1 In this chapter I use the term "United States" or "US" when I am referring to the geopolitical nation, and the term "America" when I mean the nebulous national idea that encompasses the people of the United States and their collective ideologies.

2 Thomas R. Hietala, *Manifest Design: American Exceptionalism and Empire*, Rev. ed. (Ithaca, NY: Cornell University Press, 2003).

3 Julian Go, "Introduction: Global Perspectives on the U.S. Colonial State in the Philippines," in *The American Colonial State in the Philippines; Global Perspectives*, ed. Julian Go and Anne L. Foster (Durham, NC: Duke University Press, 2003), 1–42.

4 Joseph A. Fry, "Imperialism, American Style, 1890–1916," in *American Foreign Relations Reconsidered, 1890–1993*, ed. Gordon Martel (New York: Routledge, 1994), 52.

5 "Introduction," in *Whose America? The War of 1898 and the Battle to Define the Nation*, ed. Virginia M Bouvier (Westport, CT: Praeger Publishers, 2001), 1–19.

6 Richard Hofstadter, "Cuba, the Philippines and Manifest Destiny," in *The Paranoid Style in American Politics and Other Essays*, ed. Richard Hofstadter (New York: Knopf, 1965), 145–187.

7 Kenton J. Clymer, *Protestant Missionaries in the Philippines, 1898–1916: An Inquiry into the American Colonial Mentality* (Urbana, IL: University of Illinois Press, 1986).

8 Amy Kaplan, "'Left Alone with America': The Absence of Empire in the Study of American Culture," in *Cultures of United States Imperialism*, ed. Amy Kaplan and Donald E. Pease (Durham, NC: Duke University Press, 1993), 3–21.

9 Alfred W. McCoy, Francisco A. Scarano, and Courtney Johnson, "On the Tropic of Cancer; Transitions and Transformations in the U.S. Imperial State," in *Colonial Crucible: Empire in the Making of the Modern American State*, ed. Alfred W. McCoy and Francisco A. Scarano (Madison, WI: University of Wisconsin Press, 2009), 3–33.

10 "American Imperialism? No Need to Run Away from Label," *Council on Foreign Relations*, n.d., www.cfr.org/iraq/american-imperialism-no-need-run-away-label/p5934

11 Jeremi Suri, "The Limits of American Empire: Democracy and Militarism in the Twentieth and Twenty-first Centuries," in *Colonial Crucible: Empire in the Making of the Modern American State*, ed. Alfred W. McCoy and Francisco A. Scarano (Madison, WI: University of Wisconsin Press, 2009), 523–531.

12 Thomas Bender, *A Nation among Nations: America's Place in World History* (New York: Hill and Wang, 2006).

13 Jane Burbank and Frederick Cooper, *Empires in World History: Power and the Politics of Difference* (Princeton, NJ: Princeton University Press, 2010).

14 Julian Go, "The Chains of Empire: State Building and 'Political Education' in Puerto Rico and the Philippines," in *The American Colonial State in the Philippines; Global Perspectives*, ed. Julian Go (Durham, NC: Duke University Press, 2003), 182–216; Julian Go, *American Empire and the Politics of Meaning: Elite Political Cultures in the Philippines and Puerto Rico During U.S. Colonialism* (Durham, NC: Duke University Press, 2008).

15 Missing from this collection, however, is an analysis of women's roles, and nurses' work is not addressed in the chapters on public health. Also, this collection focuses solely on the Caribbean and Pacific colonial possessions post-1898. McCoy, Scarano, and Johnson, "On the Tropic of Cancer," 3.

16 Barbara Reeves-Ellington, Kathryn Kish Sklar, and Connie A. Shemo, eds., *Competing Kingdoms: Women, Mission, Nation, and the American Protestant Empire, 1812–1960* (Durham, NC: Duke University Press, 2010).

17 Ian Tyrrell, "Woman, Missions, and Empire: New Approaches to American Cultural Expansion," in *Competing Kingdoms: Women, Mission, Nation, and the American Protestant Empire, 1812–1960*, ed. Barbara Reeves-Ellington, Kathryn Kish Sklar, and Connie A. Shemo (Durham, NC: Duke University Press, 2010), 43–66.

18 Other collections that present similar expanded ideas of historic investigation of US imperial history include Gilbert M. Joseph, Catherine C. LeGrand, and Ricardo Salvatore, eds., *Close Encounters of Empire: Writing the Cultural History of U.S.–Latin American Relations* (Durham, NC: Duke University Press, 1998); and Amy Kaplan and Donald E. Pease, eds., *Cultures of United States Imperialism* (Durham, NC: Duke University Press, 1993).

19 Nancy Rose Hunt, "'Le Bébé En Brousse:' European Women, African Birth Spacing, and Colonial Intervention in Breast Feeding in the Belgian Congo," in *Tensions of Empire: Colonial Cultures in a Bourgeois World*, ed. Frederick Cooper and Ann Laura Stoler (Los Angeles: University of California Press, 1997), 287–321.

20 Eileen J. Findlay, "Love in the Tropics: Marriage, Divorce, and the Construction of Benevolent Colonialism in Puerto Rico, 1989–1910," in *Close Encounters with Empire: Writing the Cultural History of U.S.–Latin American Relations*, ed. Gilbert M. Joseph, Catherine C. LeGrand, and Ricardo Salvatore (Durham, NC: Duke University Press, 1998), 138–172.

21 Hunt, "'Le Bébé En Brousse.'"

22 Antoinette Burton, *Burdens of History: British Feminists, Indian Women, and Imperial Culture, 1865–1915* (Chapel Hill, NC: University of North Carolina Press, 1994).

23 Catherine Ceniza Choy, *Empire of Care: Nursing and Migration in Filipino American History* (Durham, NC: Duke University Press, 2003).

24 Rudyard Kipling, "The White Man's Burden," *Modern History Sourcebook: Rudyard Kipling, The White Man's Burden, 1899*, www.fordham.edu/halsall/mod/kipling.asp

25 Eric Tyrone Lowery Love, *Race Over Empire: Racism and U.S. Imperialism, 1865–1900* (Chapel Hill, NC: University of North Carolina Press, 2004), xii.

26 Paul A. Kramer, *The Blood of Government: Race, Empire, the United States and the Philippines* (Chapel Hill, NC: University of North Carolina Press, 2006), 2.

27 Warwick Anderson, *Colonial Pathologies: American Tropical Medicine, Race and Hygiene in the Philippines* (Durham, NC: Duke University Press, 2006).

28 Carol C. Chin, "Beneficent Imperialists: American Women Missionaries in China at the Turn of the Twentieth Century," *The Society for Historians of American Foreign Relations* 27, no. 3 (2003): 327–352.

29 "Introduction," in *Competing Kingdoms: Women, Mission, Nation, and the American Protestant Empire, 1812–1960*, ed. Barbara Reeves-Ellington, Kathryn Kish Sklar, and Connie A. Shemo (Durham, NC: Duke University Press, 2010), 2.

30 Mariola Espinosa, "A Fever for Empire: U.S. Disease Eradication in Cuba as Colonial Public Health," in *Colonial Crucible: Empire in the Making of the Modern American State*, ed. Alfred W. McCoy and Francisco A. Scarano (Madison, WI: University of Wisconsin Press, 2009), 288–296.

31 Anne Perez Hattori, *Colonial Dis-Ease: US Navy Health Policies and the Chamorros of Guam, 1898–1941* (Honolulu, HI: University of Hawaii Press, 2004), 189.

32 "Cholera and the Origins of the American Sanitary Order in the Philippines," in *Imperial Medicine and Indigenous Societies*, ed. David Arnold (New York: Manchester University Press, 1988), 126.

33 Mariola Espinosa, *Epidemic Invasions: Yellow Fever and the Limits of Cuban Independence, 1878–1930* (Chicago: University of Chicago Press, 2009), 6.

34 Sheryl Nestel, "(Ad)ministering Angels: Colonial Nursing and the Extension of Empire in Africa," *Journal of Medical Humanities* 19, no. 4 (1998): 273.

35 Charles McGraw, "'The Intervention of a Friendly Power': The Transnational Migration of Women's Work and 1898 Imperial Imagination," *Journal of Women's History* 19, no. 3 (2007): 137–160.

2

WARTIME NURSING AND POWER

Kara Dixon Vuic

Wartime nurses make good Hollywood subjects. Often, they serve as romantic figures who grace the silver screen in billowing white uniforms mysteriously unsullied by work or war, while they selflessly soothe and comfort tragically wounded young men with whom they frequently fall in love. Others receive the audience's admiration as they stoically withstand their fears and the dangers of war to prove their worth as women, as nurses, and as representatives of their country. And while most film depictions of nurses blend these qualities, they consistently rely on gendered tropes to explain nurses' motivations, their work, and the meanings of their service. The 1943 production *So Proudly We Hail*, for example, undermined the tragic experiences of nurses imprisoned by the Japanese—nurses who were at the time of the film's release still living in prison camps in the Philippines—by framing the story as a wartime romance. Nearly sixty years later, the blockbuster film *Pearl Harbor* (2001) reduced the skill of nurses to their femininity, as they literally used lipstick and nylons to triage and treat the casualties of the attack on the US naval base. Admittedly, films are made to entertain. But even so, popular portrayals of wartime nurses such as these tend to paint a melodramatic picture that belies a much more complicated and even heroic story.

Historians offer a more nuanced account of wartime nursing that grounds nurses' experiences and the meanings of their work in the context of changing gender norms, the evolution of women's and men's public roles, and broad considerations of the meanings of wartime military service.[1] By placing nurses at the center of wider examinations of the history of war, women, gender, medicine, and militarization, historians reveal the ways nurses have both embodied gender ideologies and created gender change. Historians demonstrate the ways in which evolving gender norms have shaped nurses' access to warzones and battlefields, characterized their conceptions of nursing practice, and regulated their duties. They consider the ways nurses have embraced both conventional and progressive notions of gender, as well as wartime service, as tools to secure their professional status and their place in the nation.[2] Finally, historians are beginning to consider even more complicated meanings of wartime nursing as they examine the ways nursing itself has functioned as martial power.

Gender as power

Although popular images of wartime nurses usually feature fresh-faced, stylishly uniformed women sacrificially caring for wounded young soldiers, until the mid-19th century most wartime nurses were men.[3] Beginning in the Crimean War, female nurses argued for a new model of wartime nursing, one steeped in conventional understandings of women as innately suited for domestic matters and thus better qualified to be nurses. Trained and untrained nurses alike argued that allowing them to extend their feminine talents to warzone hospitals would have great benefits for medical care, while sympathetic military officials reasoned that women would domesticate the martial environment. Historians maintain that women, in harnessing traditional gender norms to smooth their entrance to the masculine environs of hospital, military, and war, contained the radical potential of their newfound work by upholding the existing class and race ideologies that defined proper womanhood and thereby excluded men and non-white women. Gender thus functioned as a form of power for women who relied on feminine ideals to justify their place as wartime nurses, and as a powerful tool of exclusion for those who did not fit an evolving mold of conventional femininity. In short, gendered rationales both united and divided nurses, in ways that simultaneously expanded and restricted the meanings of their work.

In the transformative era of the Crimean War, Florence Nightingale and her band of nurses upturned popular conceptions of the care of strangers as disreputable work for women and of warzones as dangerous, dirty sites where no respectable woman should venture. They did so, Anne Summers suggests, by arguing that women's supposed innate nurturing characteristics would transform patient care and hospital efficiency. But while notions of feminine care smoothed the entry of middle- and upper-class women to the wartime hospital, gender stunted their ability to exert authority in the wards. Accustomed to the influence their privileged class status imparted them and unwilling to be treated as servants, Nightingale's nurses struggled with the limited reception they received as medical advisors.[4] In fact, Summers maintains, Nightingale's efforts to transform medical care were not as successful as has been traditionally asserted because most nursing practice occurred "outside Florence Nightingale's jurisdiction, and without reference to her ideas of proper professional practice."[5] Still, Nightingale's gendered rationalizations of nursing as an extension of feminine nurturing began a shift in public understandings of wartime nursing and of women's wartime roles.[6]

Just as the Crimean War marked a significant change in notions of wartime nursing in Europe, the Civil War prompted transformations in the United States only a few years later. Confronted with conceptions of war as physically and morally treacherous, middle- and upper-class women extended the ideology of women's domestic sphere to justify and deem respectable their place in warzone hospitals.[7] Jane Schultz demonstrates that women characterized wartime nursing as respectable by likening nursing to their usual feminine work in the home and by characterizing soldiers as family. In this vein, women who could afford to volunteer their time argued that their work was more wholesome and meaningful than that of working-class, African American, and slave women who were assigned more physically challenging, menial, and less patient-focused tasks, and who (despite being the majority of female hospital workers) received no postwar recognition or pension.[8] Unlike nurses in Scutari, however, women in the hospitals of Antietam, Gettysburg, and Shiloh employed gender ideologies to advocate for more power in the hospital. When female nurses' assertions of medical authority brought them into conflict with physicians and military officials, Judith Ann Giesberg finds, women argued that if their feminine characteristics ideally suited them to care for the wounded, then they should have the authority to make medical decisions.[9] In Nancy Scripture Garrison's assessment, women bridged a conventional ideology of middle- and upper-class femininity with a more progressive push for medical authority by framing "nursing as an extension of their womanhood" and "an affirmation of their strength."[10]

Domestic and familial metaphors assumed new meaning during World War I, when, as Susan Grayzel indicates, national rhetoric in Britain and France defined "motherhood as women's primary patriotic role and the core of their national identity."[11] Maternal images of nurses even successfully transformed public opinion of nursing in France, Margaret H. Darrow argues, from a disreputable task to a natural extension of motherhood, feminine righteousness, and women's patriotic service to soldiers.[12] Britain's volunteer First Aid Nursing Yeomanry nurses utilized these maternal ideals to expand their nursing practice, Janet Lee attests, "by grounding their call to service in an essentialized femininity of nurturance."[13] But while maternal symbols ascribed meaning to nurses' work, complicated ties between gender, class, and professionalism divided them within the hospital. According to Janet S.K. Watson and Susan Ouditt, untrained upper-class Voluntary Aid Detachment nurses easily conformed to Britons' notions of nurses as sacrificial mothers.[14] Trained working- and middle-class nurses who required payment for their services conformed less easily to prevailing notions of sacrificial motherhood and felt compelled "to demonstrate the essential and unique skills that only graduates of recognized nursing training programs possessed" to justify their place in the wartime hospital.[15] However much professional and economic concerns divided them, Christine Hallet finds that both trained and untrained nurses believed a familial environment to be important for patient recovery and invoked notions of domesticity to guard against suspicion of their motivations.[16]

By World War II, women no longer needed to rationalize nursing as an extension of domesticity or motherhood to secure their place in war. In many ways, as the war ushered women into many previously "masculine" roles in militaries and workforces, the profession's codification as feminine protected nurses from criticism and suspicion. And yet, gendered understandings of nursing excluded many qualified nurses from wartime service. Despite a shortage so serious that the US Congress nearly drafted nurses and in spite of a qualified population of African American and male nurses, Barbara Tomblin explains, the US military resisted opening the corps to either group.[17]

According to Cynthia Toman, the Canadian military similarly excluded First Nation, black, and Asian women, as well as men.[18]

The post-World War II period witnessed remarkable changes in gender roles, and yet, my work on army nurses in the Vietnam War reveals that even after the military admitted men as nurses, gender remained a central part of the military's and the men's understanding of the work. While the army devoted considerable effort to delineating distinct roles for male and female nurses, men frequently ascribed masculine qualities to the tasks they performed in an effort to distinguish themselves from lingering associations of nursing and femininity.[19] Scholars have yet to evaluate fully the influence of gender on wartime nursing in late 20th-century conflicts, but the field is ripe for analysis. Although some, like Jan Bassett in her coda on Australian nurses in the first Gulf War, suspect that gender functions less for modern military nurses than it did for their predecessors, there is much to learn about the ways that female and male nurses conceive of gender, nursing, and power today.[20]

War as power

As nurses embraced gender to secure their place in wartime hospitals, wartime service also became a source of power for women who sought unparalleled opportunities and national recognition. Wartime service presented some women with personal experiences that most women did not have, and it allowed them to engage in a heightened and complex level of practice that escaped most nurses. Many women embraced these opportunities and sought military rank as a means of securing tangible and ideological reward for their service. As historians have convincingly shown, nurses have both reflected and shaped larger debates about acceptable and obligatory wartime roles for women. Investigating their experiences allows historians to contemplate the changing place of women in the nation and the wider world.[21]

Although domestic metaphors defined wartime nursing as merely an extension of women's nature, the reality of nurses' wartime lives "subverted the ideology of separate spheres."[22] Wartime experiences were "transitional" for women, Garrison argues in her history of Sanitary Commission nurses during the US Civil War, as they exchanged "domesticity for independence and challenge."[23] British nurses in World War I might have similarly operated within feminine convention, Summers demonstrates, but they also crossed "social and political frontiers" and helped "normalise the idea of women's war service."[24] War also facilitated a transformative professional experience for nurses pressed to perform a wider range of practice than normally expected. Toman reveals, for example, that the closer Canadian nurses in World War II were to the front, the more they were able to practice autonomously and to take on responsibilities ordinarily carried out by physicians.[25] I argue that the demands of the Vietnam War created similar situations for nurses who embraced their increased responsibilities as a sign of professional equality.[26] Ultimately, while scholars suggest that connections between conventional gender norms and nursing might have limited women's push for complete autonomy, they concede that wartime nursing allowed women to move beyond conventional propriety to participate in war, hold positions of authority, and create a "new political culture."[27]

Even as wartime demands expanded women's lives and their professional practice, military nurses continued to face restrictions and discrimination because of their gender. Initially employed as contract workers and then varyingly enlisted only in temporary or reserve services, nurses' military status remained ambiguous until the mid-20th century. Nurses were, in Summers's words, "in but not of" the military.[28] Nurses began a concerted effort to secure formal military rank during World War I, an era ripe with discussions about the expansion of women's public roles and their rights as citizens. As Susan Zeiger and Kimberly Jensen maintain, US military nurses' frustrations with their lack of hospital authority convinced them that officer rank would protect them from professional abuse and workplace harassment. Moreover, nurses began to argue not only that they needed rank for these professional reasons, but also that they had earned the benefits of such status through their work.[29] Nurses continued their efforts after the war to expand the meaning of their wartime service, arguing that their service to the nation should garner women more social and political rights. As Jensen suggests, nurses believed that their military service signaled a more progressive "civic equality and professionalism."[30]

Nurses continued to lobby for the expansion of their military status in the years following World War I, but only another war proved a compelling enough reason for belligerent nations to extend the privileges and power of rank to women. The British military granted officer commissions to nurses in the Queen Anne's Imperial Military Nursing Service in 1941, while American nurses held only relative rank until June 1944, when Congress granted temporary commissions with equal pay and benefits for the war's duration plus an additional six months.[31] Military rank provided real power for nurses, though in limited ways. Toman notes that when Canadian nurses received officer commissions in 1942, their rank facilitated a more equitable relationship with physicians than nurses experienced in civilian nursing, even though they only held authority over other women and patients and received fewer postwar veterans' benefits than men.[32] Even after the 1947 Army-Navy Nurses' Act provided permanent commissioned officer status for US military nurses, women found the benefits of militarization to be mixed.[33] The military's opening of all ranks to women in the late 1960s and the promotion of the chief of the Army Nurse Corps to the rank of general in 1970, I argue, marked profound progress for nurses and for women. And yet, even as many nurses believed that they owed martial obligations equal to men and ascribed progressive meaning to their experiences, postwar depictions once again projected a much more conservative image of nurses and the meaning of their service than the women believed they had achieved.[34]

Historians convincingly argue that nurses' wartime service has been partially to credit for women's expanding roles beyond the hospital since the mid-19th century. And while scholars have provided a solid analytical base from which to work, we know significantly less than we should about the ways that nurses in World War II or even the long Cold War era helped to shape notions of women's changing social roles. Historians suggest that women's participation in World War II planted the seeds for the growth of second-wave feminism. They also note that the postwar era was a complex time in which political fears manifested in anxieties about gender, in which women's employment opportunities multiplied, and in which the meanings and rewards of military service changed radically. We need a deeper understanding of the ways in which wartime nursing shaped, and was shaped by, each of these changes.

Nursing as power

Moving beyond strict definitions of war as a declared conflict between nations, historians are now extending their analyses to the ways nursing itself functions as a form of martial power. Rooted in studies that have demonstrated the role of medicine and gender in exerting imperial control, historians argue that nurses and nursing have functioned to extend both formal and cultural power.[35] In these ways, historians are heeding Julia F. Irwin's argument that nursing history "should not be relegated to the peripheries of U.S. international history . . . but must be made central in any historical consideration of the United States in the world."[36] These considerations of nursing as an agent of power also complicate our understanding of nursing as a humanitarian act. Although historians acknowledge the benevolence that nurses perform in the fulfillment of their medical duties, they are beginning to understand that the extension of medical care occurs within a political, social, and cultural context that gives it meaning. Nurses heal, certainly, but they do so as agents of nations, militaries, and organizations that extend services as part of a larger political ideology. In moving beyond a simplistic notion of nursing as humanitarian and of war as a military engagement, we are moving toward a more complex understanding of nursing as an element not only of waging war, but also of waging power.

Nurses have struggled with questions of nursing's powerful potential, though as scholars note, they have typically considered the matter in the context of nursing's function within wars. Military nurses in particular have struggled with whether their martial obligations conflicted with or even undermined their work as nurses. As Penny Starns explains, for example, increased militarization changed nursing practice among British World War II nurses who came to value tidy ward administration more than traditionally feminine expressions of tenderness and compassion.[37] Not all women welcomed these militarized notions of nursing. As Toman and Bassett note in their histories of Canadian and Australian nursing during the war, Commonwealth nurses in particular resisted exchanging conventional gender for militarization. Although eager to prove their worthiness of military status, nurses in both cases expressed a reluctance to salute other military officials because they associated the military tradition with masculinity.[38]

Considerations of the complex relationship between medical care and military mission extend to questions about the function of nursing for individual patients. In his examination of World War I hospital magazines, Jeffrey S. Reznick argues that soldiers viewed their regimented nursing care as an extension of war's militaristic control of their bodies.[39] Hallett maintains in her study of American and British nurses in World War I that nurses' regimented procedures "contained" instead of controlled patients, but even she acknowledges the ways that nursing practice advanced military causes.[40] Moreover, historians note that nurses in as varied wars as the two World Wars and the

Vietnam War expressed frustration over their constant efforts to heal wounded soldiers only to see them returned to battle.[41] When called upon to treat the victims of their own military's actions or prisoners of war, nurses strained even more to reconcile their medical charge to heal with their membership in the military that waged such destruction and that defined patients as enemies. Race, ideology, and language further divided nurses from these patients and frustrated nurses' efforts to bridge their medical and military motives.[42]

In addition to seeing contradictions between nurses' medical and military duties, scholars argue that nursing itself has functioned as an element of military and organizational policies. In some ways, Toman points out, nursing became an element of war as medical care assumed a strong national identity and became an essential part of militaries' efforts to wage war. As "medical units became strategic components of battle plans" during World War II, she argues, nurses' noncombatant status blurred.[43] Medicine and strategy combined in similar ways during the Vietnam War. American army nurses participated in the US government's Medical Civic Action Program, an ostensibly humanitarian aid project that delivered basic medical care to Vietnamese civilians but that also sought to create a favorable view of the American government among villagers and to craft a humanitarian image of the American military intervention. Although many nurses enjoyed the chance to work with the local population, their work undermined their own image of nursing as purely humanitarian and made the nurses complicit in government propaganda efforts.[44]

Nurses' participation in wartime policies perhaps most obviously conflicts with medical aims in the history of nurses' involvement in Nazi extermination policies. In Bronwyn Rebekah McFarland-Icke's disturbing but insightful history of psychiatric nurses' efforts to reconcile their professional aims with government sterilization efforts, she reveals the process by which nurses altered their perception of patients to rationalize their increasingly brutal and dehumanizing treatment. As nurses divorced their intent from the consequences of their actions, they relied on their place at the bottom of the medical hierarchy to acquiesce their consciences to the results of their work. Disproving the easy notion that nurses simply had little choice but to conform to Nazi policies, McFarland-Icke describes a much more disturbing process by which professional and government ideologies provided nurses "with the kind of psychological reinforcement that eased the journey down the slippery slope from treatment to complicity in murder."[45]

Studies such as these complicate the notion of wartime nursing as an apolitical, humanitarian endeavor and invite broader questions about the ways nursing has functioned as a powerful agent in cultural extensions of national power, and even as an agent of social and political control. Scholars contend that cultural imperialism frequently paves the way for more explicit political and military power, and they are beginning to understand how nursing has functioned to extend those influences. Irwin, for example, examines the work of four Red Cross nurses who traveled the world in the immediate post-World War I era to establish nurse training schools and mother/child health programs. Believing that nursing would create opportunities for women to uplift their nations and that improving public health in nations around the world was a necessary precursor for democratic society, these nurses not only paved the way for more extensive intervention on the part of the US government, but also, Irwin reveals, served as a form of diplomacy by "masking the more violent and aggressive aspects of American empire and defining U.S. influence in the world as a force for good."[46] Catherine Ceniza Choy finds similar connections between nursing, US imperialism in the Philippines, and subsequent Filipino nurse migration. Arguing that nursing concealed the unequal relationships inherent in and the more violent nature of American cultural imperialism, she demonstrates that the formation of nursing programs in the Philippines was not simply an act of American benevolence, but one that furthered the gender and racial hierarchies of American nursing and imperialism.[47]

With these fruitful works as a guide, nursing historians can continue to advance our understanding of the militarization of nursing and its use as an agent of power. Nations have waged "wars" on drugs, poverty, and terror. State organizations have employed nurses in medical work and experiments that rested on and furthered ideologies of racial hierarchy. We have much to learn about how nurses have thought about their role in such efforts and about how the subjects of such work perceived the nurses. We may not continue to imagine wartime nurses as romantic figures wiping fevered brows on foreign fields, but the story we tell can teach us much more about nursing and power in all its manifestations.

Notes

1 I do not mean to suggest that there are no melodramatic or romanticized "historical" accounts of war nursing. There are many. Here, however, I will focus on the ways analytical histories of wartime nursing investigate the subject and the interpretations they provide. Additionally, I exclude from my analysis several invaluable official military histories. These works provide a solid foundation for any nursing historian, but they do not offer an academic interpretation grounded in the scholarship of nursing history, medical history, the history of women, or the history of gender. I certainly recommend their use, though with an understanding that military-produced histories are written at least in part to advance the military's ideologies.

2 Certainly not all nursing historians agree, though I argue that most interpretations fall within Margaret R. Higonnet and Patrice L.-R. Higonnet's "double helix" metaphor, which holds that wars both enhance and retard women's status in broader society. Three works suggest the range of interpretations. In her chronicle of Australian military nurses, Jan Bassett suggests that, until very recently, military service extended the social and political limitations that women faced, in part because of economic discrimination. Even in her conservative analysis of the benefits conveyed by military service, however, she acknowledges that women serving in the Australian military enjoyed experiences beyond those that they would have faced in civilian life.

As documented by historians who have studied militaries across the globe and centuries, military women indeed faced sexual discrimination. Paid less than men, accorded limited privileges, and denied upward mobility within the ranks, women serving as military nurses have struggled for equality on many fronts. However, as Cynthia Toman argues in her study of Canadian nurses in World War II, women were not powerless within these constraints and "negotiated significant social and professional space within this traditionally male domain." Offering a similarly nuanced interpretation of the mixed opportunities and restrictions military nursing provided women, I argue in my examination of the US Army

Nurse Corps during the Vietnam War that even while retrograde gender conventions shaped nurses' work and lives in many ways, military nursing provided some opportunities that neither nurses nor women in general enjoyed outside the ranks. Vietnam-era nurses certainly negotiated power within the limitations of the military, as Canadian nurses had decades prior, but they also found that the army offered professional rewards such as equal pay and professional advancement that feminists were struggling to secure in other occupations (Margaret R. Higonnet and Patrice L.-R. Higonnet, "The Double Helix," in Margaret Randolph Higonnet et al. (eds) *Behind the Lines: Gender and the Two World Wars*, New Haven, CT: Yale University Press, 1987, pp. 31–47; Jan Bassett, *Guns and Brooches: Australian Army Nursing from the Boer War to the Gulf War*, Melbourne: Oxford University Press Australia, 1992; Cynthia Toman, *An Officer and a Lady: Canadian Military Nursing and the Second World War*, Studies in Canadian Military History, Vancouver, Canada: University of British Columbia Press, 2007, pp. 11–12; Kara Dixon Vuic, *Officer, Nurse, Woman: The Army Nurse Corps in the Vietnam War*, War/Society/Culture, Baltimore, MD: The Johns Hopkins University Press, 2010).

3 The gendered connotations of wartime nursing changed slowly even in the mid-19th century. Even as female nurses made inroads in their efforts to secure a place in the wartime hospital, Summers notes that the British military continued to use more men than women as nurses until after the Boer War, while Jane Schultz points out that more men than women nursed during the American Civil War. See Anne Summers, *Angels and Citizens: British Women as Military Nurses, 1854–1914*, New York: Routledge and Kegan Paul, 1988, pp. 1–2; Jane E. Schultz, *Women at the Front: Hospital Workers in Civil War America*, Civil War America, Chapel Hill: University of North Carolina Press, 2004, p. 18; also Vuic, *Officer, Nurse, Woman*, p. 47.

4 Summers, *Angels and Citizens*, pp. 67–96, 118–120.

5 Summers, *Angels and Citizens*, p. 46.

6 Summers, *Angels and Citizens*, pp. 29–66.

7 As Mary Denis Maher shows in her history of nuns in the war, military officials initially requested that Catholic sisters work as nurses. Nuns had performed wartime nursing care for many years and military officials were confident in their skill and experience. Moreover, the sisters' religious commitment to serving others averted the questions of propriety that other women who volunteered their service faced. Mary Denis Maher, *To Bind up the Wounds: Catholic Sister Nurses in the U.S. Civil War*, Contributions in Women's Studies, No. 107, New York: Greenwood Press, 1989, pp. 30–85. Schultz argues that military officials also requested the work of nuns because they asked for no payment. Schultz, *Women at the Front*, pp. 21, 43.

8 Schultz, *Women at the Front*, pp. 19–44, 46–63, 87–104; Judith Ann Giesberg, *Civil War Sisterhood: The U.S. Sanitary Commission and Women's Politics in Transition*, Boston: Northeastern University Press, 2000, pp. 33–52.

9 Giesberg, *Civil War Sisterhood*, pp. 113–133; also Schultz, *Women at the Front*, pp. 6, 108–141.

10 Nancy Scripture Garrison, *With Courage and Delicacy: Civil War on the Peninsula, Women and the U.S. Sanitary Commission*, Mason City, IA: Savon Publishing, 1999, p. 130.

11 Susan R. Grayzel, *Women's Identities at War: Gender, Motherhood, and Politics in Britain and France during the First World War*, Chapel Hill, NC: University of North Carolina Press, 1999, p. 3.

12 Margaret H. Darrow, "French Volunteer Nurses and the Myth of the War Experience in World War I," *American Historical Review* 101:1, February 1996, pp. 86–92.

13 Janet Lee, *War Girls: The First Aid Nursing Yeomanry in the First World War*, Manchester, UK: Manchester University Press, 2005, pp. 35, 41–42.

14 Janet S.K. Watson, "Khaki Girls, VADs, and Tommy's Sisters: Gender and Class in First World War Britain," *International History Review* 19:1, February 1997, pp. 32–51; Sharon

Ouditt, *Fighting Forces, Writing Women: Identity and Ideology in the First World War*, London: Routledge, 1994, p. 10.

15 Janet S.K. Watson, "Wars in the Wards: The Social Construction of Medical Work in First World War Britain," *Journal of British Studies* 41:4, October 2002, pp. 494, 486.

16 Christine E. Hallett, *Containing Trauma: Nursing Work in the First World War*, Cultural History of Modern War, Manchester, UK: Manchester University Press, 2009, pp. 177–180, 202.

17 The army accepted only a very small quota of black women to serve and assigned them to segregated hospitals and prisoner of war wards. Military officials contended that men could not serve as nurses in the armed forces because they would not be able to submit to authority or provide intimate care for men. Barbara Brooks Tomblin, *G.I. Nightingales: The Army Nurse Corps in World War II*, Lexington, KY: University Press of Kentucky, 1996, pp. 11, 123–124, 191–193, 197, 201, 210; Vuic, *Officer, Nurse, Woman*, p. 49; Darlene Clark Hine, *Black Women in White: Racial Conflict and Cooperation in the Nursing Profession, 1890–1950*, Blacks in the Diaspora, Bloomington, IN: Indiana University Press, 1989, pp. 162–186.

18 Toman, *An Officer and a Lady*, pp. 3, 21, 44–45.

19 Vuic, *Officer, Nurse, Woman*, pp. 47–52, 99–111.

20 Bassett, *Guns and Brooches*, pp. 207–208.

21 On the ways in which military service has conferred citizenship rights and the ways women have sought military service as a way of asserting their claim to equal citizenship, see Linda K. Kerber, *No Constitutional Right to Be Ladies: Women and the Obligations of Citizenship*, New York: Hill and Wang, 1998; Linda K. Kerber, "'May All Our Citizens be Soldiers, and All Our Soldiers Citizens': The Ambiguities of Female Citizenship in the New Nation," in Jean Bethke Elshtain and Sheila Tobias, eds., *Women, Militarism, and War*, Savage, MD: Rowman and Littlefield, 1990, 89–104; Linda K. Kerber, *Women of the Republic: Intellect and Ideology in Revolutionary America*, Institute of Early American History, Chapel Hill, NC: University of North Carolina Press, 1980; Cecilia Elizabeth O'Leary, *To Die For: The Paradox of American Patriotism*, Princeton, NJ: Princeton University Press, 1999, 30–37, 73–104; Kimberly Jensen, "Women, Citizenship, and Civic Sacrifice: Engendering Patriotism in the First World War," in John Bodnar, ed., *Bonds of Affection: Americans Define Their Patriotism*, Princeton, NJ: Princeton University Press, 1996, 139–159; Ilene Rose Feinman, *Citizenship Rites: Feminist Soldiers and Feminist Antimilitarists*, New York: New York University Press, 2000; Nina Silber, *Daughters of the Union: Northern Women Fight the Civil War*, Cambridge, MA: Harvard University Press, 2005, 263–265.

22 Giesberg, *Civil War Sisterhood*, p. 116.

23 Garrison, *With Courage and Delicacy*, p. 2.

24 Summers, *Angels and Citizens*, pp. 151, 152, also 142–153, 271–290.

25 Toman, *An Officer and a Lady*, pp. 118, 122–133.

26 Vuic, *Officer, Nurse, Woman*, pp. 73–80.

27 Giesberg, *Civil War Sisterhood*, p. 8; also Schultz, *Women at the Front*, p. 3; Garrison, *With Courage and Delicacy*, p. 2; Ouditt, *Fighting Forces, Writing Women*, p. 33; Lee, *War Girls*, p. 52.

28 Summers, *Angels and Citizens*, p. 4.

29 Kimberly Jensen, *Mobilizing Minerva: American Women in the First World War*, Urbana, IL: University of Illinois Press, 2008, pp. 117–141; also Philip A. Kalisch, "How Army Nurses Became Officers," *Nursing Research* 25:3, May–June 1976, pp. 164–177.

30 Jensen, *Mobilizing Minerva*, p. ix; also Susan Zeiger, *In Uncle Sam's Service: Women Workers with the American Expeditionary Force, 1917–1919*, Ithaca, NY: Cornell University Press, 1999, pp. 137–174.

31 Janann Sherman, "'They Either Need These Women or They Do Not': Margaret Chase Smith and the Fight for Regular Status for Women in the Military," *Journal of Military History* 54:1, January 1990, pp. 66–67; also Kalisch, "How Army Nurses Became Officers."

32 Toman, *An Officer and a Lady*, pp. 87–91, 94, 99.
33 The Army-Navy Nurses' Act of 1947 provided permanent commissioned officer status with equal pay and allowances for nurses. The 1948 Women's Armed Services Integration Act integrated women into permanent positions in the military. See Army-Navy Nurses' Act, ch. 38, United States Statutes at Large 61 Stat. 41; *Women's Armed Services Integration Act of 1948*, 62 *Stat.* 356, Public Law 80-625, June 12, 1948.
34 Vuic, *Officer, Nurse, Woman*, pp. 52–57, 66–69, 154–186.
35 For studies on the ways medicine has functioned as an extension of national power see Roy MacLeod and Milton Lewis, eds., *Disease, Medicine, and Empire: Perspectives on Western Medicine and the Experience of European Expansion*, London: Routledge, 1988; David Arnold, *Colonizing the Body: State Medicine and Epidemic Disease in Nineteenth Century India*, Berkeley, CA: University of California Press, 1993; Laura Briggs, *Reproducing Empire: Race, Sex, Science, and U.S. Imperialism in Puerto Rico*, Berkeley, CA: University of California Press, 2003; Mary-Ellen Kelm, *Colonizing Bodies: Aboriginal Health and Healing in British Columbia, 1900–1950*, Vancouver, Canada: University of British Columbia Press, 1998. On the centrality of gender to the extension of empire see Donna Alvah, *Unofficial Ambassadors: American Military Families Overseas and the Cold War, 1946–1965*, New York: New York University Press, 2007; Helen Callaway, *Gender, Culture, and Empire: European Women in Colonial Nigeria*, Urbana, IL: University of Illinois Press, 1987; Amy Kaplan, "Manifest Domesticity," in Donald E. Pease and Robyn Wiegman, eds., *The Futures of American Studies*, Durham, NC: Duke University Press, 2002, pp. 111–134; Laura Wexler, *Tender Violence: Domestic Visions in an Age of U.S. Imperialism*, Cultural Studies of the United States, Chapel Hill, NC: University of North Carolina Press, 2000.
36 Julia F. Irwin, "Nurses without Borders: The History of Nursing as U.S. International History," *Nursing History Review* 19, 2011, p. 80.
37 Penny Starns, "Fighting Militarism? British Nursing during the Second World War," in Roger Cooter, Mark Harrison, Steve Study (eds.) *War, Medicine, and Modernity*, London: Sutton, 1998, p. 198.
38 Toman, *An Officer and a Lady*, pp. 92–98; Bassett, *Guns and Brooches*, p. 3.
39 Jeffrey S. Reznick, *Healing the Nation: Soldiers and the Culture of Caregiving in Britain during the Great War*, Cultural History of Modern War, Manchester, UK: Manchester University Press, 2004, pp. 65–98.
40 Hallett, *Containing Trauma*, p. 6.
41 Zeiger, *In Uncle Sam's Service*, pp. 134–35; Toman, *An Officer and a Lady*, pp. 85–87; Vuic, *Officer, Nurse, Woman*, pp. 80–85.
42 Vuic, *Officer, Nurse, Woman*, pp. 83–84; Tomblin, *G.I. Nightingales*, pp. 147–150.
43 Toman, *An Officer and a Lady*, pp. 85, 117.
44 Vuic, *Officer, Nurse, Woman*, pp. 82–83, also Robert J. Wilensky, *Military Medicine to Win Hearts and Minds: Aid to Civilians in the Vietnam War*, Lubbock, TX: Texas Tech University Press, 2004.
45 Bronwyn Rebekah McFarland-Icke, *Nurses in Nazi Germany: Moral Choice in History*, Princeton, NJ: Princeton University Press, 1999, p. 171.
46 Irwin, "Nurses Without Borders," p. 94.
47 Catherine Ceniza Choy, *Empire of Care: Nursing and Migration in Filipino American History*, American Encounters/Global Interactions, Durham, NC: Duke University Press, 2003, p. 19.

Bibliography

Alvah, Donna, *Unofficial Ambassadors: American Military Families Overseas and the Cold War, 1946–1965*, New York: New York University Press, 2007.
Arnold, David, *Colonizing the Body: State Medicine and Epidemic Disease in Nineteenth Century India*, Berkeley, CA: University of California Press, 1993.

Bassett, Jan, *Guns and Brooches: Australian Army Nursing from the Boer War to the Gulf War*, Melbourne: Oxford University Press Australia, 1992.

Briggs, Laura, *Reproducing Empire: Race, Sex, Science, and U.S. Imperialism in Puerto Rico*, Berkeley, CA: University of California Press, 2003.

Callaway, Helen, *Gender, Culture, and Empire: European Women in Colonial Nigeria*, Urbana, IL: University of Illinois Press, 1987.

Choy, Catherine Ceniza, *Empire of Care: Nursing and Migration in Filipino American History*, American Encounters/Global Interactions, Durham, NC: Duke University Press, 2003.

Darrow, Margaret H., "French Volunteer Nurses and the Myth of the War Experience in World War I," *American Historical Review* 101:1, February 1996, 80–106.

Feinman, Ilene Rose, *Citizenship Rites: Feminist Soldiers and Feminist Antimilitarists*, New York: New York University Press, 2000.

Garrison, Nancy Scripture, *With Courage and Delicacy: Civil War on the Peninsula, Women and the U.S. Sanitary Commission*, Mason City, IA: Savon Publishing, 1999.

Giesberg, Judith Ann, *Civil War Sisterhood: The U.S. Sanitary Commission and Women's Politics in Transition*, Boston: Northeastern University Press, 2000.

Grayzel, Susan R., *Women's Identities at War: Gender, Motherhood, and Politics in Britain and France during the First World War*, Chapel Hill, NC: University of North Carolina Press, 1999.

Hallett, Christine E., *Containing Trauma: Nursing Work in the First World War*, Cultural History of Modern War, Manchester, UK: Manchester University Press, 2009.

Higonnet, Margaret R. and Patrice L.-R. Higonnet, "The Double Helix," in Margaret Randolph Higonnet et al. (eds.) *Behind the Lines: Gender and the Two World Wars*, New Haven, CT: Yale University Press, 1987, 31–47.

Hine, Darlene Clark, *Black Women in White: Racial Conflict and Cooperation in the Nursing Profession, 1890–1950*, Blacks in the Diaspora, Bloomington, IN: Indiana University Press, 1989.

Irwin, Julia F., "Nurses without Borders: The History of Nursing as U.S. International History," *Nursing History Review* 19, 2011, 78–102.

Jensen, Kimberly, "Women, Citizenship, and Civic Sacrifice: Engendering Patriotism in the First World War," in John Bodnar (ed.) *Bonds of Affection: Americans Define Their Patriotism*, Princeton, NJ: Princeton University Press, 1996, 139–159.

Jensen, Kimberly, *Mobilizing Minerva: American Women in the First World War*, Urbana, IL: University of Illinois Press, 2008.

Kalisch, Philip A., "How Army Nurses Became Officers," *Nursing Research* 25:3, May–June 1976, 164–177.

Kaplan, Amy, "Manifest Domesticity," in Donald E. Pease and Robyn Wiegman (eds.) *The Futures of American Studies*, Durham, NC: Duke University Press, 2002, 111–134.

Kelm, Mary-Ellen, *Colonizing Bodies: Aboriginal Health and Healing in British Columbia, 1900–1950*, Vancouver, Canada: University of British Columbia Press, 1998.

Kerber, Linda K., *Women of the Republic: Intellect and Ideology in Revolutionary America*, Institute of Early American History, Chapel Hill, NC: University of North Carolina Press, 1980.

Kerber, Linda K., "'May All Our Citizens be Soldiers, and All Our Soldiers Citizens': The Ambiguities of Female Citizenship in the New Nation," in Jean Bethke Elshtain and Sheila Tobias (eds.) *Women, Militarism, and War*, Savage, MD: Rowman and Littlefield, 1990, 89–104.

Kerber, Linda K., *No Constitutional Right to Be Ladies: Women and the Obligations of Citizenship*, New York: Hill and Wang, 1998.

Lee, Janet, *War Girls: The First Aid Nursing Yeomanry in the First World War*, Manchester, UK: Manchester University Press, 2005.

MacLeod, Roy and Milton Lewis, eds., *Disease, Medicine, and Empire: Perspectives on Western Medicine and the Experience of European Expansion*, London: Routledge, 1988.

Maher, Mary Denis, *To Bind up the Wounds: Catholic Sister Nurses in the U.S. Civil War*, Contributions in Women's Studies, No. 107, New York: Greenwood Press, 1989.

McFarland-Icke, Bronwyn Rebekah, *Nurses in Nazi Germany: Moral Choice in History*, Princeton, NJ: Princeton University Press, 1999.

O'Leary, Cecilia Elizabeth, *To Die For: The Paradox of American Patriotism*, Princeton, NJ: Princeton University Press, 1999.

Ouditt, Sharon, *Fighting Forces, Writing Women: Identity and Ideology in the First World War*, London: Routledge, 1994.

Reznick, Jeffrey S., *Healing the Nation: Soldiers and the Culture of Caregiving in Britain during the Great War*, Cultural History of Modern War, Manchester, UK: Manchester University Press, 2004.

Schultz, Jane E., *Women at the Front: Hospital Workers in Civil War America*, Civil War America, Chapel Hill, NC: University of North Carolina Press, 2004.

Sherman, Janann, "'They Either Need These Women or They Do Not': Margaret Chase Smith and the Fight for Regular Status for Women in the Military," *Journal of Military History* 54:1, January 1990, 66–67.

Silber, Nina, *Daughters of the Union: Northern Women Fight the Civil War*, Cambridge, MA: Harvard University Press, 2005.

Starns, Penny, "Fighting Militarism? British Nursing during the Second World War," in Roger Cooter, Mark Harrison, Steve Study (eds.) *War, Medicine, and Modernity*, London: Sutton, 1998, 189–202.

Summers, Anne, *Angels and Citizens: British Women as Military Nurses, 1854–1914*, New York: Routledge & Kegan Paul, 1988.

Toman, Cynthia, *An Officer and a Lady: Canadian Military Nursing and the Second World War*, Studies in Canadian Military History, Vancouver, Canada: University of British Columbia Press, 2007.

Tomblin, Barbara Brooks, *G.I. Nightingales: The Army Nurse Corps in World War II*, Lexington, KY: University Press of Kentucky, 1996.

Vuic, Kara Dixon, "'I'm Afraid We're Going to Have to Just Change Our Ways': Marriage, Motherhood, and Pregnancy in the Army Nurse Corps during the Vietnam War," *Signs* 32:4, Summer 2007, 997–1022.

Vuic, Kara Dixon, *Officer, Nurse, Woman: The Army Nurse Corps in the Vietnam War*, War/Society/Culture, Baltimore, MD: The Johns Hopkins University Press, 2010.

Watson, Janet S.K., "Khaki Girls, VADs, and Tommy's Sisters: Gender and Class in First World War Britain," *International History Review* 19:1, February 1997, 32–51.

Watson, Janet S.K., "Wars in the Wards: The Social Construction of Medical Work in First World War Britain," *Journal of British Studies* 41:4, October 2002, 484–510.

Wexler, Laura, *Tender Violence: Domestic Visions in an Age of U.S. Imperialism*, Cultural Studies of the United States, Chapel Hill, NC: University of North Carolina Press, 2000.

Wilensky, Robert J., *Military Medicine to Win Hearts and Minds: Aid to Civilians in the Vietnam War*, Lubbock, TX: Texas Tech University Press, 2004.

Zeiger, Susan, *In Uncle Sam's Service: Women Workers with the American Expeditionary Force, 1917–1919*, Ithaca, NY: Cornell University Press, 1999.

PART 2

New methodological approaches in the history of nursing

3

NURSES AND NURSING IN LITERARY AND CULTURAL STUDIES

Thomas Lawrence Long

Cultural representations of nursing provide historians with useful methods and insights. Like the social scientist's personal interview or focus group, cultural artifacts speak from the anecdotal and idiosyncratic experiences, perceptions, memories, and values of individuals living in specific historical conditions. Conversely, historians provide literary and cultural scholars with an understanding of the material conditions in which those discourses or artifacts were fashioned and used. If historiography describes *what* happened and explains *how* and *why* something happened, culture studies analyzes how people tried to *make sense* of what was happening and how those forms of cultural production operated within a *cultural system*.

In this survey of literary and cultural representations (and self-representations) of nursing, we see societies' concerns about the role of women in professional health care and nurses' concerns for visibility and professional autonomy, frequently configured around issues of gender, race, and social class. Although in recent years Americans surveyed have identified nursing as the most ethical profession, it is not clear that Americans also consider nursing as an analogously authoritative health profession, which may point to a representational gap. The cultural representations discussed here were selected for two reasons: First, they were available to a mass audience (in print or other media), and, second, they have achieved a canonical status in academia by becoming the objects of scholarly attention. At the same time, nurses' own self-representation in literary texts and other cultural forms seem fewer or less frequent than those by their counterparts in medicine, and nurse authors are probably less well known than comparable physician writers. For example, physician authors and their books, such as Abraham Verghese's *Cutting for Stone* (a novel), Atul Gawande's *The Checklist Manifesto* (a call for quality improvement in healthcare centers), David Servan-Schreiber's *Anticancer* (a memoir), and Siddhartha Mukherjee's *The Emperor of All Maladies: A Biography of Cancer*, all published in 2010, appeared on the *New York Times* "Best Sellers" list and received considerable acclaim in the media. Focusing on the presence of nurses' voices in news media, Bernice Buresh, Suzanne Gordon, and Nica Bell's 1991 study found a substantial gap between physicians' and nurses' representation,[1] which, Buresh and Gordon said in their *From Silence to Voice: What Nurses Know and Must Communicate to the Public*, persisted a decade later.[2]

Cultural studies and historiography

A historian might argue that literary texts and other forms of cultural production, regardless of genre, tend to be fictions, or at least are imaginative presentations of reality, so are not reliable sources of historical data. Nonetheless, literary and other cultural representations tell us something about the people who crafted them, the people who read or observed them, and the cultures in which their production and consumption occurred. As Hayden White reminds us, "the discourse of the historian and that of the imaginative writer overlap, resemble, or correspond to each other."[3] Historians, therefore, can profitably employ literary and cultural studies as part of a larger project of documenting and interpreting the history of the nursing profession and attitudes toward nurses.

Culture studies emerged in the mid-twentieth century from a variety of literary, philosophical, and political schools of thought (and conversely literary studies at the same time has been influenced by culture studies). Traditional literary studies, with its roots in Plato's discourses on written language and poetry and Aristotle's treatises on tragedy (*Poetics*) and public discourse (*Rhetoric*), had become by the mid-twentieth century focused primarily on formal, stylistic, and aesthetic dimensions of literary art. The approach of literary studies might be exemplified in a famous phrase of Victorian critic Matthew Arnold, for whom culture was "a pursuit of our total perfection by means of getting to know . . . the best which has been thought and said in the world,"[4] with Arnold providing his readers with the touchstones of "the best." In contrast, culture studies in its origins saw its role as illuminating all that has been thought and said (not just "the best"), and not just in literary texts, defining "culture" much more broadly. Clifford Geertz's influential *The Interpretation of Cultures* defines the term *culture* as "an historically transmitted pattern of meanings embodied in symbols, a system of inherited conceptions expressed in symbolic forms by means of which men [*sic*] communicate, perpetuate, and develop their knowledge about and attitudes toward life," and Geertz explores the ways in which culture is a text to be interpreted.[5] In their introductory essay to the anthology *Cultural Studies*, Cary Nelson, Paula A. Treichler, and Lawrence Grossberg note the relationship between anthropology and cultural studies, but underscore the latter's emergence from progressive political commitments.[6] Although Michel Foucault's methodological weaknesses as a historian have been frequently noted, his *The Birth of the Clinic: An Archeology of Medical Perception* remains an important theoretical foundation for culture studies' examination of healthcare discourses and practices.[7] Taking Foucault's analysis as a starting point, Robert Hodge's social semiotic *Literature as Discourse: Textual Strategies in English and History* illuminates the "social processes that flow through and irresistibly connect literary texts with many other kinds of texts, and social meanings that are produced in different ways from many social sites."

Adopting Foucault's concept of *discourse*, Hodge sees "literature as a process rather than simply a set of products; a process which is intrinsically social, connected at every point with mechanisms and institutions that mediate and control the flow of knowledge and power in a community."[8] Historicizing literary studies, Anthony Easthope's *Literary into Cultural Studies* analyzes the dissolving of a distinction between literary "high culture" (such as fiction, poetry and drama) and popular "low culture" (such as film and television).[9]

Culture studies' object of study is everything and anything that has been thought, said, done, performed, manufactured, crafted, fashioned, communicated, and mediated. These "discourses" (a pliable term that includes phenomena beyond the printed page) can include traditional literary forms, but also personal correspondence, diaries, scrapbooks, pamphlets, performances, and audio and video recordings, among other popular mass media. Some of these "artifacts" of culture are well known to historians as documentary evidence, so the question might arise: How differently does a scholar in culture studies interpret them? To start with, culture studies asks different questions from the historians' questions: What is the larger cultural system in which these artifacts are produced and how do they shape that system? How do these artifacts appropriate existing discourses or shape existing discourses? What cultural or ideological work do these artifacts perform? In what ways do these artifacts uphold cultural structures and in what ways do they subvert them? What claims do these artifacts make about reality and how do they argue those claims? How are these artifacts produced and circulated within a society? The literary text may be qualitative evidence for the historian, who asks if the text is credible or reliable as historical evidence or who uses the literary text to humanize the documentary record, but for culture studies the literary text (or a mass media form) is a component of larger systems about which culture studies theorizes.

By appropriating contemporary critical theory and by democratizing literary criticism and analysis, culture studies is concerned with political and material dimensions of culture, particularly the ways in which marginal cultures interact with dominant cultures. Culture studies is concerned with power, with the ways that cultural production creates social identity, and the ways that it legitimates, resists, or subverts existing structures of power, and leverages economic, social, or cultural capital. Culture studies strips away the cultural facades of political, social, and economic structures in order to reveal their disguised operations (which it assumes are always there regardless of a creator's or society's intentions). It is no wonder that culture studies approaches have often been adopted by scholars with commitments to underrepresented groups, such as women, sexual minorities, ethnic and racial minorities, and the disabled, which resonates with nursing historiography. As nurse historian Patricia D'Antonio has observed, nursing historiography is both an account of "the myriad ways in which women and some men reframed the most traditional of gendered expectations—that of caring for the sick" while it is also an account of the history of women.[10] The result is a complex subjectivity in the nurse and a paradox in the profession, what historian Susan Reverby has called the "dilemma of American nursing" in its first century, namely that being "ordered to care" nurses confronted "a series of limitations—of imagination, of cultural ideology, of economics, and ultimately of political power—in their efforts to care."[11] One other theme of the narrative of the nursing profession is "nurses' desires to differentiate their work from other health-related pursuits, and for professional autonomy and visibility."[12] Buresh and Gordon refine that theme by noting that nurses' invisibility is less the problem than nurses' silence. To bridge this gap, culture studies provides the historian with useful insights into how societies have thought of nursing and how nurses have thought of themselves.

In the second half of the twentieth century culture studies began to examine the elaborate systems whereby certain groups were culturally as well as politically and economically marginalized. *Self-representation*, a term that has a decidedly political sound, becomes an important cultural resource for groups accustomed to being the objects of another's literary or artistic representations, often by means of stereotyping. Solidarity or liberation movements among marginalized groups often undertake a campaign of cultural self-representation, both by cultivating artists and authors and by creating an infrastructure for making those self-representations public (e.g. establishing publishing venues such as periodicals or small presses). A culture studies approach to nursing history, then, is keenly interested not only in how others represent nursing (in novels, films, television, or advertising, for example), but also in how nurses represent themselves in cultural forms.

The twentieth century: conflict and competing narratives of ambiguity, agency, and autonomy

Literary representations of nursing in the twentieth century inherited from Victorian culture a range of archetypal images and stereotypes of nurses ranging from the benign to the malevolent. Nineteenth-century fiction and non-fiction depicted nurses as angels of mercy or as heroic healers (particularly in war narratives) or as the silent ancillaries of physicians or as young seductresses or as old battle axes. Nursing was represented as a noble profession but also as a romantic opportunity for adventure, particularly in novels whose lack of realism Florence Nightingale, herself a prolific writer, vigorously condemned.[13] Skilled and dedicated care of the sick was a major preoccupation of Victorian fiction in the hands of distinguished writers such as Charles Dickens, Jane Austen, Anne Brontë, Charlotte Brontë, Emily Brontë, George Eliot, and Elizabeth Gaskell.[14] These nursing characters and narratives were widely read, often published initially in mass-circulation periodicals that also featured the debates of the day, including articles and editorials concerning nursing,[15] which in turn were discourses that shaped literary texts, representing the period's concerns with "relationships between men and women, upper and lower classes, employers and employees, professionals and laypeople."[16] These social fault lines would deepen after the Victorian era in a period of accelerated change.

The twentieth century witnessed catastrophic war technologies and convulsive social movements, both on unprecedented scales, and both affecting nursing.[17] Nurses saw their professional roles expand, but not without controversy, and their increased visibility occasioned sometimes ambivalent responses. As a largely female health profession, nursing was affected by the woman suffrage movement in Europe and North America in the early twentieth century. A dominantly (though far from exclusively) White profession, US nursing also had to come to terms with the growing social and political movements for Black equality.

Nurses during World War I wrote about their experiences from a variety of motives and often may have believed that their role was to uphold morale, particularly in their letters home. For example, Pauline McVey asserted for an American readership:

> The spirit of the boys was wonderful. They had a few desires which constantly obsessed them. The predominant one was to be mended as soon as possible so that they could get back to their units. They were of the opinion that to lose connections with their outfits was even more to be regretted than the missing of a limb, or a severe operation of some other nature.[18]

However, not all nursing representations of World War I military hospitals were as uncritical of the war's conduct. Two writers, Ellen Newbold La Motte (a professional nurse, administrator, and specialist in tuberculosis care) and Mary Borden (a wealthy philanthropist and volunteer nurse whose initial frustration with the war's wasted medical resources prompted her to fund and establish her own frontline medical unit, which La Motte joined), wrote narratives representing the full moral ambiguity of the war. Both La Motte and Borden drained their narratives of the sentimentality or even sensationalism that had tended to characterize earlier nurse war texts from the Crimean War and the American Civil War, and both employed the concise genre of the sketch. La Motte's *The Backwash of War*, published during the war, "was so frank and powerful that it could not be distributed in England or France. By 1918, with American troops finally going over to France, the U.S. government inked out advertisements for the book in the *Liberator*, a monthly on whose editorial board La Motte was serving."[19] In *The Forbidden Zone*, published after the war, Borden asserts: "I have not invented anything in this book. The sketches and poems were written between 1914 and 1918, during four years of hospital work with the French Army. The five stories I have written recently from memory; they recount true episodes that I cannot forget."[20] In eerily paired accounts of the same patient, La Motte in "Heroes" and Borden in "Rosa" relate the case of a soldier who has attempted suicide in order to escape the horrors of war but who must be saved in order to try him for desertion, a capital crime for which he will be found guilty and executed. As the editor of a recently published anthology of Borden and La Motte's wartime writings, Margaret Higonnet, notes: "Military hospitals preoccupied with detecting fake wounds suppressed suicide reports,"[21] and, as Joanna Bourke documents, self-inflicted wounds could account for as many as one-quarter of a division's casualties not directly attributable to enemy fire.[22] Both of these nurse writers represented the horror, irrationality, and mendacity of the war with the same indignation as many of the war's greatest poets, such as the British-born Wilfred Owen and Siegfried Sassoon.

While wartime nurses were acutely aware of combat's horrors, they might also have been excited by the opportunities that nursing provided: a wider scope of action, an opportunity to contribute to a larger national cause, learning needed technical skills, and having occasions for leadership. In contrast to depictions of the horrors that wartime nurses witnessed, at mid-century young female readers were introduced to popular literary representations of nursing as an exciting, varied, and personally fulfilling career. Popular career narratives featuring the characters Sue Barton (in books written by Helen Dore Boylston after World War I) and Cherry Ames (in a book series initially authored by Helen Wells during World War II, with subsequent books written by Julie Tatham, before Wells returned to writing the series), these fictions reflect changing gender expectations, representing young women as energetic, autonomous, adventurous, and career-minded. Boylston, a World War I nurse, also wrote *Sister: The War Diary of a Nurse*[23] and *Clara Barton: Founder of the American Red Cross*.[24] Although Boylston's character Sue Barton had a steady romantic interest (Bill Barry, MD), their marriage was continually deferred from one book to the next while Sue climbed the nursing career ladder, from student nurse to hospital superintendent of nurses. Along the way she practiced nursing in a variety of settings: home visiting, rural, urban, hospital, and public health nursing. By the time Barton finally married Dr Barry (who had become a hospital director), her husband developed pneumonia and was bed-ridden, leaving Barton to run the hospital in his absence. As Deborah Philips observes, "Nursing is consistently constructed in the Sue Barton novels as an appropriate means for a young woman to achieve some measure of financial independence and professional status and to contribute to the social good."[25] Viewing themselves as candidates for meaningful careers outside the home, young female readers might see nursing as rewarding and varied work that did not necessarily preclude marriage.

If Barton was a focused and ambitious career professional, advancing in rank from one position to the next, her plucky counterpart Cherry Ames had more in common with the better known adventurous youth-literature characters, the Hardy Boys and Nancy Drew. In a series of 27 books published between the early 1940s and the late 1960s, Ames was alternatively depicted as contributing to the war effort during World War II (and encouraging the books' readers to do the same, in the books written by Helen Wells), as an adventurous amateur sleuth in the immediate post-war years (in the sequels written by Julie Tatham), and as a glamorous lifestyle figure in the final novels (which marked the return of Helen Wells's authorship). As Anita G. Gorman and Leslie Robertson Mateer observe: "Changes in authorship, Cherry's character, Cherry's vocation and relationships all reflect the shifting paradigms of a series adapting to changing conditions in both the world around it and the world it so assiduously portrays."[26] As much representations of historically contingent social norms changing over time as they are of the changing realities of nursing, the books and their different authors were responding to young readers' interests (or at least the publisher's understanding of them). Unlike Sue Barton, Ames had no steady love interest, although each novel has a romantic subplot, and her multiple and varied jobs (*Country Doctor's Nurse, Dude Ranch Nurse, Jungle Nurse, Department Store Nurse*) do not seem to constitute a career trajectory but are opportunities for adventure. Across two and a half decades and two authors, the Cherry Ames series "broke ground by depicting a woman with a career, a woman who did not see marriage as her immediate or ultimate goal, a woman who showed some independence and insubordination as well as the more conventional qualities of beauty, compassion, and adherence to hierarchical organization."[27] Betting on these novels' enduring popularity, in 2005 the health science publisher Springer reissued the books in boxed sets, aiming for a seemingly discrepant demographic by announcing on one hand, "Cherry Ames is back, just as you remember her! The books are just as you remember them," while on the other hand claiming Cherry's timeless youthfulness and appeal for today's younger readers: "making friends, pushing the limits of authority, leading her nursing colleagues, and sleuthing and solving mysteries. Smart, courageous, mischievous, quick-witted, and above all, devoted to nursing, Cherry Ames meets adventure head-on whereever [sic] she goes. Springer Publishing Company is delighted to be bringing Helen Wells's beloved heroine back into print for a new generation of younger readers."[28] Perhaps as well the publisher is counting on the series' innocent and uncomplicated depictions of nursing as a welcome tonic to readers after the darker, more conflicted nurse characters of the past fifty years.

The rewards of submitting oneself to an ordered profession, joining a community engaged in noble work, and even having opportunities for global travel occurred not only in wartime or civilian settings, but also in Catholic religious life. In Kathryn Hulme's *The Nun's Story*[29] (later adapted into Fred Zinneman's 1959 film of the same name and Zoe Fairbairns's radio play *The Belgian Nurse*), events in the life of Mary-Louise Habets (1905–1986) were novelized and dramatized. Habets, a nurse, entered the Roman Catholic religious order Soeurs de la Charité de Jesus et de Marie in Ghent, Belgium, in the late 1920s, and was trained for tropical nursing in the Belgian Congo where she served through much of the 1930s, returning to Belgium shortly before its invasion by the Germans and the onset of World War II. Chafing under the strict rule of the order and growing more conflicted at the order's neutrality during the Nazi occupation, she left the convent in 1944. Hulme and Habets met in Europe after the war, thereafter becoming lifelong companions, as well as literary collaborators in *The Nun's Story*, with Habets's work as a nurse subsidizing the household while Hulme pursued a literary career. When Zinneman proposed turning the book into a film, Hollywood studio executives were not receptive until Belgian-born actress Audrey Hepburn expressed her interest in the role (into which she was cast). In one of the extraordinary instances of life imitating art, Habets later helped nurse the actress who played her dramatized self, Hepburn, after the actress experienced a riding accident. Debra Campbell in a conference paper on the book and film observes:

> Catholic readers/moviegoers and Catholic historians alike have trouble knowing what to do with *The Nun's Story*. Like most contemporary reviewers of the book and film, we do not quite know how to read and evaluate a narrative that feels like fiction but claims to be "true in its essentials." Do we dare to treat *The Nun's Story* like an authentic life-writing, even perhaps a personal narrative?[30]

Historians might ask that question concerned primarily with the text's reliability as a historical document. However, from the perspective of culture studies, as Campbell concludes, "we need more life studies of twentieth-century Catholics and how the study of personal narrative takes historians of Catholicism to places that we could reach in no other way." So might historians of nursing, appropriating culture studies, concur about *The Nun's Story*. In other words, for culture studies, the novel's very ambiguity is an occasion for an open-ended discussion about representation or self-representation and its relationship to historical context. What readers of the book come to see, for example, is the extent to which the culture of Catholic religious orders prior to the reforms of the Second Vatican Council in the 1960s had a martial quality, with an extended and rigorous basic training, a uniform code of conduct, and strict adherence to hierarchy and regulations. This same rigor would not have been unfamiliar to nurses who trained in the 1940s and 50s, so that the profession of nursing and profession of religious vows appear to coexist as twins of each other in certain respects, which reminds us of Nightingale's admiration for Catholic women religious in healthcare vocations.[31]

A kind of martial discipline—creating and sustaining order on behalf of patients' wellbeing in the midst of chaos and attending to details, even being a stickler for policies and procedures—may have been characteristics of a competent nurse through the middle of the twentieth century.[32] However, in the ethos of the 1960s at a time when all institutions and conventions came under scrutiny, not least the healthcare establishment, Ken Kesey's representation of Nurse Ratched (or "Big Nurse") in the novel *One Flew Over the Cuckoo's Nest*[33] (later made into the 1975 film of the same title) sounded a responsive chord with its caricature of a castrating female and clinical dictator. Mental health professions had often been the subject of dramatic or melodramatic representations: *Spellbound*, Hitchcock's 1945 tribute to Freudian analysis; *The Snake Pit*, Anatole Litvak's 1948 castigation of mental asylums; *The Three Faces of Eve*, Nunnally Johnson's 1957 quasi-documentary dramatization of multiple personality disorder; and *Suddenly, Last Summer*, Joseph L. Mankiewicz's 1959 film version of Tennessee Williams's play in which a psychiatrist finds himself pressured by a wealthy benefactor to lobotomize her daughter, quickly come to mind. In each instance, the mental health professionals believe themselves to be well-intentioned but are, in fact, emotionally conflicted and ethically confused. In Kesey's counter-cultural ethos, Nurse Ratched personifies all that is wrong with contemporary America (conformity, intolerance of difference, adherence to unjust laws), but what makes her malevolent (rather than merely a comic foil) is her absorption and manipulation of power, against the patients, her staff, and the physicians. In Leslie Fiedler's analysis:

> In part Kesey's attitude can be explained by the age which bred him and whose spokesman he became: a revolutionary time, when all hierarchal institutions, not least the hospital, had come to be despised, and all professions, specialties—especially, perhaps, medical ones, and most especially psychiatry—were regarded with hostility and suspicion. After all, in the late sixties, as reading R. D. Laing reminds us, madness had come to be venerated in many quarters as a higher kind of sanity.[34]

For the post-Freudian Kesey, who had worked in a psychiatric hospital during his graduate studies and had volunteered in a CIA-funded study of LSD at a veterans hospital, Nurse Ratched is all Superego and castrating female. However, she is not alone among nurses in the novel, all of whom (including the "little" Japanese nurse and the Catholic nurse) seem the object of Kesey's contempt. As Leslie Horst notes:

> The women [including the wives of the male patients] . . . seem lost all along, hopelessly imprisoned in the narrowest of sex-roles or in projections of male fantasy . . . Not only is the portrayal of women demeaning, but considerable hatred of women is justified in the logic of the novel. The plot demands that the dreadful women who break rules men have made for them become the targets of the reader's wrath.[35]

Anxieties among nurses about their role and scope of practice in the 1960s appear to have collided, at least in the United States, with broader social anxieties about the role and scope of women's work in society and about the unquestioned authority of healthcare professionals. These anxieties would become amplified in the 1970s over the emerging gay rights movement and feminist movement, and in the 1980s at the beginning of the HIV/AIDS epidemic, when health research and healthcare became, to an unprecedented degree, contested and politicized.

In the early 1980s HIV/AIDS did not initially affect a broadly defined "general population" since its two most common vectors of transmission are IV drug use (sharing infected needles) and unprotected or "unsafe" sexual practices, usually with multiple partners and often in anal sex between men. The stigma associated with these behaviors and a recently visible and vocal Christian conservative political activism combined to circulate a rhetoric of apocalyptic vehemence in which a public health issue became inflected as a biblical plague, God's judgment on sinners.[36] Because the initial cases of AIDS were documented by epidemiologists and represented in the media as a problem of two marginalized groups (gay men, Afro-Caribbean Haitians), individual nurses caring for AIDS patients would have been challenged in their own attitudes about minorities and proscribed behavior.[37] In the first decade and a half of the epidemic, social dissent, political dissent, and epidemiological dissent emerged, influencing both the research agenda and the provision of healthcare.[38]

One of the more important cultural representations of the epidemic, Tony Kushner's two-part epic drama *Angels in America*,[39] depicting the AIDS epidemic in the 1980s during the Reagan Administration, is conspicuous in its featuring a nurse as a central character, Norman Arriaga (also known by his drag name as "Belize"), an Afro-Puerto Rican gay man who is the faithful friend to (and former lover of) the play's protagonist, Prior Walter, and who is the play's moral center of gravity. In doing so, Kushner subverted what had become a common AIDS narrative in which a physician (either angelic or demonic or some mixture of the two) was the representative healthcare professional, nurses generally being either absent or spectral (visible, but wielding little professional power or influence on the narrative). Campy, witty, and sharp-tongued, Belize provides his patients with both competence and care. Visiting Prior in the hospital, Belize massages him:

PRIOR: This is not Western medicine, these bottles . . .

BELIZE: Voodoo cream. From the botanica 'round the block.

PRIOR: And you a registered nurse.

BELIZE (*Sniffing it*): Beeswax and cheap perfume. Cut with Jergen's Lotion. Full of good vibes and love from some little black Cubana witch in Miami.[40]

Later, preparing to leave Prior's hospital room:

BELIZE: I have to go. If I want to spend my whole lonely life looking after white people I can get underpaid to do it.

PRIOR: You're just a Christian martyr.

BELIZE: Whatever happens, baby, I will be here for you.

PRIOR: Je t'aime.

BELIZE: Je t'aime. Don't go crazy on me, girlfriend, I already got enough crazy queens for one lifetime. For two. I can't be bothering with dementia.[41]

The historical figure of Roy Cohn (right-wing Republican power broker and closeted homosexual who rose to fame as an assistant to Senator Joe McCarthy in the 1950s) appears throughout the play, a character of almost Shakespearian evil. Diagnosed with AIDS (which he denies because only "fags" get AIDS), Cohn is eventually hospitalized and becomes Belize's patient:

BELIZE: This didn't come from me and I don't like you but let me tell you a thing or two: They have you down for radiation tomorrow for the sarcoma lesions, and you don't want to let them do that, because radiation will kill the T-cells and you don't have any you can afford to lose. So tell the doctor no thanks for the radiation. He won't want to listen. Persuade him. Or he will kill you.

ROY: You're just a fucking nurse. Why should I listen to you over my very qualified, very expensive WASP doctor?

BELIZE: He's not queer. I am.[42]

Here Belize gestures to two phenomena: first, a utopian assertion that the difference of queer identity may transcend differences of class, race, and ideology; second, that healthcare professionals at the time (with some improvement in the intervening three decades) were conflicted at best about their patients' non-normative sexual behaviors and could not always be trusted to provide care in the patients' interest. As though to emphasize the latter point, Belize also advises Cohn to pull strings in order to secure medications from federal AZT trials but advises him not to sign up for the trial itself, where he might only receive a placebo: "You'll die, but they'll get the kind of statistics they can publish in the *New England Journal of Medicine*."[43] This generosity on Belize's part is rewarded later in the play after Cohn dies, when Belize takes possession of Cohn's stash of AZT in order to provide it to Prior: "He was a terrible person. He died a hard death. So maybe . . . A queen can forgive her vanquished foe. It isn't easy, it doesn't count if it's easy, it's the hardest thing. Forgiveness. Which is maybe where love and justice finally meet."[44] This last statement, consistently enacted throughout the play by Belize's refusal to abandon either his friend Prior or the despicable Roy Cohn, by his subordinating his own personal feelings and political commitments on behalf of the wellbeing of the patient Cohn, and by his willingness to tell the truth (to Cohn and to Prior's boyfriend Louis, who has left Prior after learning of his AIDS diagnosis), summarizes the play's central theme in which Belize has served as the moral exemplar: the meeting of love and justice.

Angels in America's representation of one nurse evokes the questions of personal visibility and professional autonomy that have been dominant themes in the nursing literature throughout the twentieth century. As a gay man, as an Afro-Caribbean, as a nurse, and as a man in nursing, Belize is multiply constrained in regard to visibility and autonomy. In addition, Kushner depicts a profession that is still considered culturally and professionally contingent on and ancillary to medicine and that is self-consciously concerned with questions of social justice and ethical ambiguity. At the same time, the character of Belize also raises issues about a marginalized minority within a frequently professionally marginalized healthcare field: men. Stereotypes of men in nursing (only gay men go into nursing; men in nursing are a new phenomenon) belie the complex (and sometimes invisible) history of gender in the nursing profession.[45] Although it is unclear why Kushner chose to write Belize as a nurse, he has expressed his own ambivalence about the character and the politics of representation: "I was wrestling, and I'm still wrestling, with the whole question of representation and the rights of representing different people's experience. The issue of a white writer writing a black character is so loaded. And I made mistakes when I started the play in 1988 and if I were doing it over again I probably wouldn't make him a nurse; having read Toni Morrison's *Playing in the Dark* I would have avoided that."[46] Kushner refers to Morrison's "Disturbing Nurses and the Kindness of Sharks," one of her William E. Massey Sr Lectures in the History of American Civilization at Harvard,[47] in which Morrison limns the paradox of the ubiquity and invisibility of race in American culture and associates it with gender. In an analysis of Hemingway's fiction, Morrison sees a preoccupation with nurturing people of color (men and women) who attend to the white male protagonists. Thus Kushner's multiple anxiety about his representing Otherness (the Afro-Caribbean male nurse), inflected through a cultural stereotype of servitude with its long pedigree, supports a culture studies refusal of facile or naïve notions of representational realism. Culture studies helps the historian to ask the right questions about any text without begging the question of a text's representational authority.

As seen on TV

Although fiction, drama, and film have been important forms of cultural production for nursing, in the second half of the twentieth century television probably exerted more widespread cultural influence than any other medium in the Western world on how people imagined themselves and saw others. Seeking cultural validity in the 1950s, television producers aspired to present serious drama and documentary reporting, but by the 1960s television's commercial success had led to the establishment of commercially safe genres, such as half-hour situation comedies, daytime serialized dramas (soap operas), and hour-long evening dramatic or adventure programs. Their ensemble casting did not require new exposition each week, and the characters rarely developed over the course of a season. The success of one network's programming spawned imitations by the others (like the proliferation of Westerns in the 1950s).

In the 1980s meticulous analysis of nursing representations in popular media came from the groundbreaking interdisciplinary research of Philip Kalisch, a professor of history, politics, and economics in the Center for Nursing Research at the University of Michigan, and Beatrice Kalisch, a professor of nursing at the University of Michigan, using social science methods of content analysis. In one longitudinal study of television from 1950 to 1980, the researchers characterized the predominant representations of nursing: the nurse appears as a resource to other healthcare providers and an emotional support for families and patients, but rarely as a professional providing education or demonstrating a scholarly or expanded role. This longitudinal study also noted that an emphasis on nursing's contribution to patient welfare and television's emphasis on professional nursing peaked in the 1960s, and declined precipitously in the 1970s.[48] The researchers identified a similar pattern in popular fiction, though novels seem to have been a leading indicator with researchers noting that fictional representations of nursing reached a pinnacle in the 1940s and early 1950s, followed by a precipitous decline in the later 1950s and 1960s when nurses tended to be relegated to two familiar stereotypes: the frigid unmarried authoritarian nurse and the sexually available young nurse (both female).[49] More recently a Kalisch study of representations of nursing on Internet websites in 2001 and 2004 suggested a more mixed picture, including declines in representations of the characteristics of nurses as authoritative, scientific, creative, and powerful.[50] While such quantitative analyses might be familiar to the historian, they do not constitute a culture studies approach, but they can be the occasion for the culture studies scholar to theorize more broadly about the cultural systems in which they were produced and the ways in which other discourses of gender and professions were imbricated in the same period.

Hospital and medical dramas featuring nurses have been a perennial television genre, though their representations of the nursing profession have often been subordinated to the requirements of melodramatic or humorous plots. And television may be a representation of the culture's Id at certain historical moments, telling us more about the times than about nursing. For example, ABC's *General Hospital*, launched in 1963, is now the longest-running daytime drama on American television. Although professionally ancillary to physicians, nurses in the show have been represented in a variety of dimensions and relationships, both professional and personal. In another instance, although professionally competent and a stickler for the rules, the character of Major Margaret "Hot Lips" Houlihan, RN, in *M*A*S*H* (which aired for over a decade and was based on the 1970 feature film adapted from Richard Hooker's 1968 novel *MASH: A Novel about Three Army Doctors*), underwent a transformation from harridan to sharing "in the audience sympathy for the irreverent, iconoclastic, yet utterly humane doctors who work in a field hospital," while nursing itself was presented "more forcefully and positively in [the show's] last two seasons."[51]

The proliferation of cable television changed the media landscape, drawing some contrasts between older broadcast shows and new cable network programming. Perhaps the contrast between *Nurse* (a critically acclaimed but short-lived CBS drama of the early 1980s) and *Nurse Jackie* (a production of cable television's Showtime starting in 2009) tells us more about changes in social norms and what was permissible in media production at the times each was made. The star of *Nurse*, actress Michael Learned (famous as the beloved and wise mother in *The Waltons*), won an Emmy Award for her performance as Mary Benjamin, RN, in *Nurse*; the show's premise was that Benjamin had returned to her nursing career after the death of her husband, a physician, and she became a supervising nurse. The program suggested to viewers that nursing might be a career that is interrupted and returned to later (although it also leveraged some of the stereotypes of nurse–physician romance). As a network program aired in prime time, *Nurse* was required to observe broadcast standards of the day. In contrast, *Nurse Jackie* (which features Edie Falco in the title role) offers a darkly complicated and unsentimental view of the nurse. A highly skilled health professional, Jackie Peyton is also drug addicted, with a densely cluttered psychological landscape. Because subscriber-based cable programs are not constrained by the Federal Communications Commission's decency regulations as CBS had been, cable programming such as Showtime's can present edgier dramas than those of broadcast networks such as CBS. However sensationalist the plot summary of *Nurse Jackie* may appear, the show's depictions of nursing have prompted the organization The Truth About Nursing, in its website's reviews of television programs and films, to characterize it as "the most thoughtful and persuasive treatment of nursing issues on U.S. television."[52] The New York State Nurses Association, however, has been less happy with the character, requesting the display of a disclaimer before each episode,[53] a request that was denied. The American Nurses Association likewise issued a call to action to its members, providing a sample letter of protest.[54] Thus the nursing profession finds it difficult to shape others' representations of it, in part because the profession does not always speak with one voice and has limited resources for corporate self-representation.

Where are nurse writers?

The problem of cultural self-representation is a consistent theme of nursing's history. The title of Nightingale's classic book formulated the problem clearly (without permanently resolving it): *Nursing, What It Is and What It Is Not*. Nurses still need to explain that. And even today, if you were to ask a well-read friend to name a physician writer, your friend probably could name several (Jerome Groopman, Oliver Sacks, Atul Gawande come quickly to mind) who appear regularly in popular print publications. If you ask your friend to name a nurse author, however, you might be met with abashed silence. Where are the nurse writers in popular forums?

Several explanations for this relative invisibility come to mind. First, nursing has disproportionately employed women, and women's sometimes precarious position in the cultural politics of writing and publishing may account for the seeming absence. However, the claims of gender disparity should not be hardened into a stereotype, since in significant instances over the past two centuries women writers' enormous popular success has been the lament of male writers (such as Nathaniel Hawthorne's famous complaint about the "damn'd mob of scribbling women" who edged him out of the literary marketplace). The cultural visibility and commercial success of women writers in the second half of the twentieth century and in the early twenty-first also complicate this explanation. However, Virginia Woolf's famous observation that writing requires a room of one's own (both in the literal sense of a space reserved for writing and in the metaphorical sense of enjoying the leisure of time to write)[55] may be apposite. In addition, women in nursing often leave their physically, mentally, and emotionally demanding roles as health caregivers to go home, where they are engaged in the physically, mentally, and emotionally demanding roles in caregiving to spouses and children or aging parents. For them there is little time or energy for writing. Another explanation may derive from the discrete historical roles of physician and nurse (which are not without their historically gendered dimensions): the physician who ponders, diagnoses and prescribes (then leaves the bedside) in contrast to the nurse who provides a variety of forms of care, carries out the physician's "orders," and keeps continuous vigil with the patient at the bedside. The physician's role historically has also included reporting on interesting cases, published in professional or scholarly journals. Literary writing by physicians (the essays and narratives published in popular magazines and books, which often entail case studies written for a general audience) may be an extension of that tradition of professional writing.

Educational attainment might also provide an explanation for cultural under-representation. All physicians have completed a baccalaureate curriculum, graduate training in medical school, and a residency; the majority of nurses have not. While educational attainment does not preclude a writing career, advanced education is probably conducive to it, at least by providing role exemplars and professional mentors. Also, an ethos of nurses' self-effacement (combined with a cultural script that celebrates the heroic physician) may render less successful the work of those nurses who do publish. Finally, Buresh and Gordon suggest an even more tenaciously ingrained reticence among nurses, who "often seem as hesitant to tell their friends and relatives about their work as they are to tell the *New York Times* or the *Globe and Mail*."[56] Alone or in combination, these conditions may have created an ethos in which nurses either do not write about their experiences or are discouraged from doing so, thus limiting cultural self-representation.

The irony is that the nineteenth-century founder of modern professional nursing was herself a prolific writer on a variety of topics in a variety of forms. Who are Florence Nightingale's literary heirs today? Among them are men and women. They are working in a variety of genres, and their work has achieved canonical status in anthologies. Cortney Davis and Judy Schaefer's two collections, *Between the Heartbeats: Poetry and Prose by Nurses*[57] and *Intensive Care: More Poetry and Prose by Nurses*,[58] have brought nurse writers to a wider audience. Schaefer's more recent anthology, *The Poetry of Nursing: Poems and Commentaries of Leading Nurse-Poets*,[59] gives 15 nurse poets the space to present and to comment on three or four of their own poems, an unusual and engaging meta-analysis. An accomplished poet, Davis is also a talented essayist, whose recently published

The Heart's Truth: Essays on the Art of Nursing encapsulates the relationship between clinical practice and writing, not as conflicting but as mutually supportive:

> I find that when I'm not seeing patients, it's a struggle for me to write. It seems that for me, nursing and writing have become, over the years, inextricably bound. That intimate connection that links us, human to human, is essential both to my vocation and my avocation.[60]

Nurse writers such as Davis and Schaefer, Jeanne Bryner, Theodore Deppe, and Veneta Masson have published their work in distinguished literary journals, such as *Minnesota Review, Prairie Schooner, Hudson Review, Poetry, The Sun,* and *Kenyon Review,* as well as in their own books published by respected presses. One more recent welcome development is that Theresa Brown, RN, a former professor of English and author of *Critical Care: A New Nurse Faces Death, Life, and Everything in Between,*[61] has moved from regular blogger for the *New York Times* to one of its regular columnists, for "Bedside," the paper's new op-ed feature that promises to represent nurses.

The uneven quality of representations of nursing in literature and mass media suggests the ways in which the nursing profession is wise to advocate on behalf of fairness and accuracy. Moreover, the unevenness is consistent with a cultural history in which these depictions have often been out of the control of nurses themselves. Culture studies can offer an account of nurses' efforts at cultural self-representation and advocacy and can suggest why some have succeeded while others have not.

Future directions for scholars of nursing and its history should include the further recovery of nursing's texts and cultural artifacts, both published and unpublished. Although the situation may have improved in the past twenty years, Susan Reverby's observation in 1987 is still probably valid to a great extent: "Much of nursing's history still lies buried in attics, slowly disintegrating in forgotten hospital file cabinets, or fading in the memories of older nurses."[62] Using diverse sources, cultural studies scholarship over the past decade or more has produced some exemplary work, such as literary scholar Jane Schultz's documentation and analysis of American Civil War female nurse narratives, Margarete Sandelowski's study of the material culture of nursing and its visual representations in the use of technology, and comparative literature scholar Margaret Higonnet's groundbreaking work with twentieth-century Modernist-era nurse authors. Schultz, a professor of English, meticulously historicizes published and unpublished diaries and memoirs of women who served in Civil War military hospitals, documenting their production and reception.[63] Sandelowski, a nurse and American studies scholar, employs archival sources (including ephemera), professional publications, biographical and autobiographical literature, and interviews to read between the lines, filling in gaps and silences in the discourse.[64] Higonnet's work is remarkable both for her editing works long out of print and for her perceptive literary analysis in which she has moved these figures from the background to the foreground of literary history. In addition to making available for readers today the World War I writings of Ellen La Motte and Mary Borden,[65] Higonnet has argued persuasively for the ways that those writers influenced and were influenced by more famous Modernist figures.[66]

Building on their work and learning from their methods, nurse historian Jennifer Casavant Telford and I in an article in the British Medical Journal's *Medical Humanities* apply sociologist Daphne Spain's critical analysis of gendered spaces to the physical space of the Union Civil War hospital and the literary "spaces" of the pages of subscription-published nurse narratives.[67] Since academic nursing, unlike most fields in the humanities, has a robust tradition of co-authorship in joint studies, nursing historians and cultural studies scholars might profitably collaborate in this research.

Furthermore, nursing leaders, educators, scholars, and professionals should consider why nursing seems under-represented in the literary marketplace (or the larger cultural forum), at least when compared to its medical colleagues, many of whom are well established in the literary canon. They might start by supporting mentors for nurses' writing and publishing and providing incentives for nurses to encourage their writing. Remedying that imbalance would be a worthy project because the stories and insights of nursing practice are indispensable to advancing human health and to our understanding of wellness and illness, of health and disease, and of the gendered dimensions of work. Scholars in cultural studies, along with historians, can also elucidate for nursing leaders nationally and globally the cultural and historical mechanisms whereby nurses' and the public's perceptions of nursing have been shaped, and can suggest strategies for the profession's more accurate and visible self-representation.

Notes

1 B. Buresh, S. Gordon, N. Bell 1991, "Who counts in news coverage of health care?" *Nursing Outlook*, vol. 39(5), pp. 204–208.
2 B. Buresh, S. Gordon 2000, *From silence to voice: What nurses know and must communicate to the public*, Canadian Nurses Association, Ottawa, Canada.
3 H. White 1978, "The fictions of factual representation," *Tropics of discourse: Essays in cultural criticism*, Johns Hopkins University Press, Baltimore, MD, pp. 121–134; p. 121.
4 M. Arnold 1869, *Culture and anarchy: An essay in social and political criticism*, London, p. viii.
5 C. Geertz 1973, *The interpretation of cultures*, Basic Books, New York, p. 89.
6 C. Nelson, P.A. Treichler, L. Grossberg 1992, "Cultural studies: An introduction," in L. Grossberg, C. Nelson, P. Treichler (eds.), *Cultural studies*, Routledge, New York, pp. 1–22.
7 M. Foucault 1973, 1994, *The birth of the clinic: An archeology of medical perception*, A.M. Sheridan, trans., Vintage, New York.
8 R. Hodge 1990, *Literature as discourse: Textual strategies in English and history*, Johns Hopkins University Press, Baltimore, MD, p. viii.
9 A. Easthope 1991, *Literary into cultural studies*, Routledge, London.
10 P. D'Antonio 2010, *American nursing: A history of knowledge, authority, and the meaning of work*, Johns Hopkins University Press, Baltimore, MD (Barnes and Noble Nook Edition), p. 11.
11 S.M. Reverby 1987, *Ordered to care: The dilemma of American nursing, 1850–1945*, Cambridge University Press, Cambridge, UK, p. 2.
12 M. Sandelowski 2000, *Devices and desires: Gender, technology, and American nursing*, University of North Carolina Press, Chapel Hill, NC, p. 179.
13 F. Nightingale 1860, 1969, *Notes on nursing: What it is and what it is not*, Dover Publications, New York, pp. 134–135.

14 See C. Judd 1998, *Bedside seductions: Nursing and the Victorian imagination, 1830–1880*, St Martin's Press, New York; J.E. Schultz 2004, *Women at the front: Hospital workers in Civil War America*, University of North Carolina Press, Chapel Hill, NC; T.A. Baker 1984, *The figure of the nurse: Struggles for wholeness in the novels of Jane Austen, Anne, Charlotte, Emily Brontë, and George Eliot*, dissertation, Purdue University, West Lafayette, IN; J.J. Fenne 2000, *"Every woman is a nurse": Domestic nurses in nineteenth-century English popular literature*, dissertation, University of Wisconsin, Madison, WI.

15 A. Young 2008, "'Entirely a woman's question'?: Class, gender, and the Victorian nurse," *Journal of Victorian Culture*, vol. 13, 18–41.

16 Fenne, *Domestic nurses*, p. 12.

17 See D'Antonio, "Race, place, and professional identity," *American nursing*, pp. 119–141; Sandelowski, "The utensils and materials at hand," *Devices and desires*, pp. 44–66.

18 "Our U.S. boys" 1919, *The Trained Nurse and Hospital Review*, vol. 62, 291–293.

19 M.R. Higonnet, ed. 2001, *Nurses at the front: Writing the wounds of the Great War*, Northeastern University Press, Boston, p. xiv.

20 M. Borden 1929, "The preface," *The forbidden zone*, William Heinemann, London.

21 Higonnet, *Nurses at the front*, p. xii.

22 J. Bourke 1996, *Dismembering the men's bodies, Britain, and the Great War*, University of Chicago Press, Chicago, p. 86.

23 H.D. Boylston 1927, *Sister: the war diary of a nurse*, Washburn, New York.

24 H.D. Boylston 1955, *Clara Barton: Founder of the American Red Cross*, E.M. Hale, Eau Claire, WI.

25 D. Philipps 1999, "Healthy heroines: Sue Barton, Lillian Wald, Lavinia Lloyd Dock and the Henry Street Settlement," *Journal of American Studies*, vol. 33, pp. 65–82; p. 68.

26 A.G. Gorman, L.R. Mateer 2008, "Measuring up to the task: Cherry Ames as nurse and sleuth," in M.G. Cornelius and M.E. Gregg (eds.), *Nancy Drew and her sister sleuths: Essays on the fiction of girl detectives*, McFarland Publishing, Jefferson, NC, pp. 124–139, p. 125.

27 *Ibid.*, p. 137.

28 Springer Publishing 2012, *Cherry Ames* Boxed Set 1–4, www.springerpub.com/product/9780977159741

29 K. Hulme 1956, *The nun's story*, Little Brown, Boston.

30 D. Campbell 2010, "Work in progress: The nun and the crocodile," American Catholic Historical Association, www.achahistory.org/2010/08/work-in-progress-the-nun-and-the-crocodile (accessed 1 December 2011).

31 Nightingale, *Notes on nursing*, pp. 134–135.

32 See D'Antonio, "Competence, coolness, courage—and control," *American nursing*, pp. 45–69.

33 K. Kesey 1962, *One flew over the cuckoo's nest*, Viking Press, New York.

34 L. Fiedler 1983, "Images of the nurse in fiction and popular culture," *Literature and Medicine*, vol. 2, pp. 79–90, p. 89.

35 L. Horst 1977, 1996, "Bitches, twitches, and eunuchs: Sex-role failure and caricature," *Lex et Scientia*, vol. 13, nos. 1–2, pp. 14–17; reprinted in *One flew over the cuckoo's nest: text and criticism*, J.C. Pratt, ed., Penguin Books, New York, pp. 464–471; p. 471.

36 See T.L. Long 2005, *AIDS and American apocalypticism: The cultural semiotics of an epidemic*, State University of New York Press, Albany, NY; and S. Palmer 1997, *AIDS as an apocalyptic metaphor in North America*, University of Toronto Press, Toronto, Canada.

37 R.C. Fox, L.H. Aiken, C.M. Messikomer 1990, "The culture of caring: AIDS and the nursing profession," *The Milbank Quarterly*, vol. 68, Supplement 2 (Part 2), *A Disease of Society: Cultural Responses to AIDS*, pp. 226–256.

38 T.L. Long 2010, "AIDS and the paradigms of dissent," in Z. Li and T. L. Long, eds., *The meaning management challenge: Making sense of health, illness and disease*, Inter-Disciplinary Press, Oxford, UK, pp. 147–157.

39 T. Kushner 1992, 1993, *Angels in America part one: Millennium approaches*, Theatre Communications Group, New York; T. Kushner 1992, 1994, *Angels in America part two: Perestroika*. Theatre Communications Group, New York.

40 Kushner, *Millennium approaches*, p. 59.

41 *Ibid.*, p. 61.

42 Kushner, *Perestroika*, p. 29.

43 *Ibid.*, p. 30.

44 *Ibid.*, p. 124.

45 C.E. O'Lynn, R.E. Tranbarger, eds. 2007, *Men in nursing: History, challenges, and opportunities*, Springer, New York.

46 B. McLeod 1998, "The oddest phenomenon in modern history," in *Tony Kushner in conversation*, Robert Vorlicky, ed., University of Michigan Press, Ann Arbor, MI, pp. 77–84; p. 80.

47 T. Morrison 1992, "Disturbing nurses and the kindness of sharks" in *Playing in the dark: Whiteness and the literary imagination*, Vintage Books, Nook Edition, New York, pp. 47–64.

48 P.A. Kalisch, B.J. Kalisch, J. Clinton 1982, "The world of nursing on prime time television, 1950 to 1980," *Nursing Research*, vol. 31, pp. 358–363.

49 P.A. Kalisch, B.J. Kalisch 1982, "The image of nurses in novels," *American Journal of Nursing*, vol. 82, pp. 1220–1224.

50 B.J. Kalisch, S. Begeny, S. Neumann 2007, "The image of the nurse on the Internet," *Nursing Outlook*, vol. 55, pp. 182–188.

51 P.A. Kalisch, B.J. Kalisch 1982, "Nurses on prime-time television," *American Journal of Nursing*, vol. 82, pp. 264–270; p. 270.

52 The Truth about Nursing 2012, "Nurse Jackie," www.truthaboutnursing.org/media/tv/nurse_jackie.html (accessed 2 January 2012).

53 New York State Nurses Association 2009, "NYSNA responds to 'Nurse Jackie' series," www.nysna.org/general/communications/nursejackie.htm (accessed 1 February 2013).

54 American Nurses Association 2009, "Call to action: Protesting negative portrayals of nursing in 'Nurse Jackie' and 'Hawthorne,'" www.nursingworld.org/HomepageCategory/NursingInsider/Archive_1/2009-NI/June-09-NI/Negative-Portrayal-of-Nursing-.html (accessed 1 February 2013).

55 V. Woolf 1929, *A room of one's own*, Hogarth Press, London.

56 Buresh and Gordon, *From silence to voice*, p. 4.

57 C. Davis, J. Schaefer, eds. 1995, *Between the heartbeats: Poetry and prose by nurses*, University of Iowa Press, Iowa City, IA.

58 C. Davis, J. Schaefer, eds. 2003, *Intensive care: More poetry and prose by nurses*. University of Iowa Press, Iowa City, IA.

59 J. Schaefer, ed. 2006, *The poetry of nursing: Poems and commentaries of leading nurse-poets*. Kent State University Press, Kent, OH.

60 C. Davis 2009, *The heart's truth: Essays on the art of nursing*, Kent State University Press, Kent, OH, p. 98.

61 T. Brown 2010, *Critical care: A new nurse faces death, life, and everything in between*, HarperStudio, New York.

62 Reverby, *Ordered to care*, p. 275.

63 Schultz, *Women at the front*.

64 Sandelowski, *Devices and desires*.

65 Higonnet, *Nurses at the front*.

66 M.R. Higonnet 2002, "Authenticity and art in trauma narratives of World War I," *Modernism/modernity*, vol. 9, pp. 91–107.

67 C. Telford, T.L. Long 2012, "Gendered spaces, gendered pages: Union women in Civil War nurse narratives," *Medical Humanities*, vol. 38, pp. 97–105.

4

COMMEMORATING CANADIAN NURSE CASUALTIES DURING AND AFTER THE FIRST WORLD WAR

Nurses' perspective[1]

Dianne Dodd

The First World War looms large in Canadian national consciousness, not least because of the staggering death toll of over 66,000 in a country of less than 8 million people. Canada became a nation in 1867, through an act of the British Parliament that brought together several British North American colonies that had long resisted the pull of the American republic to their south, including what would become the predominantly French-Catholic province of Quebec. Joining the defense of the motherland in August 1914, Canadian troops played a decisive role in the Great War, earning Canada a prominent place in the British Empire and forging a new identity as a truly autonomous nation – a colony no more.[2] During this five-year trial by fire which ended in November 1918, over 3,000 Canadian nurses, whose official title was Nursing Sister and who entered the military with the relative rank of second lieutenant, served in the Canadian Army Medical Corp (CAMC), caring for the sick and wounded.[3] More than 60 of them died, 21 as a result of enemy action. This chapter examines the ways in which this first generation of Canada's military nurses were remembered, and forgotten, in the great outpouring of memorializing in postwar Canada.

Analysts of gender and war have pointed out the profound unease toward women's presence in or near war zones in the interwar period, and this is clearly evident in nurse memorials.[4] Kathryn McPherson and Natalie Riegler provide early studies on the Canadian Nurses Association's prominent marble relief erected in the Parliament Buildings in 1926, showing how Canadian nursing leaders successfully used nurses' wartime service to win rare recognition for women/nurses in the commemorative terrain.[5] Indeed, secular, religious and military nurses appear relatively early and frequently in prestigious public places devoted to historic memory.[6] However, this Parliamentary war memorial is generic in nature and avoids a direct acknowledgement of nurses' sacrifice of life, placing them in the traditional feminine role of mourner and/or nurturer.[7] This has led Canadian historian Susan Mann to declare a postwar amnesia regarding nurses' wartime service and sacrifice.[8]

This chapter revisits these and other studies within a larger context, examining all major national commemorations[9] – including statues, plaques, books, posters, and the naming of streets, institutions and geographic features – of nurse casualties in Canada, beginning in wartime and continuing to the present day. Similar to Katie Pickles' study of the martyred First World War British nurse, Edith Cavell,[10] the study finds that changes in the commemorative message over time reveal nuances not always evident in a static snapshot of any one memorial. During the war, nurses were applauded for their bravery, albeit often in the service of wartime propaganda, while the interwar period shows ambivalence and reluctance to acknowledge nurses' military role. Recent memorials show a more soldierly role for the nurse, particularly in those sponsored by nurses themselves, reflecting the perception, recently confirmed by analyses of their wartime writings, that military nurses saw themselves as soldiers.[11] As well, military organizations belatedly recognized nurses as pioneers in opening the doors of the military to women,[12] an acknowledgement that also served the military's recruitment needs.

The chapter also places commemorative initiatives within the context of recent literature on historic memory. Successful public memorials, particularly those at the national level, are sufficiently ambiguous to allow meanings to vary according to the viewer's perspective.[13] The dominant or mainstream message is meant to unify all citizens in common celebration or remembrance, and to foster national loyalty across gender, class or ethnic divides. First World War commemorations erected all across Canada in the 1920s and 1930s, as Jonathon Vance has convincingly argued, met a very real need to give meaning to immense human suffering and loss.[14] Beyond this dominant message, however, there is a minority discourse that speaks to nurses' experience. Like other non-elites, women have been largely invisible in the commemorative terrain. Their bodies traditionally appear as allegories of abstract principles such as liberty or peace,[15] and they are seldom accorded an active role. Even more rarely do they achieve the status of real, named heroines. A middle ground is evident in many modern nurse memorials where the military nurse fulfills a symbolic role as "representative woman," standing at the apex of women's wartime contributions. A common strategy in historic recognition of women is to recognize them as part of a generic group, such as pioneer mothers.[16] In the case of military nurses, this serves to neutralize the threat to gender roles that nurses' military rank and professional stature posed, and to downplay their actual work. Still, when examined within the sphere of commemorating women's role in history, it is clear that nurses assume a large and symbolic role vis-à-vis their gender. Further, despite the dominant message directed at all Canadians, especially women, nursing leaders' realized their goal of speaking to nurses through depictions of their own work, largely by highlighting the all-important symbol of the uniform,[17] as well as other markers previously overlooked.

Llandovery Castle, Edith Cavell and the propaganda value of dead nurses

In 1904, Canadian Nursing Sisters were integrated into the Canadian Army Medical Corp (CAMC) as officers with the relative rank of second lieutenant.[18] This made them the first nurses in the British Empire and allied countries to gain military rank. Also, it made the Great War the first major conflict in which women played an official role, with access to military funerals and having their names recorded on official casualty lists. Thus their deaths could not be ignored. As many scholars have noted, this challenged longstanding gendered conceptions of warfare in which women played the role of "other."[19] The resulting ideological turmoil found early expression in the outrage over the execution of British nurse Edith Cavell in October 1915, for her role in helping Allied soldiers escape German-occupied Belgium, followed by a wave of commemorative initiatives, including several in Canada. Later that year, Canadian Prime Minister Sir Robert Borden and the Premier of British Columbia, Sir Richard McBride, named a majestic mountain in Jasper National Park, Mount Edith Cavell.[20] This made the British-born Cavell the first named, wartime nurse to be commemorated in Canada – an unusual honor. With the Dominion Parks Branch just established in 1911 to administer Canada's emerging national parks system, the naming of Mount Cavell also boosted tourism.[21] Reflecting Cavell's enduring symbolic value, a church in Jasper holds a service in her honor each year on the Sunday nearest Remembrance Day.

British authorities used the outrage over Cavell's execution to bolster sagging recruitment for a war bogged down in static trench warfare. Similarly, the Canadian government exploited the deaths of 14 nursing sisters to motivate battle-weary troops in 1918. The Canadian hospital ship, *Llandovery Castle,* was torpedoed by the German U-86, 114 miles off the coast of Ireland on 27 June 1918. Its crew, medical officers, nursing sisters and orderlies had been returning to England after bringing 644 convalescing patients to Halifax. The ship took a hit to its engine room, lost power, could not call for help, and quickly sank. Although most passengers were evacuated onto lifeboats, the Germans rammed, shelled and fired on them. Only one boat, with 24 passengers aboard, escaped. The death toll of 234 included all 14 nursing sisters aboard. Typical of the tone of wartime propaganda, Sergeant A. Knight, who was in the lifeboat with the nurses, portrayed an uneasy mix of bravery and helplessness:

> Unflinchingly and calmly, as steady and collected as if on parade, without a complaint or a single sign of emotion, our fourteen devoted nursing sisters faced the terrible ordeal of certain death – only a matter of minutes – as our lifeboat neared that mad whirlpool of waters where all human power was helpless.[22]

Knight tells us it was doubtful "any of them came to the surface again, although I myself sank and came up three times, finally clinging to a piece of wreckage and being eventually picked up by the captain's boat."[23] In this masculine narrative, the reader is left to presume that the nurses were overwhelmed by the water's powers.

The Government of Canada/CAMC's commemorative booklet on the sinking also praised the nurses:

> Through it all nothing stands out more brilliantly than the coolness and courage of the 14 Canadian nursing sisters, every one of whom was lost, and whose sacrifice under the conditions about to be described will serve to inspire throughout the whole Empire a yet fuller sense of appreciation of the deep debt of gratitude this nation owes to the nursing service.[24]

Knight crafted nurse sacrifice in terms of selfless nurture, noting that one of the 14 nurses, Matron Margaret Marjorie ("Pearl") Fraser, had served in a casualty clearing station, where she had provided care to all, including German prisoners of war. He reported "Many times had she been the first to give a drink of water to these parched enemy casualties. Many a time had she written down the dying statements of enemy officers and men, transmitting them to their relatives through the Red Cross."[25]

Canadian military officials used *Llandovery Castle* as a battle cry for the critical Battle of Amiens on 8 August 1918, which began the German army's retreat and ultimately ensured Allied victory. Led by its shock troops, who over five years of war had developed a reputation that inspired fear in the enemy, the Canadian Corps of the British First Army advanced an unprecedented eight miles in one day,[26] eventually pushing through to Mons in a series of battles on the Western Front called the Last Hundred Days.[27] Exploiting soldiers' identification of nurses with feminine nurture, rest and recovery – the antithesis of mud, violence and death[28] – Brigadier General George Tuxford gave instructions to his brigade that the cry of *Llandovery Castle* "should be the last to ring in the ears of the Hun as the bayonet was driven home."[29] Tragically, nurses were used to motivate rank and file soldiers in a campaign that they and Canadian historians later criticized as unnecessarily costly in human lives.[30] The *Llandovery Castle* also inspired war posters such as one for Canadian Victory Bonds (Figure 4.1), which shows a drowned nurse in the arms of a Canadian soldier who shakes an angry fist at the villainous Hun who would kill "innocent" women.[31] Although the buoy clearly identifies the ship as the *Llandovery Castle*, the nurse, who wears the Red Cross on her uniform, is inaccurately identified. The use of this international symbol of wartime humanitarian aid was meant to highlight the heinous crime of attacking a clearly marked hospital ship.

Edith Cavell, the first high-profile nurse casualty of the war (1915), was memorialized in numerous ways not only in Canada but all across the British Empire. Her death symbolized for many the dangers of having women/nurses near the front. However, by war's end, the shock value of nurse casualties had dissipated somewhat and the 14 nurses of *Llandovery Castle* were largely forgotten.[32] No major memorial was erected to them, although in 1924 their names were included among 415 soldiers, sailors and merchant seamen on a Halifax memorial, known locally as the "sailors' memorial."[33] The Imperial War Graves Commission (IWGC), which was formed early in the war to bury and later to commemorate soldiers, developed policies guided by the principle of absolute equality among the war dead. Repatriation of bodies was prohibited, as were

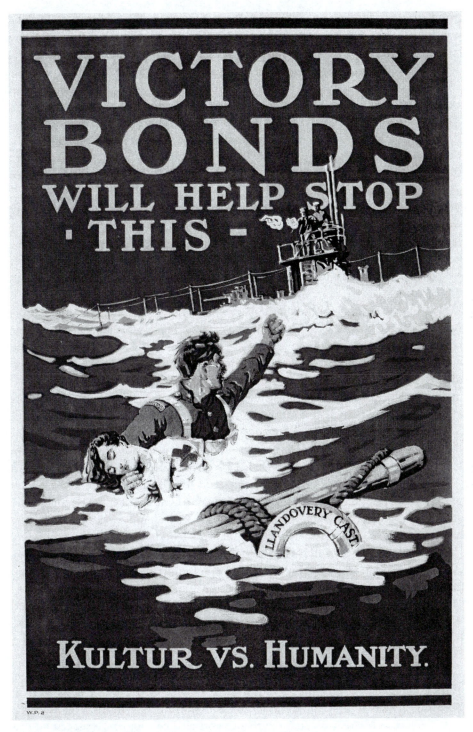

Figure 4.1 First World War Victory Bond poster.

Source: Canadian War Museum.

private markers. Headstone and military gravesites were uniform, and once a person was named, either on a grave or, if no body was found, on a memorial, they could not be named again, at least not at the national level.[34] Once named in Halifax, the nurses could not be named again and they were not included on the impressive Vimy Memorial in France, unveiled in 1936. It listed 11,285 Canadian soldiers for whom no graves existed.

Despite military nurses' obvious elite role in women's wartime work, art historian Kristine Huneault points out a similar absence in the "home front" collection of the Canadian War Memorial Fund (CWMF).[35] This collection was created by Max Aitken (Lord Beaverbrook), an expatriate Canadian businessman in London, who obtained an official mandate to document the participation of Canadians in the Great War.[36] Beaverbrook began by taking charge of the war records department and expanded this work to include the commission of art works. While the latter focused on the troops, the attention given to women's patriotic work at home pushed him to record the "home front" as well. For this, he hired primarily female artists, to produce works that valorized women's war work and encouraged more women to take on critical labor in munitions and agriculture.

One of these artists was the American-born Florence Wyle, who had studied at the Art Institute of Chicago, where she met fellow sculptor Frances Loring. The two became lifelong companions and collaborators, moved to Toronto in 1913 and did home front war art. They and other artists portrayed female war workers engaged in active labor, often displaying an unusual sense of purpose and muscular strength.[37] As Huneault notes, this potentially radical gender equality was rendered acceptable through the ideology of patriotism. Interestingly, like nurses' wartime sacrifice, these images of strong, active working women were largely forgotten after the war.[38]

They were not immediately forgotten, however, as we see in Wyle's depiction of Edith Cavell in a privately funded memorial erected at the Toronto General Hospital (TGH) (Figure 4.2) in 1918–19. As often occurs with community initiatives, there was no unveiling and there is little surviving documentation, leaving the monument's origins obscure. We do know that by December 1918, the Edith Cavell Memorial Fund had raised $4,000, much of it coming from schoolchildren who apparently found Cavell's feminine bravery and patriotism appealing.[39] It may have been linked to nurses at TGH, a leading centre of nurse education and home to several nursing leaders, including Mary Agnes Snively, president of the Canadian National Association of Trained Nurses (CNATN) from 1908 to 1912. In the spring of 1919, Sir Edmund Walker, a prominent banker, philanthropist and art lover, served as assessor and chose Florence Wyle to carve this relief. Jules F. Wegman of the prominent architectural firm Darling and Pearson designed the frame in which it sits.[40]

Wyle's work also reflects the postwar evolution of Cavell's wartime propaganda image of youthful innocence (despite her actual age of 49) to a more mature, heroic ideal of British womanhood more closely associated with nursing.[41] Wyle portrayed Cavell as an individual, rather than a generic type, her portrait-like appearance suggesting that the artist used one of the earlier sculptures or portraits of Cavell as a model.[42] She is placed in three-quarter view, between two soldiers in profile, "against a neutral,

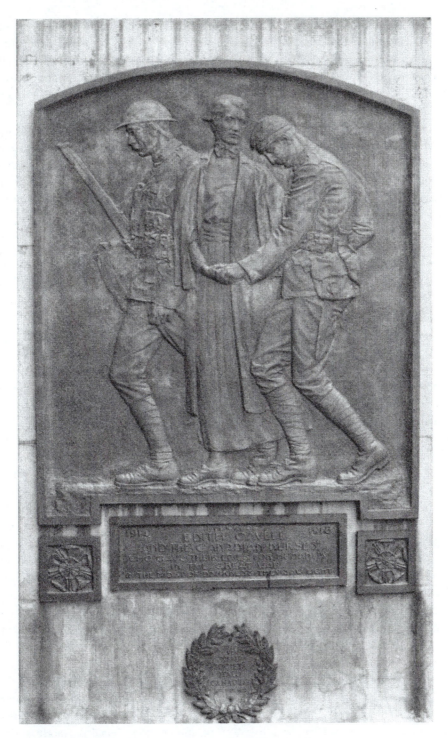

Figure 4.2 Relief of Edith Cavell, Toronto General Hospital.

Source: M. Moher.

undefined and timeless space."[43] The soldiers move slowly, bent with fatigue, whereas Cavell stands tall and holds the injured soldier's hand. Symbolizing the ideals of humanity and conveying the compassion of the nursing profession, it also depicts Cavell's strength and courage.[44] It is a fitting tribute to the only named, heroic military nurse memorialized in the period.

The inscription, which links British-born Cavell with Canadian nurses, is dedicated to: "Edith Cavell and the Canadian nurses who gave their lives for humanity in the Great War. In the midst of darkness they saw light." Curiously, another layer of meaning was added in 1922 when an Italian-Canadian organization, for reasons completely unknown, added a small round plaque at the bottom, with the more conventional inscription "Lest we forget." In this case there was an unveiling at which flowers were placed at the cenotaph at Toronto City Hall.

Cenotaphs, or empty tombs, were erected to honour those whose remains lie elsewhere, serving as sites of public and private mourning in most Canadian communities. Dr Harley Smith, former Italian consul, also linked the "sacrifice of Miss Cavell" to the Italian community. In his remarks, he gave a resume of the Italian military campaign, while another speaker made a generic tribute to women, praising the "wonderful work of womanhood, at home and as nurses on the field."[45]

The memorial in Parliament, 1926

Although the connections are not always clear, this Toronto memorial (and a proposal for another one in Ottawa) appears as a prelude to the truly Canadian memorial, the impressive high relief made of Italian Carrara marble unveiled in the Canadian Parliament (Figure 4.3) in 1926. At their 1919 annual meeting, the CNATN, later the Canadian Nurses Association (CNA), discussed a proposal to erect a memorial dedicated to Cavell in Ottawa on which the names of nurse casualties were to be inscribed. This one does not appear to have made it past the discussion stage. Nonetheless, it pushed Canadian nurses to make a decision to erect a war memorial "distinct from any association with Cavell" (CNATN, 1919), reflecting the nascent Canadian nationalism typical of commemorative initiatives in this period.[46] Many of the same people were connected with the two initiatives. Jean Gunn, Superintendent of Nursing at TGH, assumed the chair of the nursing association's memorial committee.[47] Architects from Darling and Pearson, who designed both frames in which the two reliefs were placed, had done architectural work for both the TGH and the Parliament Buildings, rebuilt following a 1916 fire. The latter incorporated a memorial Peace Tower which contains Books of Remembrance, on which the names of casualties were listed, alphabetically, by year of death, including the names of nursing sisters.

Gunn chaired the memorial committee responsible for raising funds and liaising with those who negotiated the site. In 1922, on the advice of Frank Darling,[48] the nurses appointed a business committee to collect designs and transact business. It was composed of three men: C. Barry Cleveland from Darling and Pearson, Gerald R. Larkin, son of a hospital trustee, and Lawren Harris, a prominent Canadian artist. The nurses had initially asked the government for space in the Centre Block of the Parliament Buildings

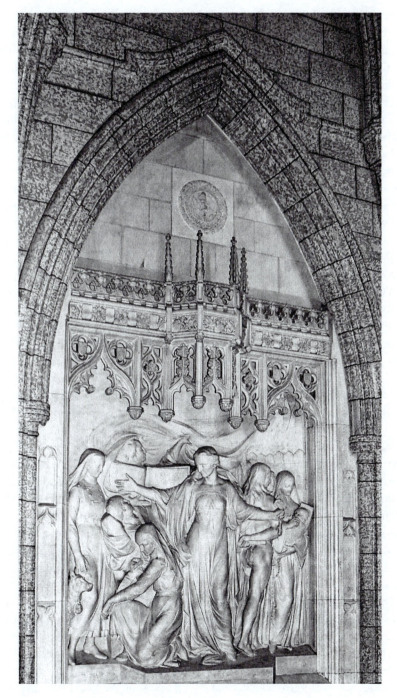

Figure 4.3 Nurses' Memorial, House Of Commons, Ottawa.

Source: © Parks Canada, M. Trépanier.

but were offered a site in nearby Major's Hill Park instead. They would likely have accepted this, except that the business committee pressed for a site in Parliament.[49] As criteria and precedent reserved this space for statuary of Canadian statesmen and historic figures, Cleveland and Larkin met with Prime Minister William Lyon Mackenzie King, asking him to place the memorial in the "Hall of Fame" outside the Parliamentary Library, where it could be accommodated within an historic theme. King agreed, despite strong objections from the speakers of the Senate and House of Commons, and several ministers, including Charles Murphy who had been acting Minister of Public Works when the initial request was refused.[50] King was aware that the government's 1917 imposition of military conscription had badly divided English and French Canadians.[51] A large majority of English-speaking Canadians supported the war; indeed, many of the numerous military recruits, including nursing sisters, and/or their families were relatively recent arrivals from Great Britain. By contrast, many French-speaking Canadians, angry over recent incidents hostile to their language and culture, took a more isolationist stance.[52] While for the nurses the relief was a war memorial, for King it was an opportunity to link the impeccable wartime service of military nurses, most of them English-speaking, with the heroic past of Catholic, French-speaking nuns from hospital orders, who helped found New France in the 17th century.[53] Indeed, Pearson and Darling's preliminary sketches of the memorial gave prominence to the nuns.[54]

Having acquired the space, the nurses' memorial committee appears to have given its advisors a lot of latitude, particularly in the choice of artist. Initially, Gunn negotiated a method for choosing the design with the national nursing association's provincial affiliates. Reflecting Canada's federal government, the Canadian Nurses Association was composed of provincial branches that were responsible for registration of individual nurses.[55] However, the business committee persuaded the nurses that "sculptors of recognized talent" would not enter designs unless guaranteed that they would be judged by their peers. As a result, the provincial affiliates voluntarily waived their selection rights, leaving the business committee to appoint a board of assessors, another all-male committee, composed of prominent artists David N. Brown, James Edward Hervey MacDonald and Ernest Ross Rolph, to make the final choice.[56] The latter were unanimous in choosing a model submitted by George W. Hill, a Paris-trained sculptor from Montreal who had built his reputation on war memorials and statues of politicians. Assuming the nurses wanted a high-quality, conventional work of art, the business committee's choice was a good one. However, it also served the interests of artists and architects who preferred peer review. It also left little room for the nurses to pursue, had they wanted to, excellent female sculptors such as Wyle or Loring.[57] Perhaps the nurses did not want to jeopardize their precarious foothold in the military (or prestigious space in Parliament) by embracing images of gender equality or aligning themselves too closely to the women's movement.

This raises the question as to what the nurses did want. We know that they wanted to ensure that nurses' sacrifices were remembered in the larger enterprise of historic/war remembrance, and that they deliberately raised the money entirely from nurses. The national committee also expressed the hope that the memorial would "present some visible expression of the nursing sister and her work."[58] But the inscription, written by

King, reflects a generic tribute that fails even to mention nurses: "Led by the spirit of humanity across the seas woman by her tender ministrations to those in need has given to the world the example of an heroic service embracing three centuries of Canadian history." Still, the nurses were accorded sponsorship: "Erected by the nurses of Canada in remembrance of their sisters who gave their lives in the Great War, nineteen fourteen–eighteen, and to perpetuate a noble tradition in the relations of the old world and the new." The historic reference was made necessary by the memorial's placement in the "Hall of Fame" or history hall. While King's generic tribute hardly reflected longstanding efforts of nursing leadership to dissociate generic feminine caregiving with skilled, professional nursing, it did accord nurses a leadership role *vis-à-vis* women.

In her insightful analysis of the memorial's images, Kathryn McPherson shows how the artist used gender and race to highlight an historic, nation-building discourse in which a few elite, white, uniformed women were allowed to play a minor role.[59] But Hill's highly symbolic memorial reveals other layers of meanings when looked at through the nurse's eyes. In the centre of the relief a female allegorical model representing humanity links the religious nurses on the right with First World War military nurses on the left. History, a male allegorical figure in the background, holds the Book of Records from 1639 to 1918 which reveal, as Hill recounts in his explanatory text, "the great deeds of heroism and martyrdom of the early nurses." On the left, one military nurse kneels beside a wounded soldier. McPherson does not use the word *pietá* to describe her mournful pose, yet the image clearly brings to mind the powerful Christian image of Mary cradling the crucified Christ. Here, the artist uses familiar Christian imagery to express the nation's grief, common to memorials of the period in which a soldier's sacrifice often paralleled that of Christ.[60] Indeed the mourning pose is so dominant that, McPherson declares, "neither nurse is actually doing anything."[61] However, Hill tells us that the military nurses are caring for a wounded soldier, and on closer examination we see that the kneeling nurse is unravelling a bandage. In depicting her changing a dressing, the artist highlights a typical, representative military nursing task. In light of King's generic tribute, this draws an unspoken, symbolic link between nurses' work and that of millions of women throughout the empire who made bandages and other supplies to send to the troops through patriotic organizations such as the Red Cross. While it remains striking that a memorial to remember dead nurses assigns them the role of mourning the soldier[62] and the image is far removed from earlier depictions of strong, working women, the nurse does reflect the important Christian figure of Mary.

The nurse standing behind the kneeling nurse conforms to traditional depictions of the *pietá* in which other mourning figures often surround Mary and Jesus. However, she also fulfils a more practical function in providing a full-length view of the nurses' uniform. Clearly marking nurses as officers in the previously all-male military hierarchy is the uniform, a highly valued symbol of professional (and military) status.[63] While it is not clear whether the Canadian Nurses' Association or the artist chose to have the nurses wear their service or work uniform rather than their formal, or "walking out" uniform, it is certainly in keeping with the nurses' association's expressed preference for a work theme. This uniform, with its distinctive blue dress, white veil, brass buttons and two stars to denote lieutenant rank, had earned Nursing Sisters the soldiers' affectionate nickname "bluebirds," which the nurses valued highly. The nurse also holds back a dog, the meaning of which McPherson suggests may relate to death,[64] allowing it to provide balance to the opposing image of the nun holding a baby, as nurses are present during birth and death. The dog could also suggest loyalty. However, given the preference for Red Cross imagery in military nurse memorials, and the pouch that the dog carries around his neck, it was likely meant to refer to the Red Cross's use of dogs on the battlefield to help bring back the wounded for care and treatment.[65] Although CAMC nurses did not get close enough to the front to use dogs themselves, nor is there any evidence the CAMC used them, they are a symbol of care of the wounded during wartime and search and rescue.

Vancouver Memorial Window: A soldier among soldiers

One commemorative initiative sponsored by the Canadian Nursing Sisters Association, a group of former military nurses formed after the war, shows the nurse in a somewhat more egalitarian, soldier-like posture. The Canadian Memorial Church was built in Vancouver in 1928 as a war memorial. In its vestibule are four stained glass windows honouring the soldier, sailor, airman and nursing sister, the last of these funded by the Nursing Sisters Association (Figure 4.4).[66] It shows the nurse posed in a similar manner to that of the other military representatives, implying a measure of equality. However, in contrast to the airman who holds a propeller; the sailor a rope; and the soldier who leans on his rifle; the nurse does not hold any tools or symbols of her work except that she wears her service uniform. Rather, she folds her hand over her heart, likely to signify compassion. Nurses held this memorial in high regard. A commemorative booklet notes, "For years the surviving members of the Nursing Sisters have attended Remembrance Day services in a body."[67]

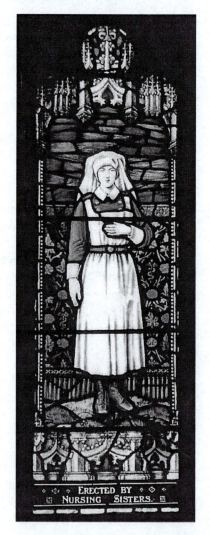

Figure 4.4 The Nurse Memorial Window, Canadian Memorial Church, The United Church of Canada, Vancouver.

Source: BC History of Nursing Society.

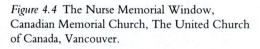

Nurses and the National Cenotaph

Historian Susan Hart suggests that there is a reluctance to show nurses at work in Canada's National Cenotaph (Figure 4.5, overleaf).[68] Located in the nation's capital, this symbolic tomb represents the graves of soldiers buried overseas and serves as the site for National Remembrance Day services each 11 November. Unveiled in 1939, "The Great Response" by British sculptor Vernon March depicts 22 figures marching purposefully through a triumphal arc, with female allegorical figures representing Peace and Freedom above it. Dressed in historically correct uniform and equipment, with the infantrymen in front, each represents its branch of the military.[69] At the rear, with the support services are two uniformed nursing sisters, of whom Hart has this to say:

> Whereas the male figures are all heavily burdened with the instruments typical to their branch of service, such as rifles and machine guns, one nurse carries a small handbag and the other one appears to be holding her gloves. As well, the glove-carrying figure has one hand pressed into the side of her abdomen as if she might be experiencing a stitch in her side as a result of the brisk pace set by the male figures ahead. While the two nurses have no attributes of their service, the near-by stretcher bearer, in addition to the stretcher he carries, has a medical kit bag over his shoulder clearly marked with a Red Cross emblem.[70]

Here, the marching nurses are dressed in their official military or walking uniform. Wearing short skirts and short-brimmed hats, one of the Nursing Sisters sports a greatcoat while the other wears a cape which flies up into the wind in a shape suggestive of an angel's wings, invoking popular images of nurses as ministering angels. Still, nurses' presence with the troops in a national monument gave high profile to Nursing Sisters' role in the military's medical system.

One can only speculate as to what input nurses had into these two memorials, but the uniform appears to have served as a symbol of professional work. How do we read the hand over the heart, however? Military nurses, as their wartime writings reflect, hoped that their war service would demonstrate the worth of professional nurses.[71] And, although they identified themselves as soldiers, they also drew upon the "safe" gender roles favoured by society, acting as sisters or mothers, and often extolled the bravery of their "boys" ahead of their own.[72] Many spent their own funds buying comforts for their patients, grieved those who died, attended their funerals and even decorated their graves.[73] Canadian nurse Warner relates, for example, "I put some roses on the grave of one of our Saint John boys. I wish his mother could see how well cared for it is."[74]

A belated acknowledgement: Recent depictions of military nurses

With the recent resurgence in interest in First World War nurses and the acceptance of women in the military, we are seeing new commemorative initiatives that recognize Nursing Sisters (later Nursing Officers) as soldiers, and as pioneers for women in the

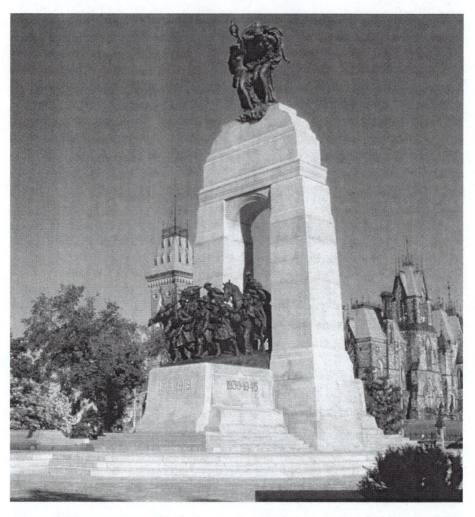

Figure 4.5 (above) National Cenotaph, Ottawa.

Source: © Parks Canada, A. Guindon.

Small photos *(below)* show nurses at the rear of the memorial's arch.

Source: © Parks Canada, D. Dodd.

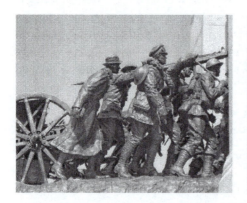
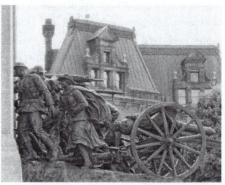

military. In 1998, more than 80 years after the naming of Mount Edith Cavell, a mountain was named for Canadian Nursing Sister Gladys Wake: Mount Wake near Pemberton, British Columbia.[75] Nursing Sister Wake died in Étaples, France during the Germans' 1918 spring offensive when one of two hospitals there was bombed by German air gunners, taking the lives of six Canadian nurses along with many more medical personnel and patients. As with the *Llandovery Castle*, news reports extolled the nurses' bravery as they attended to the wounded, while German planes flew low attacking with machine guns. Wake's last words served well as propaganda: "Tell them not to be sorry, but glad, and tell them to carry on."[76]

A provincial war memorial on the grounds of the Province of Saskatchewan's legislative buildings in Regina was unveiled in 2007 (Figure 4.6), joining an earlier statue depicting an infantryman. Together they mark the entranceway to panels listing the names of 5,348 First World War casualties from the province.[77] Canadian nurses, including Loretta Miller, head nurse at Winnipeg General Hospital, and the Anglican sister Hannah Grier Coomes from Toronto, were the first to serve with the military in Saskatoon, Saskatchewan during the 1885 North West Rebellion.[78] Thus, the province staked a claim as the birthplace of Canada's military nurses. The Saskatchewan War Memorial Committee decided in 2006 that "recognition of the women's role in armed conflict had been long overdue and that the most recognizable role played by women in the early years had been that of the Nursing Sister."[79] The committee raised the funds, obtaining a major contribution from the Saskatchewan Registered Nurses Association, whose maquette (small model of the statue) was unveiled by Princess Anne in July 2007. Alberta artists Don and Shirley Begg modelled the sculpture on a photograph of Saskatchewan Nursing Sister Elizabeth Matheson. Born in Onion Lake, Saskatchewan in 1892, Matheson was the daughter of Doctor Elizabeth Beckert Matheson and Rev. John Matheson. Before interrupting her nurse training to help her parents with their health care and missionary work, Matheson enlisted in 1917 and served in France and England. Her story is told on the Saskatchewan Nurses' Association website.[80] In the unveiling, Second World War Nursing Sister, Lt Col. (retired) Hallie Sloan proudly exclaimed that it was perfect in every detail, right down to the boots that nurses wore.[81] Symbolizing the acceptance of women in the military, the Nursing Sister wears her official uniform and stands with her arms at her side, beside the soldier.

A less lasting tribute, Veterans Affairs Canada and the National Capital Commission produced an ice sculpture in 2011 for Ottawa/Gatineau's winter festival, *Winterlude*. Although we are reminded that, as Canada was then active in Afghanistan, acknowledgement of nurses as pioneers for women in the military also served recruitment goals, this project did acknowledge their pioneering role. The ice sculpture replicated the 1926 nurse memorial, and text on accompanying panels extolled women's long wartime role beginning with the 1885 North West Rebellion, when "women bravely stood in harm's way to nurse wounded soldiers." It continues, "since then women have taken part in a variety of aspects of military life, now joining their male counterparts on the frontiers, operating submarines, providing necessary intelligence support and patrolling battlefields."[82]

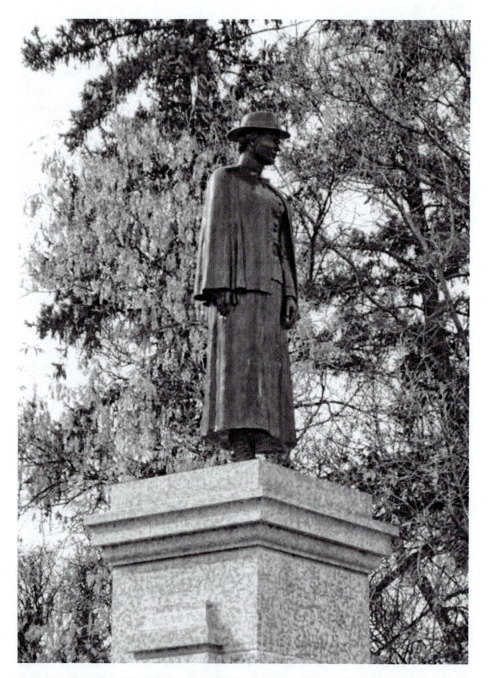

Figure 4.6 First World War Memorial, Regina, Saskatchewan.

Source: John G. Connors, RCAMC/CFMS (Retired), unidentified photographer.

Conclusion

Changing values are revealed in this progression from wartime exploitation of nurses for their propaganda value to postwar forgetting and generic tributes, to acceptance of nurses as pioneering military women. Nurses actively remembered their heroism by erecting memorials, and these reveal minority discourses in which nurses depicted their work through symbols such as the uniform. As the success of any public monument should be measured in its ability to elicit a response, more research is needed into how the Canadian nursing body used these memorials to create their own traditions and rituals of remembrance.[83]

Do these memorials also shed light on the question asked by numerous scholars: "Did nurses/women make gains through their wartime service?"? The military was an exclusive organization, accepting only males, and at the time of the First World War predominantly white males. Women were excluded, based on the gender ideology that suggests they were in need of protection. In return for their war service, veterans were ensured full political rights, public honors – indeed the families of war dead often made further demands of the state.[84] Although less successful, some ethnic minorities tried to gain military admission and to subsequently use their war service to gain enfranchisement and other political rights previously denied them.[85]

How did women fare in this exchange? Some scholars assert that war left conventional gender ideology unchanged.[86] One can certainly point to the forgetting of nurses' sacrifices through generic memorials in the immediate postwar years to support such a claim. However, other scholars point to nurses' postwar professional gains.[87] In Canada, for example, most provincial nurses' associations gained registration legislation and saw the launching of university-based educational programmes. Women in Canada, as did women in many Western democracies, also obtained the right to vote at or immediately following the war. Indeed, many historians have observed that women's wartime services, from knitting socks to nursing, gave politicians a face-saving "reason" to finally accede to women's longstanding suffrage demands. As nurse casualties played an important symbolic role in "representing" all women in postwar memorials, one might conclude that military nurses' presence among the nation's war heroes helped undermine the longstanding objection to women's full political equality: that they could not fight and die in the defense of their homeland(s).

Notes

1 The author would like to thank Rhona Goodspeed for helping me to find new ways to look at visual images, and to Monique Trepannier, Parks Canada, for her invaluable photographic support.
2 David MacKenzie, 2005, *Canada and the First World War: Essays in Honour of Robert Craig Brown*, University of Toronto Press, Toronto.
3 Geneviève Allard, 2005, "Caregiving on the Front: The Experience of Canadian Military Nurses during World War I," *On All Frontiers: Four Centuries of Canadian Nursing*, ed. Christina Bates, Dianne Dodd and Nicole Rousseau, University of Ottawa Press and Canadian Museum of Civilization, Ottawa.

4   Margaret T. Higgonet, ed., 2001, *Nurses at the Front: Writing the Wounds of the Great War*, Northeastern University Press, Boston; Sharon Ouditt, 1994, *Fighting Forces, Writing Women: Identity and Ideology in the First World War*, Routledge, New York; Angela K. Smith, 2000, *The Second Battlefield: Women, Modernism and the First World War*, Manchester University Press, Manchester; Susan R. Grayzel, 1999, *Women's Identities at War: Gender, Motherhood and Politics in Britain and France During World War I*, University of North Carolina Press, Chapel Hill, NC.

5   Kathryn McPherson, 1996 "Carving Out a Past: The Canadian Nurses' Association War Memorial," *Histoire Sociale/Social History*, vol. XXIX, no. 58, pp. 417–429; Natalie Riegler, 1992, "The Work and Networks of Jean I. Gunn, Superintendent of Nurses, Toronto General Hospital, 1913–1941: A Presentation of Some Issues in Nursing during her Lifetime, 1882–1941," PhD Thesis, University of Toronto, pp. 291–327.

6   Dianne Dodd, 2009, "Canadian Historic Sites and Plaques: Heroines, Trailblazers, the Famous Five," *CRM: The Journal of Heritage Stewardship*, vol. 6, no. 2, pp. 29–66; Eileen Eagan, 2003, "Immortalizing Women: Finding Meaning in Public Sculpture," *Her Past Around Us: Interpreting Sites for Women's History*, eds. Polly Welts Kaufman, Katharine T Corbett, Krieger Publishing Company, Malabar, FL, pp. 31–68.

7   Denise Thomson, 1995–96, "National Sorrow, National Pride: Commemoration of War in Canada, 1918–1945," *Journal of Canadian Studies*, vol. 30; David W. Lloyd, 1998, *Battlefield Tourism: Pilgrimage and the Commemoration of the Great War in Britain, Australian and Canada, 1919–1939*, Berg Publishing, Oxford, UK.

8   Susan Mann, 2001, "Where Have All the Bluebirds Gone? On the Trail of Canada's Military Nurses, 1914–1918," *Atlantis*, vol. 26, no. 1, p. 36.

9   Although the national level tends to exclude women, elite, white nurses are an exception. The local level of commemoration will be the focus of another study.

10 Katie Pickles, 2007, *Transnational Outrage: The Death and Commemoration of Edith Cavell*, Palgrave Macmillan, Basingstoke, UK.

11 Christine E. Hallett, 2009, *Containing Trauma: Nursing Work in the First World War*, Manchester University Press, Manchester; Hallett, 2010, "Portrayals of Suffering: Perceptions of Trauma in the Writings of First World War Nurses and Volunteers," *Canadian Bulletin for the History of Medicine*, vol. 27, no. 1, pp. 65–84; Hallett, 2007, "The Personal Writings of First World War Nurses: A Study of the Interplay of Authorial Intention and Scholarly Interpretation," *Nursing Inquiry*, vol. 14, no. 4, pp. 320–329; Cynthia Toman, 2007, *An Officer and a Lady: Canadian Military Nursing and the Second World War*, University of British Columbia Press, Vancouver.

12 Barbara Dundas, 2000, *A History of Women in the Canadian Military*, Art Global, Montreal.

13 Jay Winter, 1995, *Sites of Memory, Sites of Mourning: The Great War in European Cultural History*, Cambridge University Press, p. 78.

14 Jonathon Vance, 1997, *Death So Noble: Memory, Meaning, and the First World War*, University of British Columbia Press, Vancouver.

15 Martha Norkunas, 2002, *Monuments and Memory: History and Representation in Lowell, Massachusetts*, Smithsonian Institution Press, Washington, DC; Marina Warner, 1985, *Monuments and Maidens: The Allegory of the Female Form*, Weidenfeld and Nicolson, London.

16 Eagan, 2003; Norkunas, 2002.

17 Christina Bates, 2010, "Looking Closely: Material and Visual Approaches to the Nurse's Uniform," *Nursing History Review*, vol. 18, pp. 167–188.

18 G.W.L. Nicholson, 1975, *Canada's Nursing Sisters*, A.M. Hakkert, Amsterdam, p. 44.

19 Margaret R. Higgonet, Jane Jenson, Sonya Michel, Margaret Collins Weitz, eds., 1987, *Behind the Lines: Gender and the Two World Wars*, Yale University Press, New Haven, CT; Higgonet, 2001; Smith, 2000; McPherson, 1996; Ouditt, 1994, p. 10.

20 Pickles, 2007, pp. 111, 117.

21 Ibid. pp. 188, 201.

22 "The Sinking of Llandovery Castle by German Submarine," 9 July 1918, *Canadian Daily Record*, File 9-28C Llandovery Castle and Bombings, RG 24, Department of National Defense. Library and Archives Canada.

23 Ibid.

24 Director General, Canadian Army Medical Corps, n.d., "Llandovery Castle," File 9-28C RG 24, p. 2. Library and Archives Canada.

25 Ibid., p. 3.

26 S.F. Wise, 1999, "The Black Day of the German Army: Australians and Canadians at Amiens, August 1918," *Defining 1918 Victory*, eds. Peter Dennis, Jeffrey Grey, Army History Unit, Department of Defence, Canberra; James McWilliams, James R. Steel, 2001, *Amiens: Dawn of Victory*, Dundurn Press, Toronto.

27 In Canada, Belgium and France, this series of victories is called Canada's Hundred Days, in recognition of the Canadian contribution. Tim Cook, 2008, *Shock Troops: Canadians Fighting the Great War, 1917–1918*, Viking Canada, Toronto, p. 579.

28 Desmond Morton, 1993, *When Your Number's Up: The Canadian Soldier in the First World War*, Random House, Toronto, pp. 181–206.

29 Tuxford, as cited in Cook, 2008, p. 417.

30 Desmond Morton, J.L. Granatstein, 1989, *Marching to Armageddon: Canadians and the Great War, 1914–1918*, Lester & Orpen Dennys, Toronto, p. 228.

31 Canadian War Museum, n.d.

32 Mann, 2001, p. 36.

33 Their names included 50 sailors lost at sea or in the Halifax Explosion of 1917 when two ships, one carrying explosives, collided in the Halifax harbor; 177 merchant seamen who died as a result of enemy action; and 188 soldiers and Nursing Sisters buried or lost at sea. Dominique Boulais, Deputy Secretary-General, Canadian Agency, Commonwealth War Graves Commission, 23 August 2011, personal communication.

34 While rules at the national level often precluded naming, local communities usually engraved the names of nurses along with other war casualties on their memorials. Peter Longworth, 1985, *The Unending Vigil: The History of the Commonwealth War Graves Commission*, Commonwealth War Graves Commission, Maidenhead.

35 Kristina Huneault, 1994, "Heroes of a Different Sort: Representations of Women at Work in Canadian Art of the First World War," MA Thesis, Concordia University; Huneault, 1993, "Heroes of a Different Sort: Gender and Patriotism in the War Workers of Frances Loring and Florence Wyle," *Journal of Canadian Art History*, vol. XV, no. 2, pp. 26–49; Christine Boyanoski, 1987, *Loring and Wyle: Sculptors' Legacy*, Art Gallery of Ontario.

36 Laura Brandon, 2006, *Art or Memorial? The Forgotten History of Canada's War Art*, University of Calgary, Calgary.

37 Huneault, 1994, pp. 29, 38, 64.

38 Ibid., pp. 46, 29.

39 Pickles, 2007, pp. 129–132.

40 Boyanoski, 1987, pp. 24, 27.

41 Pickles, 2007, pp. 86–107.

42 It most resembles Sir George Frampton's memorial in London. Pickles, 2007, p. 132.

43 Boyanoski, 1987, p. 25.

44 Rhona Goodspeed, 2010, "Frances Loring (1887–1968) and Florence Wyle (1881–1968)," Historic Sites and Monuments Board of Canada Submission Report 2010–18.

45 Italian Consul Chevalier Victor Gianelli as cited in Pickles, 2007, p. 132.

46 Thomson, 1995–96.

47 Riegler, 1992, pp. 291–327.

48 Besides being a partner in Darling and Pearson, Frank Darling had been appointed in 1920 as one of three professional assessors to the Canadian Battlefield's Memorial Commission.

49 Riegler, 1992, p. 305.

50 Riegler, 1992, p. 306.

51 J.L. Granatstein, "Conscription in the Great War," in MacKenzie, 2005, pp. 62–75.

52 Patrice A. Dutil, "Against Isolationism: Napoléan Belcourt, French Canada, and 'La grande guerre,'" in MacKenzie, 2005, pp. 96–137.

53 McPherson, 1996, p. 424.

54 J.B. Hunter, Deputy Minister of Public Works to Acting Minister of Public Works, 24 Feb. 1922, Briefing Note, File D-155 Department of Public Works, RG 11, House of Commons.

55 Diana Mansell and Dianne Dodd, "Professionalism and Canadian Nursing," Bates et al., 2005, pp. 199–200.

56 Riegler, 1992, pp. 309–319.

57 In the United States, army nurses commissioned Frances Luther Rich to create a monument to nurses who died in the war, located in Arlington Cemetery, Washington. However, their first choice had been Gutzon Gorglum, who sculpted the presidents at Mount Rushmore. Mary T. Sarnecky, 1999, *A History of the U.S. Army Nurse Corps*, University of Pennsylvania Press, Philadelphia, PA, pp. 165–166.

58 "Report of the Memorial Committee," 1922, *Canadian Nurse*, vol. 18, no. 5, p. 263.

59 McPherson, 1996, p. 427.

60 Robert Shipley, 1987, *To Mark Our Place: A History of Canadian War Memorials*, NC Press, Toronto; Vance, 1997.

61 McPherson, 1996, p. 425.

62 Thomson, 1995–96, p. 12; John R. Gillis, ed., 1994, *Commemorations: The Politics of National Identity*, Princeton University Press, Princeton, NJ, p. 12; Alan Young, 1989–90, "'We throw the torch': Canadian Memorials of the Great War and the Mythology of Heroic Sacrifice," *Journal of Canadian Studies*, vol. 25, no. 4, pp. 5–28.

63 Bates, 2010; Ouditt, 1994, p. 17.

64 McPherson, 1996, pp. 426–427.

65 John Hutchinson, 1996, *Champions of Charity: War and the Rise of the Red Cross*, Westview Press, Boulder, CO, p. 276.

66 B.C. History of Nursing Professional Practice Group, 2005, "The Nurse Memorial Window, Canadian Memorial Church, The United Church of Canada," B.C. History of Nursing Society.

67 It is also well cared for. In 1989 the Vancouver unit of the Nursing Sisters Association published several editions of note cards to raise funds to restore the window and provide perpetual care and maintenance. With aging membership of the Nursing Sisters Association, the B.C. History of Nursing Society has now assumed this responsibility. Ibid., p. 12.

68 Susan Hart, 2000, "Traditional War Memorials and Postmodern Memory", MA Thesis, Concordia University, Montreal; Susan Hart, 2006, Universities Art Association of Canada Annual Conference, Nova Scotia College of Art and Design, Halifax, Nova Scotia; Hart, 2008, "Sculpting a Canadian Hero: Shifting Concepts of National Identity in Ottawa's Core Area Commemorations", PhD Dissertation, Concordia University, Montreal.

69 Veterans Affairs Canada, 1982, *The National War Memorial*, p. 16.

70 Hart, 2000, p. 51.

71 Hallett, 2010, p. 80.

72 Ibid., p. 68.

73 Shawna M. Quinn, 2010, *Agnes Warner and the Nursing Sisters of the Great War*, Goose Lane Editions and New Brunswick Military Heritage Project, Fredericton, pp. 99, 104.

74 Ibid., p. 116.

75 The designation came about through the efforts of archivist and local historian Sherri K. Robinson. Marjorie Barron Norris, 2002, *Sister Heroines: The Roseate Glow of Wartime Nursing 1914–1918*, Bunker to Bunker Publishing, Calgary, pp. 146–147.

76 Wake as cited in Debbie Marshall, 2007, *Give Your Other Vote to the Sister: A Woman's Journey into the Great War*, University of Calgary Press, p. xxiii.

77 Gordon Goddard, 27 June 2011, interview with author.

78 Elizabeth Domm, 2010, "From the Streets of Toronto to the Northwest Rebellion: Hannah Grier Coome's Call to Duty," in *Caregiving on the Periphery: Historical Perspectives on Nursing and Midwifery in Canada*, ed. Myra Rutherdale, McGill-Queen's Press, Montreal, pp. 109–126; Nicholson, 1975, pp. 18–27.

79 Goddard, 2011.

80 Saskatchewan Registered Nurses' Association website, n.d., www.srna.org

81 Hallie Sloan as cited in Heather Polischuk, "New Statue Honours Nurses in War," *Regina Leader-Post*, 1 October 2007.

82 Veterans Affairs Canada, consulted online 12 July 2011, "Canadian Nursing Sisters," www.veterans.gc.ca/eng/history/other/nursing

83 For example, the CNA lays flowers at the Parliamentary memorial every Remembrance Day and conducts an informal service to "acknowledge and pay respects to the nurses who died as a result of war service." June Weber, 4 July 2011, interview with author; *Canadian Nurse*, 2011, vol. 197, no. 1, p. 14.

84 Lara Campbell, 2000, "'We who have wallowed in the mud of Flanders': First World War Veterans, Unemployment and the Development of Social Welfare Canada, 1929–1939," *Journal of the CHA*, New Series, vol. 11, pp. 125–149; Morton, 1993, pp. 181–206.

85 Lyle Dick, 2010, "Sargeant Masumi Mitsui and the Japanese Canadian War Memorial," *Canadian Historical Review*, vol. 91, no. 3, pp. 435–463.

86 Smith, 2000, p. 91; Sandra L. Gilbert, 1987, "Soldiers' Heart: Literary Men, Literary Women, and the Great War," in Higgonet et al., pp. 197–226; Ouditt, 1994; Margaet R. Higgonet, 1993, "Not So Quiet in No-Woman's Land," *Gendering War Talk*, eds. Miriam Cooke and Angela Woollacott, Princeton University Press, Princeton, NJ.

87 Meryn Stuart, 1999, "War and Peace: Professional Identities and Nurses' Training, 1914–1930," *Challenging Professions: Historical and Contemporary Perspectives on Women's Professional Work*, eds. Elizabeth Smyth, Sandra Acker, Paula Bourne, and Alison Prentice, University of Toronto Press.

5

SEARCHING FOR CONNECTIVITY

Using historical methods and social network analysis to uncover new discoveries in community organizing

J. Margo Brooks Carthon and Katherine Abbott

The time has come for more social science historians to join the ranks of . . . theory builders, who modify social theory in the laboratory of the past.[1]

On January 8, 2011, the American Historical Association (AHA) convened its 125th Annual Meeting in Boston. Among the conference's offerings was a panel entitled, *Historical Social Network Analysis: A Practicum*.[2] Round table discussants included four university-based international scholars, who each presented on subjects ranging from institutional change in the colonial economy of Buenos Aires to Klan violence in the post-reconstruction American South. For some conference attendees the two-hour practicum served as an initial introduction to Social Network Analysis (SNA); for others it demonstrated the wide range of software and data management tools available to current and nascent users. Social network analysis refers to "a distinctive set of methods used for mapping, measuring and analyzing the social relationship between people, groups, and organizations."[3] In recent decades SNA has grown in use and is currently employed across an array of disciplines ranging from sociology to medicine and business.[4]

Advances in technology and widening training opportunities are opening doors for the use of SNA for historical research purposes. Many historians, however, are unfamiliar with SNA, hence the purpose of this chapter is to introduce the SNA method and describe how it might be applied to a historical case study. Drawing on our respective backgrounds in history, social work, sociology, and health services research, we explore what historical data sources are required to employ a network approach, examine whether the applicability of SNA is better suited for large data sets or equally beneficial to smaller localized historical or cultural studies, and discuss how a network analytic approach might enhance the arguments or results of a historical investigation.

The chapter begins with an overview of the theoretical and analytic underpinnings of SNA, followed by a review of examples of studies employing history and SNA. Finally, we present an illustration of this integration with a case study of the Starr Centre, a settlement association with deep civic roots in Philadelphia's early 20th century ethnic immigrant and black communities. The case study was drawn from a historical research study originally conducted by Dr Brooks Carthon. Using the original study we describe how the use of a network perspective facilitated new understandings of how individuals and organizations historically mobilized to disseminate important social and health information in local minority communities. The chapter ends with a discussion of the limitations associated with combining SNA and history and with recommendations to future users.

An introduction to social network analysis

Social network analysis is a term that not only describes a method of analysis, but equally refers to a set of theories which take into account how people are interconnected.[5] It has developed over the past century as an area of inquiry encompassing a broad range of disciplines including social psychology, business, geography, political science, economics, and physics.[6] SNA traces its roots in the early 20th century to the fields of anthropology and sociology.[7] SNA users are interested in understanding how social interactions are patterned by the structure of the network in which individuals are embedded. By helping to understand the patterns of interactions, SNA can elucidate how individuals become susceptible to infectious diseases, obtain information, and influence or are influenced by others.[8]

Early researchers employing SNA include Jacob L. Moreno, who conducted a study at Sing Sing Prison in 1932 and another at the Hudson School for Girls in 1934. In his Hudson School study Moreno sought to understand the reasons behind a rapid increase in runaways among the pupils at the New York school. To answer his question, Moreno graphically represented relationships between students and their social positions with one another.[9] He concluded that social proximity and influence between pupils determined whether and when a girl ran away rather than the girls' personalities or other motivations. Moreno's findings were published in the *New York Times* and in book form in 1934. His scholarship, along with that of other early SNA pioneers such as researchers at the Group Networks Laboratory at the Massachusetts Institute of Technology (MIT) and that of anthropologist Radcliffe Brown, helped to launch the discipline.[10] Later research conducted in the 1980s and early 1990s affirming that HIV/AIDS was transmitted through a network process added credibility to SNA and attracted research funds for SNA, contributing to its further evolution throughout the 20th century.[11]

The name "SNA" implies that it is only a method of analysis, but it has a strong foundation in theory as well. Social theorists Emile Durkheim and Georg Simmel were the first to discuss the role of social integration or isolation on a variety of outcomes. Today, SNA theories focus on understanding how ties are formed or dissolved, how actors come to occupy positions, and how networks come to have properties, such as a core or periphery structure. SNA goes beyond simply identifying how actors are connected to one another, to examining how the structure of relations and the position of actors within a social structure help to determine the opportunities or the constraints that an actor encounters.[12] This represents a shift from solely using attributes of the individual, such as race, gender, and health status, as explanations for social position to a focus on relationships and interactions with others, thereby adding situational and environmental factors to the list of attribute variables that can be studied.

The social network analyst attempts to evaluate the multidimensional aspects of human interactions through the mapping and measurement of social ties. Social ties are defined as the linkages between two or more persons, groups, or institutions and are viewed as the essential unit of analysis. Network analysts focus specifically on the relational or social cohesion aspects of social structures by examining the direct ties or interactions between actors. Depending on the data used, ties can have different strengths, represent asymmetrical relations, and carry values that reflect multiple aspects of relationships.[13] Network analysts look for relational tie patterns and social cohesion developments such as the formation of very strong, dense, and relatively isolated social networks, which facilitate the formation of subgroups or cliques. Because SNA studies frequently include measures of strength of social ties, the final analysis yields a wealth of information on the relational aspects of social structures.

Sociologist Mark Granovetter examined the implicit meaning of tie strength and posited that while information spreads rapidly through densely knit groups because the actors are strongly connected to one another, they are less apt to gain access to new information since they frequently share the same set of social contacts and are more likely to hold similar views and opinions. This feature of densely knit groups is frequently exemplified in ethnic enclaves or social cliques. Alternatively, Granovetter suggests that weaker ties, defined as contact with extended non-intimate ties, inject innovations and novel ideas into groups that would otherwise be more homogeneous in their views and opinions.[14] Weak ties may be identified as individuals with whom less is shared in common, but who nonetheless may indirectly connect individuals or serve as bridges between isolated social groups (or individuals).

To better understand the influence of tie strength, let us take an example of a nurse working in a Hispanic migrant community. Ties between members of the migrant community may be very strong and dense, with the community itself being ethnically and culturally homogeneous and relatively isolated. The nurse is not of Hispanic origin nor is she a resident of the immediate community. Hence, the affiliation between the nurse and clients could be defined as comprising weaker "ties" due to cultural, socio-economic, residential, and perhaps racial differences. The nurse in this example nonetheless serves as an important link between migrant residents and the healthcare community, providing access not only to health resources but also to social services and perhaps employment opportunities. According to Granovetter's theory, which specifies the "strength of weak ties," these seemingly more fragile connections may (in the end) serve as conduits for increased diversity of thought and widening opportunities for social mobility.

Depending on the research question of interest, researchers employing SNA examine a number of key network features about their social ties such as size (number of network members), density (the extent to which the members are connected to each other), composition (the degree to which they are defined on the basis of traditional group structures such as kin, co-worker, neighbor); and homogeneity (the extent to which individuals are similar to each other in a network, such as age, gender). In addition, they can examine the frequency of contact between ties and determine the content of what is flowing through ties. The extent to which exchanges or transactions are reciprocated is also an example of a network characteristic that can be explored.[15]

The three primary approaches to analyzing network data are the whole network (WN), personal/egocentric network (EC), and affiliation network.[16] The WN approach seeks to capture all essential connections among actors in a defined group, such as all patients in a unit of a hospital. Determining who will be studied is fundamental to research employing whole networks. When using the WN approach all members of the network are ideally included and all possible ties are documented and analyzed. In contrast the egocentric (EC) approach seeks to examine an individual and the multiple ties that he or she relies upon for support, such as discussing important matters, borrowing money, or the receipt of emotional support. Networks can also be constructed using affiliation data, such as organizations and the members of their board. This approach will likely be the most applicable approach for historians, who can use archival records to infer relationships among people who serve together as board members. There are a variety of mathematical algorithms and software programs, such as UCINET, that offer comprehensive SNA data analysis capability. In order to generate network models, analysts apply mathematical and graphical techniques to illustrate and understand the complexity of human and organizational relationships.[17]

Merging SNA and historical methods

Over the past decade access to SNA software and training has improved, increasing its accessibility to historians.[18] This section provides a number of examples of studies that have simultaneously employed historical and social network research methods. We end it with a discussion of the possibilities and limitations of such endeavors.

One of the best-known examples of SNA use with historical materials is the 1993 work of John Padgett and Christopher Ansell, who analyzed marriage and financial transactions to examine how the Medici family rose to power in early 15th century Florence based on their network position. In their work, Padgett and Ansell employ the concept of structural equivalence to identify "the family, economic, and patronage networks that constituted the Medicean political party" and their rivals, the "oligarchs."[19] Using archival data such as marital and economic records as well as personal corres-pondences, the researchers were able to produce an overall relational picture of Florence's social structure within a 92 family ruling elite. Through their analysis they were able to predict and reveal connections among networks, groups, and party membership. They concluded that "rather than [political] parties being generated by social groups . . . both parties and social groups were induced conjointly by underlying networks."[20] More specifically, the researchers reveal that there was no simple way to map groups into parties simply based on social status, but instead contend that attributes such as social class are "cognitive categories" that party affiliation, networks, and actions crosscut.[21] In this application of SNA using archival records, Padgett and Ansell reject categorical affiliation as motivation for political party association, but instead demonstrate how the complex interplay of marriage, finances, residential affiliation, and other social determinants served as precursors and motivators to political allegiances.

Another example of the use of SNA and historical archival data is the work of Naomi Rosenthal et al., whose research examined women's social reform activities in New York State between 1840 and 1914.[22] Through their use of organizational records, Rosenthal and her associates mapped out the organizational affiliations of 202 prominent women reformers and developed a detailed portrait of the multiorganizational field of social movement activity during this period. Using measures of centrality they were able to detect the role and functions of particular groups that were more important to the network of reform activities. In addition, using a "directional flow" analysis they were able to detect the movement of individuals across organizations. The results of this study aided researchers in mapping the interorganizational networks operating in women reform efforts and revealed the complex interplay between reform movements and civic association affiliation.

An additional example of the combined application of historical sources and SNA includes research conducted by historians Michael Alexander and James Danowski in 1990.[23] The aim of the study involved the content textual analysis of 280 letters written by Cicero, to study the personal communication and social structure of the Late Roman Republic (68–50 BC). Central to their research were questions about frequency and distance between knights and senators, two groups who functioned as social and political elites within ancient Roman society. To answer these questions, Alexander and Danowski completed a network analysis of all actors, including their ranks, in order to generate a complete representation of the network structure and how individual position or status within the network influenced network role.

To examine the role of "centrality," the researchers performed cross-tabulations of seven categories of social status in Roman society (including citizen, freedman, slave, knight) by network role. Centrality reflects relational power and control over information in a network. Results from the analysis revealed that individuals on the periphery of the network were somewhat more likely to be of lower status and that information within a group tended to flow through more central figures. However, the study also revealed that while status frequently served as a barrier to group entry, once accepted within the central group position, the individual was no longer defined by formal status. This finding suggested that while centrality reflected a type of relational power *between* "in-group" and "out-group" members, once accepted into the in-group all members were viewed as socially equivalent. Hence, social structure of Cicero's ancient Roman society was much like that of a club, fraternity, or sorority; all outsiders were viewed as social subordinates, until they were formally accepted into the organization.

When used alongside traditional historical methods, SNA allows users to reconstruct the structure and properties of social networks and examine relational interactions within and between individuals, groups, and organizations. While historians have always recognized that social interactions have influenced the development of institutions and communities, few have quantified frequency of interactions between individuals or measured the influence of people within networks and systems as the central feature of their work. Moreover, the chronological order that generally gives structure to historical narratives and the dependence on words rather than (graphic) images emphasizes temporal over spatial and structural patterns.[24]

To better understand the importance of spatial and structural patterns, let's return to our example of the nurse working in the Hispanic migrant community. As noted, the analysis of spatial and structural patterns relies in part on the measurement of relational ties and proximity. A straightforward assessment of this case study might focus on the cultural discordance existing between the nurse and community and the importance for the nurse to understand the specific beliefs and values of community residents in order for health promotion to occur. The application of SNA, however, prompts us to examine not only the individual nurse–client interactions but also the nurse in relationship to her contacts *outside* of the migrant community. If for instance this nurse is connected socially to individuals from a local parish, and is a neighbor of a city council board member, and sits on a board for her professional nursing organization, then we are able to visualize how she is uniquely positioned to serve as a bridge to the migrant community from a public health, social, political, and advocacy perspective. Analyses that focus solely on direct individual–individual interactions, without taking into consideration the full social network and all possible connections, may miss the important impact of these simultaneous relations. Hence the application of SNA principles may allow us to view relational patterns in unexpected and more complex ways.

A social network approach also provides a means to test theories and may enhance the arguments or results of a historical investigation by helping to either support or challenge conclusions made through historical inquiry alone. As an example, one of the primary archival sources used in Alexander and Dankowski's work was Cicero's personal letters. While Cicero's letters are recognized as the best evidence for ancient Roman society during that period, it is undeniable that they are from his vantage-point only. Hence, a reliance on this body of evidence alone may render the results flawed due to the limited representativeness of the source.[25] However, Alexander and Dankowski's use of the content analysis of Cicero's letter in addition to quantitative methods helps to substantiate their final conclusions.

Using a database management system, each of Cicero's letters was compiled and an entry was recorded for each personal contact that Cicero mentioned. This resulted in 1914 observations involving 524 individuals with four items recorded for each entry, namely the name and rank of the two individuals involved. The database records recorded each mention of a contact named in a Cicero letter.[26] The researcher's use of quantitative methods helped to create a multidimensional picture of organizational or relational patterns. The use of textual analysis retained rich qualitative information about human interactions, while the use of SNA methods allowed the researchers to quantify the position and status of actors in the network and statistically test hypotheses.

SNA limitations

As with all methods, SNA has its limitations. While SNA may do well to determine structural components of networks such as frequency of interactions and the distance between individuals, this method alone is unable to determine the texture and quality of these relationships. While SNA illuminates structural patterns, it cannot explain why such patterns occur and how social processes change over time. For instance, in the historical SNA study conducted by Rosenthal et al., the researchers were able to delineate early 19th century women's reform activities. While the analysis did well to reveal these activities, the study culminates in the reproduction of static map configurations and relational snapshots of network patterns.[27] Missing from the analysis is a full explanation of the social and political processes underlying such reform involvement; instead these processes are viewed as exogenous variables and are not fully explored or explained by the researchers.

Critics of SNA also contend that SNA does not concern itself with "ideals" or "discursive frameworks" although such abstractions are indeed generally difficult to quantify in "concrete" ways.[28] In their critique of social network analysis, Mustafa Emirbayer and Jeff Goodwin assert that SNA's tendency to objectify social relations through its use of technical tools drains relations "of their active, subjective dimensions and their cultural elements and meanings."[29] Finally, due to its focus on the structure of networks, the motivations behind individual human behavior may not fully be examined or explained using an SNA only model. However, if other aspects of human agency, choice, and volition are measured using historical methods then the two may be used together effectively.

SNA applied to the early history of the Starr Centre

Our own attempt to bring together historical and SNA methods utilized a whole network analytic approach and was drawn from a case study of the Starr Centre, a Philadelphia-based civic association founded in the late 19th century. The primary historical sources used for this analysis were extracted from research conducted previously by Brooks Carthon for a study that examined community and health organizing among blacks living in Philadelphia during the early 20th century.[30] During this period the Starr Centre launched an ambitious campaign to address social inequities and illness among poor blacks and ethnic immigrants living in South Philadelphia, an impoverished area of the city.

The primary aim of the project was to integrate SNA and historical methods in an effort to explore how the theoretical and methodological tools of SNA might help to augment or extend conclusions revealed during the original historical process. The SNA methodology used for this study included three main stages: (1) describing the set of actors and members of the network; (2) characterizing the relationships between and across members of the network; and (3) analyzing the structure of the civic association. The historical sources used for this case study included Starr Centre annual reports, pamphlets, and meeting minutes. SNA tools allowed us to measure and quantify the structural relationships operating across a range of Starr Centre constituents, while our historical records helped to establish the organization's goals, missions, and programmatic changes over time.

Starr Centre: Historical background

Our case study begins in late 19th century Philadelphia, which at the time was in the midst of cataclysmic changes due to mass industrialization and migration.[31] Brooks Carthon captures the transformation in Philadelphia, noting that "the population of Philadelphia was in particular flux as huge swells of immigrants from Eastern Europe and rural Southern migrants entered the city during the opening decades of the twentieth century."[32] Between 1890 and 1910, the city's black population increased more than 100 percent to 84,000 in a city with a total population of 1.5 million, and by 1920 it had expanded to 134,000 in a population of 1.7 million.[33] In search of jobs and increased social freedoms, the city's newest residents packed into cramped dwellings, which resulted in rapidly deteriorating housing conditions and the spread of infectious diseases.[34] To address the growing threat of infectious illness and urban decay, progressive reformers waged a battle through settlement houses and other charities.[35] During this turbulent time, Theodore Starr, a white businessman and philanthropist with deep roots in Philadelphia's black community, established the Starr Centre to address concerns of residents living in some of the poorest and most segregated neighborhoods in the city.[36]

During his lifetime, Theodore Starr's concern for the social welfare of local residents led to the development of a number of initiatives, including building public playgrounds and gardening centers for neighborhood children. By the time of this death in 1884, Starr's social-welfare initiatives were well entrenched within Philadelphia's black community. After his death, Susan P. Wharton, a well-to-do white social progressive, took over management of Theodore Starr's collective philanthropic interest and served as the Centre's first chairperson and president. In addition to Wharton, the Starr Centre comprised a broad constituency of ethnically and culturally diverse individuals. The association's organizational structure included a Board of Directors, donors, various committees, trained visitors, and neighborhood residents.[37]

Local blacks became Starr Centre "members" and gained access to the association's programs by contributing one dollar annually.[38] White well-to-do civic workers served as organizers or trained paid visitors, who made house calls to Centre members to assess housing and health conditions.[39] The heterogeneous nature of the Starr Centre Association's social network fostered connections between people from diverse backgrounds and made concrete the association's desire to come into intimate contact with those they were attempting to help in the local community. The Starr Centre's first charter and bylaws document the association's mission as one that would: "provide for and promote by practical methods, the educational and social improvement of those poor neighborhoods; primarily in the vicinity of the Starr Garden."[40] Starr Centre organizers put this vision into practice by organizing a range of widely attended programs, including classes on housekeeping, carpentry, and health.

Brooks Carthon describes the efforts of the Starr Centre in her account of early 20th century urban community health efforts:

> Starr Centre leaders were particularly interested in health promotion and disease prevention. In 1905, the Starr Centre created a medical department and contracted the services of the Visiting Nurses Association of Philadelphia to provide care to sick children and adults in clinics and homes. Despite the excessive illness present in the black community, many families were forced to juggle their participation in health programs and visits to local clinics with more quotidian domestic concerns, such as finding coal to warm their homes or food to fill their children's hungry stomachs. Even as infectious disease rates spiked among blacks, poor families were frequently obliged to work long hours instead of seeking medical care. Starr Centre board members saw this dilemma and realized that any efforts to curtail excess sickness had to address the limited material resources of community members first.[41]

The Starr Centre coordinated its services with local blacks through frequent visits to the homes of club members. While in the home, Starr Centre visitors were charged with collecting dues, learning about members' living conditions, and offering assistance or referrals when needed. By building relationships and offering "constant sympathy and care," trained visitors hoped "to help, to advise, to inspire."[42] In 1911, the black membership in the Starr Centre totaled more than 900 paid members, and visitors that year made more than 41,000 home visits.[43] Members frequently asked visitors to "please call on my aunt, who wants to join" or "my cousin or friend."[44] The Starr Centre's philosophy of "active touch" between the trained visitors and black Starr Centre members helped to foster a "mutual understanding and confidence," resulting in an "inspiring" partnership that would endure.[45]

The results of the historical study revealed that the establishment of these trusting relationships served as prerequisites for the later success of the Centre's health promotion initiatives. Our application of SNA helped to make these relationships and the roles of stakeholders within the Starr Centre organization more concrete, and revealed potential alternative pathways for resource and informational flow.

Defining organizational ties and determining meaning

The initial application of SNA using historical sources began with understanding the organizational features of the Starr Centre and learning which members of the civic association were likely to engage or form "ties" with one another. Individual affiliates from the Starr Centre used in this example include Theodore Starr, Susan Wharton, two Starr Centre employed visitors and Annie (a black member of the local community and Starr Centre member). To do this with the historical data we constructed a matrix where zeros (0) and ones (1) are used to show the presence or absence of a relationship between a set of actors (see Table 5.1). Thus, there are two sets of items: the rows correspond to individuals who were affiliates of the Starr Centre and the columns reveal if individual affiliates had known interactions with one another.

Table 5.1 Relational data matrix

ID	Starr	Wharton	Visitor 1	Visitor 2	Ms Annie
Starr	0	1	0	0	0
Wharton	1	0	1	1	0
Visitor 1	0	1	0	1	1
Visitor 2	0	1	1	0	1
Annie	0	0	1	1	0

The data in this matrix can also be used to determine the "direction" of the relation-ships between organization members. Directional ties are oriented ties such as charities giving money to recipients, but recipients not giving money to the charity. Nondirectional ties are not oriented and a tie is either present or absent. In the Starr Centre example we created a nondirectional matrix based on the historical documents that inferred a relationship between Theodore Starr and Susan Wharton. As seen in Table 5.1, there is a tie indicated in the cell from Theodore Starr to Wharton and also from Wharton to Starr. On the other hand, there are no ties linking Annie to Wharton or to Starr, which suggests that elites within the organization had more interactions with one another. Annie's most frequent contacts came through interactions with Starr Centre visitors. At first glance this may appear to suggest that Annie had little inter-action with elites within the Starr Centre organization. Given their intermediary roles, however, Starr Centre visitors represented an important feature of the network, providing Annie with potential access to powerful members of the Starr Centre executive board with very few degrees of separation.

To answer our question related to how the members of the Starr Centre were positioned in relation to one another, we created a network visual based on the data presented in Table 5.1. It is through visualizing the network that the structure of the Starr Centre network is revealed. Figure 5.1 presents a visual representation of the Starr Centre social network computed from data in Table 5.1 and integrating attribute data such as gender and race found in Starr Centre records.

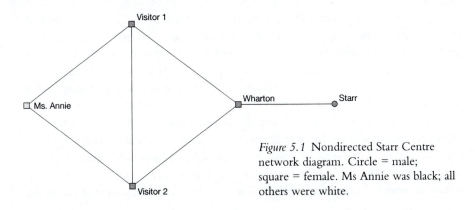

Figure 5.1 Nondirected Starr Centre network diagram. Circle = male; square = female. Ms Annie was black; all others were white.

In viewing the structure of the diagram we can see the various roles and groupings in the Starr Centre network. Wharton plays a classic bridging role between Starr and the Centre staff (Visitors 1 and 2) given her position between two important constituencies in this network. In this capacity Wharton also had great influence over what flowed or did not flow through the network. Remove Wharton and the network falls apart. This is not to suggest that another person could not fill Wharton's role. However, SNA's focus on organizational structure demonstrates Wharton's strategic position and function as the transmitter of upstream and downstream information between association benefactors and members. In this example we were able to capture Annie's interactions with the Starr Centre Visitors, but we know little about Annie's social network outside of those interactions. If, for instance, we had data linking Annie to a local church or sorority, then she too would represent a bridge between the Starr Centre and other facets of the black community.

Visitor 1 and Visitor 2 also appear to hold important, structurally equivalent roles within the network. The Starr Centre visitors are viewed as structurally equivalent because they are connected in the same ways to other structurally related points such as to Annie and Susan Wharton. As structurally equivalent actors in the network, the visitor's roles are viewed as substitutable, meaning if Visitor 1 was unavailable, then Visitor 2 could assume her responsibilities. The presence of structurally equivalent network actors would have been particularly important when serving large numbers of Starr Centre members as, for example, visitors could help to support one another with caseloads and could also provide enhanced coordination of services. SNA visualization also helps to reveal alternatives to traditional organizational flow diagrams. If Figure 5.1 were to be shifted 90 degrees the visualization structure would be a traditional top-down organizational structure, where information flows in one direction (top to bottom). Our representation, which incorporates attribute and relational data from the historical record, introduces a competing explanation where the role and function of a variety of stakeholders influence the flow of information within the Starr Centre network.

Analyzing the structure of the Starr Centre

Centrality is another core concept in SNA that answers critical questions about which individuals occupy positions of power, prestige, and visibility. Highly central individuals can be influential in the spread of diseases, ideas, or behaviors. Three of the most widely used measures of centrality are degree, closeness, and betweenness centrality. Degree centrality is a measure of individual or local network activity and is calculated by the total number of ties to and from an individual. A person who has a high degree centrality is connected to many people in the group.

Both closeness and betweenness centrality are measures of centrality that take account of the pattern of ties of the overall network. Closeness centrality is a measure of a person's communication role, or how reachable an individual is to all other people in the network, and is calculated by measuring the average distance (or paths) an individual is from all other individuals (or "nodes"). This measure of social distance would be useful

Table 5.2 Centrality measures for the Starr Centre members

	Degree centrality (total no. of ties)	Closeness centrality (average distance between members)	Betweenness centrality (information control)
Starr	1	0.125	0.000
Wharton	3	0.200	3.000
Visitor 1	3	0.200	1.000
Visitor 2	3	0.200	1.000
Annie	2	0.143	0.000

if you needed to know who could rapidly communicate information through a network because you would want to start with the person who can reach all other ties through the fewest number of people. For example, a person with high closeness centrality would be the ideal person to discuss important health information with Starr Centre members. The final centrality measure, betweenness centrality, measures information control. A person with a high betweenness centrality is strategically located with ties to other people who have high centrality values, but may not necessarily have a large number of ties. The person with high betweenness centrality can function as a gate-keeper by allowing or not allowing information to flow to ties with lower betweenness centrality. Centrality for the five individuals in the Starr Centre example is derived from the data provided from Table 5.1 and is shown in Table 5.2. Here we illustrate how each individual captures slightly different aspects of centrality. As can be seen from Table 5.2, Wharton, Visitor 1, and Visitor 2 have the highest degree and closeness centrality. However, Wharton stands out when we examine betweenness centrality values. Wharton occupies a strategic position in the network connecting the visitors, executive Board members and black members of the Starr Centre.

Measures such as centrality often serve as proxies for social distance and may illuminate class structure and power dynamics between and among group members. While our records do not permit a nuanced exploration of class within and between Starr Centre members, the application of SNA using historical sources reveals a clear pattern of power and prestige evidenced through Wharton's role as the "gate-keeper" and central organizer for Starr Centre mission, vision, and programming. In this capacity she was a central figure for the control of critical information and resources. Our results also reveal the equally critical roles of Visitors 1 and 2. Due to their high degree of centrality evidenced through their frequent contact with a range of members across the Centre's network, they were highly visible and more apt to interact with Starr Centre members at different levels of the organization.

Discussion

Our application of SNA to historical sources helped to support many of the findings of the Brooks Carthon original historical research. Relational and structural patterns that were evident in the historical record were made more explicit through the application of a network perspective. In particular, SNA helped to reveal how the structure and composition of Starr Centre membership networks influenced the flow of resources and how an individual's receipt of information shifted depending on their position in the Centre. Our use of historical methods and SNA also helped us to affirm who the most central person(s) working in the Starr Centre were, which aided in facilitating our understandings of the role of stakeholders and provided insight into the paths that information may have traveled in order to reach constituents. In addition, we were able to challenge a top-down narrative related to the flow of information within the Starr Centre network through visualization techniques to demonstrate how the structurally equivalent roles of some actors served as support mechanisms, thereby enhancing coordination of care, increasing communication, and reducing social distance between Starr Centre affiliates.

This endeavor was not without its challenges. We did not for instance have access to data about all individuals in the Starr Centre network, which in some cases prevented comprehensive analysis of all actors. The absence of these records limited our ability to draw conclusions about potential interactions between Starr Centre constituents and may have particularly silenced the voices of black members of the Starr Centre, who were often mentioned only briefly in annual reports. Since the application of SNA was completed retrospectively, we were restricted to data that was previously collected, hence our ability to formulate questions might have been altered had the methods been applied simultaneously at the outset of the original project.

Data limitations also prevented us from examining the formation of subgroups and cliques within the Starr Centre network. While the historical records indicated that Starr Centre visitors made over 41,000 visits to the homes of black Starr Centre members in 1911, the individual records for each of these visits were not present in the archive. If we had all relationships between all Starr Centre affiliates accounted for we could have also looked to see where cliques existed and who was in them, the number of bridges (individuals who, if removed, would break the single network into two unconnected networks), how many people individuals had to go through to reach other individuals (geodesic distance), who was in the core or center of the network, and who was on the edges or periphery. Notwithstanding these limitations, a number of interesting findings emerged from the given data, which reinforced results revealed in the original historical evaluation.

Consideration for future users

Successful application of historical SNA hinges on the researcher's ability to access archival data that can infer relationships among a group of individuals or larger entities, such as hospitals or organizations. The use of a variety of archival records such as newspapers, court records, membership rosters, patterns of citations among scholars, and other publicly available information is needed to create data matrices for SNA. The extent to which one can collect information such as the types of ties, similarity or difference of those ties, quality of tie (strong/weak), what is transmitted across ties (information/beliefs), and how it is transmitted (talking/sexual activity) are important aspects to explore in archival materials. However, the historical record is often incomplete, hence gaining access to complete sources and inferring network specific information may be difficult unless one is working with data from multiple sources.

Further limiting the integration of SNA with historical methods is the lack of researcher knowledge in using SNA software programs, such as UCINET and NetDraw. Most graduate-level history students receive limited course work in quantitative methods. Schools with quantitative courses rarely include historical research within the coursework, hence students often do not see how such an integration might work and are subsequently forced to seek training outside their university.[46] However, many sources of training are now being offered, including free online materials (see Node XL and http://faculty.ucr.edu/~hanneman/nettext). We also highly recommend collaborating with colleagues who perform SNA in other disciplines.

Conclusion

This chapter examined both the benefits and the limitations of an integration of historical and SNA methods and theories. Our exploration of the early decades of the Starr Centre offers an illustration of this merger in action. While data limitations present a challenge to broad usage of SNA by many historians, it presents an innovative method, which may add interesting and provocative insights to the historical research and analytic process.

Notes

1 C. Wetherell, 1999, "Theory, method, and social reproduction in social science history: A short Jeremiad," *Social Science History*, vol. 24, no. 4, p. 494.
2 American Historical Association, 2011, *Historical social network analysis: A practicum*. American Historical Association Annual Meeting. Boston: American Historical Association, 86.
3 K. Blanchet and P. James, 2012, "How to do (or not to do) . . . a social network analysis in health systems research." *Health Policy and Planning*, vol. 27, no. 5, p. 439.
4 M. Emirbayer and J. Goodwin, 1994, "Network analysis, culture, and the problem of agency," *American Journal of Sociology*, vol. 99, no. 6, pp. 1411–1454.
5 S. Wasserman and K. Faust, 1994, *Social network analysis: Methods and application*, Cambridge University Press, New York.
6 L. Freeman, 2004, *The development of social network analysis: A study in the sociology of science*, Empirical Press, Vancouver, p. 244.
7 L. Freeman, 2004, *The development of social network analysis*, p. 244; J. Moreno, 1934, *Who will survive?*, Nervous and Mental Disease Publishing Company, Washington, DC; S. Wasserman and K. Faust, 1994, *Social network analysis*; C. Wetherell, 1994, "Network analysis comes of age," *Journal of Interdisciplinary History*, vol. 19, no. 4, pp. 645–651.
8 S. P. Borgatti, A. Mehra, D. J. Brass, and G. Labianca, 2011, "Network analysis in the social sciences," *Science*, vol. 323, pp. 892–895.

9   L. Freeman, 2004, *The development of social network analysis*, p. 244; J. Moreno, 1934, *Who will survive?*

10 S. P. Borgatti et al., 2011, "Network analysis in the social sciences."

11 A. A. Adimora and V. J. Schoenbach, 2005, "Social context, sexual networks, and racial disparities in rates of sexually transmitted infections," *Journal of Infectious Diseases*, vol. 191, no. 1, pp. S115–S122.

12 D. Knoke and J. H. Kuklinski, 1982, *Network analysis*, Sage, Beverly Hills, CA.

13 C. Wetherell, 1999, "Theory, method, and social reproduction in social science history." See also M. S. Granovetter, 1973, "The strength of weak ties," *American Journal of Sociology*, vol. 78, no. 6, pp. 1360–1380. C. Wetherell, A. Plakans, and B.Wellman, 1995, "Social networks, kinship, and community in Eastern Europe," *Journal of Interdisciplinary History*, vol. 24, no. 4, pp. 639–663.

14 M. S. Granovetter, 1973, "The strength of weak ties," pp. 1360–1380.

15 L. F. Berkman, T. Glass, I. Brissette, and T. E. Seeman, 2000, "From social integration to health: Durkheim in the new millennium," *Social Science & Medicine*, vol. 51, no. 6, pp. 843–857. For other readings on the relationship between social networks and health see: L. F. Berkman, 1986, "Social networks, support and health: Taking the next step forward," 1986, *American Journal of Epidemiology*, vol. 123, no. 4, pp. 559–562; S. Cohen, 1989, "Psychosocial models of the role of social support in the etiology of physical disease," *Health Psychology*, vol. 7, no. 3, pp. 269–297; J. Holt-Lundtad, T. B. Smith, and J. B. Layton, 2010, "Social relationships and mortality risk: A meta-analytic review," *PLOS Medicine*, vol. 7, no. 7, p. e316; D. A. Luke and J. K. Harris, 2007, "Network analysis in public health: history, methods, and applications," *Annual Review of Public Health*, vol. 28, pp. 69–93; T. W. Valente, 2010, *Social networks and health: Models, methods, and application*, Oxford University Press, New York.

16 B. H. Erickson, 1997, "Social networks and history: A review essay," *Historical Methods*, vol. 30, no. 3, pp. 149–157.

17 K. Blanchet and P. James, 2012, "How to do (or not to do) . . . a social network analysis in health systems research," pp. 438–446.

18 C. Lipp, 2005, "Kinship networks, local government, and elections in a town in southwest Germany, 1800–1850," *Journal of Family History*, vol. 30, no. 4, pp. 347–365.

19 J. F. Padgett and C.K. Ansell, 1993, "Robust action and the rise of the Medici, 1400–1434," *American Journal of Sociology*, vol. 98, no. 6, pp. 1259–1619, quote on page 1260.

20 Ibid., p. 1277.

21 Ibid., p. 1278.

22 N. Rosenthal, M. Fingrutd, and M. Ethier, 1985, "Social movements and network analysis: A case study of nineteenth-century women's reform in New York State," *American Journal of Sociology*, vol. 90, no. 5, pp. 1022–1054.

23 M. C. Alexander and J. A. Danowski, 1990, "Analysis of an ancient network: Personal communication and the study of social structure in a past society," *Social Networks*, vol. 12, no. 4, pp. 313–335.

24 A. Hillier, 2010, "Invitation to mapping: How GIS can facilitate new discoveries in urban and planning history," *Journal of Planning History*, vol. 9, no. 2, pp. 122–134.

25 M. C. Alexander and J. A. Danowski, 1990, "Analysis of an ancient network," pp. 313–335.

26 Ibid.

27 M. Emirbayer and J. Goodwin, 1994, "Network analysis, culture and the problem of agency, pp. 1411–1454.

28 Ibid., p. 1428.

29 M. Emirbayer, and J. Goodwin, 1994, "Network analysis, culture and the problem of agency," pp. 1411–1454.

30 M. B. Carthon, 2011, "Making ends meet: Community networks and health promotion among Blacks in the city of Brotherly Love," *American Journal of Public Health*, vol. 101, no. 8, pp. 1392–1401.

31 A. F. Davis, 1973, *The peoples of Philadelphia: A history of ethnic groups and lower class life, 1790–1940,* Temple University Press, Philadelphia.

32 M. B. Carthon, 2011, "Making ends meet."

33 U.S. Bureau of the Census, 1968, *Negro population in the United States, 1790–1915.* Government Printing Office, Washington, DC, pp. 350–351.

34 S. T. Mossell, 1921, The standard of living among one hundred negro migrant families in Philadelphia," *Annals of the American Academy of Political and Social Science,* vol. 98, pp. 174–175.

35 W. E. B. Dubois, 1899, *The Philadelphia negro: A social study.* University of Pennsylvania Press, Philadelphia, pp. 147–163; V. P. Franklin, 1979, *The education of black Philadelphia: The social and educational history of a minority community, 1900–1950,* University of Pennsylvania Press, Philadelphia.

36 Starr Centre Association, Charter and Bylaws of the Starr Centre Association, 1905, Starr Centre Collection, Box 9, Folder 105, p. 4, The Barbara Bates Center for the Study of the History of Nursing Archives, University of Pennsylvania; Starr Centre Association, Constitution, by-laws, and minutes of Annual and Board of Directors, 1900–1906, Starr Center Collection, Box 1, Folder 1, The Barbara Bates Center for the Study of the History of Nursing Archives, University of Pennsylvania.

37 E. J. G. Beardsley, 1911, "The value of the intelligent direction of the sick poor – A story of the Starr Centre Association of Philadelphia," *Therapeutic Gazette,* vol. 3, no. 27, pp. 400–403.

38 S. P. Wharton, 1903, Starr Centre First Annual Report, Starr Centre Collection, Box 4, Folder 41, pp. 2–4, The Barbara Bates Center for the Study of the History of Nursing Archives, University of Pennsylvania.

39 Starr Centre Association, *A Few Facts about the Starr Centre,* nd, Starr Centre Collection, Box 6, Folder 109, The Barbara Bates Center for the Study of the History of Nursing Archives, University of Pennsylvania; Starr Centre Association, untitled pamphlet, 1907, Starr Centre Collection, Box 9, The Barbara Bates Center for the Study of the History of Nursing Archives, University of Pennsylvania.

40 Starr Centre Association, Charter and Bylaws of the Starr Centre Association, 1905, p. 4; Starr Center Association, Annual Board of Directors Meeting Minutes, 1900, Box 1, Folder 5.

41 M. B. Carthon, 2011, "Making ends meet," pp. 1392, 1394. See also S. P. Wharton, 1903, Starr Centre First Annual Report, Starr Centre Collection, Box 4, Folder 41, pp. 2–4.

42 S. P. Wharton, 1909, "Negro Branch of the Starr Centre," Starr Centre Collection, Box 6, Folder 104, p. 4, The Barbara Bates Center for the Study of the History of Nursing Archives, University of Pennsylvania.

43 Starr Centre Association, 1911, "Annual Report," Starr Centre Collection, Box 4, Folder 42, p. 7, The Barbara Bates Center for the Study of the History of Nursing Archives, University of Pennsylvania.

44 Starr Centre Association, 1909, "Annual Report," Starr Centre Collection, Box 4, Folder 41, pp. 4–5, The Barbara Bates Center for the Study of the History of Nursing Archives, University of Pennsylvania.

45 M. B. Carthon, 2011, "Making ends meet," p. 1392. See also Starr Centre Association, 1909, "Annual Report."

46 Ibid.; A. Hillier, 2010, "Invitation to mapping: How GIS can facilitate new discoveries in urban and planning history," *Journal of Planning History,* vol. 9, no. 2, pp. 122–134.

PART 3

The politics of nursing knowledge

6

"INTELLIGENT INTEREST IN THEIR OWN AFFAIRS"[1]

The First World War, *The British Journal of Nursing* and the pursuit of nursing knowledge

Christine E. Hallett

The development and transmission of nursing knowledge was a significant, but messy and inchoate process during the late nineteenth and early twentieth centuries. While a number of authors have commented on the ways in which the social and cultural origins of nursing as a female, practice-based and low-status occupation impeded the advance of nursing knowledge,[2] very few have attempted to trace the ways in which knowledge and skill emerged in spite of these impediments.[3] This chapter provides one example of a way in which this gap in our understanding might be addressed. By tracing the written, British nursing response to the medical treatment dilemmas created by the traumatic injuries of the First World War, it presents a case study of one way in which a few elite nurses were arguing that nursing knowledge was scientific knowledge. The chapter thus traces a significant phase in the development of nursing as a discipline.

In the first decades of the twentieth century, the argument (put forward primarily by Florence Nightingale) that nursing knowledge was sanitary knowledge was complicated by the newly emerging perspective (espoused by Ethel Bedford Fenwick and her professional circle) that nursing knowledge was, in fact, scientific knowledge. The chapter argues that, by claiming scientific knowledge as part of the foundation of their own practice base, these writers were consciously contributing to the development of nursing both as a discipline and as a profession. Sanitary knowledge and practical competence remained important in the early twentieth century. Yet the emergence of an interest in science within the writings of nurses cannot be ignored. Nor can its coincidence with the battle that had been raging since the late 1880s to secure the professionalization of nursing, through recognized standards of training. While the focus of this chapter will be on the nurses' claims to the relevance of scientific knowledge for their practice, it will also consider the links between these claims and the fight for professional recognition.

Three professional nursing journals were significant during the early twentieth century and appear to have had wide circulation among both trained nurses and volunteers: *The British Journal of Nursing*, *The Nursing Mirror and Midwives Journal* and *The Nursing Times*. The chapter focuses, in particular, on *The British Journal of Nursing* (*BJN*) which, as a deliberate organ of professionalization, was distinct from the other two in both content and aspirations – and considers the ways in which its editors attempted to develop a corpus of knowledge suitable for nurses. Its owner and editor, Ethel Bedford Fenwick,[4] promoted this work, even as she emerged as the best known and most persistent of campaigners for nurse registration in Britain. The chapter further looks at one particular nurse-author, Violetta Thurstan, who is interesting because she was both one of the most powerful advocates for scientific knowledge in nursing and an energetic campaigner for the education and registration of nurses. Her book *A Text Book of War Nursing* was highly technical in its content and was enthusiastically promoted by the *BJN*.[5]

While this chapter argues that the *BJN* was acting as an agent of knowledge development within the discipline of nursing during the First World War, it does not claim that the journal's project was entirely successful. Many of its attempts to translate medical knowledge and scientific discovery into material that was demonstrably part of a nursing corpus of knowledge were limited in scope, while claims to any exclusivity of nursing knowledge were infrequent. Fenwick appears to have used three distinct approaches: firstly, the verbatim presentation of medico-scientific material; secondly, the publication of invited papers authored by medical scientists; and, thirdly, the publication of material with scientific content, written by nurses, often in response to essay-writing competitions.

The struggle for professionalization and the advent of *The British Journal of Nursing*

The *BJN* was first established as *The Nursing Record* in 1888. Its foundation was part of a forceful drive from within the nursing profession in Britain to place itself on an autonomous and independent footing.[6] Central to this process, which is usually considered to have begun with the formation of the British Nurses' Association (BNA) in 1887, was the thirty-two-year struggle for a single, closed and legally defined British professional nurses' register. The creation of the *BJN* took place rapidly after the formation of the BNA and was heavily influenced by the BNA's founding members. Indeed, it was both edited and, later, financed by Ethel Bedford Fenwick. Hence, it is probable that the foundation of this new journal, which came to represent the interests of the professionalizing group in Britain, and which frequently published both medico-scientific and pro-registration articles in its pages, represented a clear link between the claim to scientific knowledge and the aspirations of the pro-registrationists.

Historians have been somewhat divided over the nature of the so-called "struggle" for professionalization. In 1960, Brian Abel-Smith offered what has been viewed as the first real analysis of the process, seeing it as one in which a professional elite fought to put in place a middle-class nursing workforce that mirrored its own aspirations. More nuanced interpretations came later.[7] Anne Marie Rafferty, focusing on the inescapable link between knowledge and professional power, emphasized the anti-intellectualism that impeded the professionalizers' efforts.[8] Susan McGann explored the differing perspectives of individuals such as Isla Stewart, Matron of St Bartholomew's Hospital and a strong supporter of registration and examination, and Eva Luckes, Matron of The London Hospital, who shared the view of Florence Nightingale that a register based on the passing of a written examination would fail to test the moral suitability of women that entered the profession, and who argued that moral capacity was more important than scientific knowledge.[9]

Recently, Carol Helmstadter refocused attention onto the class interests of those who fought for professional status, arguing that the professionalizing project became imbued with the values of the upper and middle classes.[10] Conversely, Arlene Young argued that powerful class and gender forces inhibited the nursing profession's quest for independence.[11] Anne Summers had already demonstrated that these forces were particularly powerful in slowing the development of professional military nursing in the three decades prior to the First World War.[12] Christopher Maggs and Sue Hawkins both argued that there was greater social fluidity within the nursing profession than had previously been acknowledged.[13] Others have argued that the struggle for professionalization, a prolonged and, at times, destructive one, was characterized by the efforts of nurses to free themselves from the controlling influence of hospital administrators, particularly within the powerful London and provincial voluntary hospitals.[14] Few have examined the significance of nurses' claims to scientific knowledge as an element in this process. The focus on moral responsibility has overshadowed any examination of the profession's knowledge base.

Although the earliest impetus for a nurses' register came from Henry Burdett, an influential spokesman for the Hospitals Association, it seemed to some nurses that his purpose was to guarantee a large and stable workforce rather than to safeguard quality.[15] This led to an irresolvable conflict between the forces for professionalization led by Ethel Bedford Fenwick and influential matrons such as Isla Stewart and Catherine Wood on one hand, and powerful hospital administrators such as Henry Burdett and Sydney Holland on the other. Some matrons – notably Eva Luckes – aligned themselves with the anti-registrationists, for both professional and ideological reasons. Some feared that a single professional register would lower, not raise, standards of nursing care.

Arguments for a better-educated nursing workforce were bound to become enmeshed in issues relating to class, because lower-class women in Britain had few educational opportunities. Some matrons may have been fighting for a better-educated workforce rather than an intrinsically higher-status one. Women's drives for the professionalization of nursing were accompanied by the demands for better political and educational opportunities which were particularly espoused by the suffrage movement. Evidence for Fenwick's support of this movement can be found in the weekly column devoted to women's issues, entitled "Outside the Gates", in her journal.[16] It was perceived that the foundation of the *BJN*, which both promulgated nursing knowledge and promoted the arguments of the registrationists, provided a vehicle to represent the wider interests of the nursing profession. Identifying scientific knowledge as part of the foundation for intelligent – and therefore effective – nursing practice was the keystone of this project.

In an article published in *The American Journal of Nursing* in 1907, Mary Burr, Director of the National Council of Trained Nurses of Great Britain and Ireland, argued that the *BJN*'s inception was part of an attempt to counter the adverse publicity against the professionalization of nursing that was being propagated by *The Hospital*, a journal owned and edited by Henry Burdett.[17] Burr argued that a prolonged and vitriolic campaign had been waged against the nascent journal. Some hospitals had forbidden their nurses to purchase or read *The Nursing Record*, and sponsors had been persuaded not to advertise within its columns. As a result the journal ran at a loss for many years and two successive publishers abandoned the enterprise. In 1893 Dr and Mrs Bedford Fenwick purchased *The Nursing Record* in order to keep it in business, continuing to publish at a loss for a further eight years, and changing its name to *The British Journal of Nursing* in July 1902. Following the publication of a significant report by a Select Committee of the British Parliamentary House of Commons on the Registration of Nurses in 1905,[18] the tide of opinion began to turn. Rank and file nurses became more accepting and less wary of a journal that openly promoted both knowledge and professional status, and the *BJN* won more widespread support.[19] Nevertheless, its circulation figures remained lower than those of other nursing journals. *The Nursing Mirror and Midwives Journal*, created as an offshoot of *The Hospital* and edited by Henry Burdett, was deliberately promoted as a journal that would appeal to the mass of nurses. It did enjoy a larger circulation than any other nursing journal during the first half of the twentieth century.[20] *The Nursing Times*, founded in 1905, was also a successful commercial venture. It came to support the interests of the College of Nursing, a significant professional organization founded in 1916.[21] The Fenwicks, nevertheless, argued that the *BJN* was the only journal that really spoke for nurses. It was clearly the only one that took an overtly professionalizing stance. It was adopted as the official journal of the International Council of Nurses (of which Fenwick was President) in 1901.[22] It claimed to speak for those nurses who were well educated and capable both of assimilating scientific knowledge and of appreciating arguments for professional status (of which the centrepiece was the claim to a register).

The history of *The British Journal of Nursing* was presented by many of those who lived to see it come to prominence as one of extraordinary struggle, determination and "pluck". Burr presented its development to a United States audience as part of an immense struggle for survival. The language she used was powerful – if a little florid – and resonates with the tone of class struggle in a way that seems to contradict those historians who have seen the professionalizers as a middle-class elite:

> Order–Organisation–Unity– by them alone is it possible for a class of workers to succeed, to be strong, to have liberty of speech and conscience, to live decently, and withstand the almost overwhelming pressure of industrial conditions, which in the furious competition for abnormal wealth, grinds the individual to powder.[23]

The language of this text offers a powerful sense of the forces of elite wealth, political power and industrialization in the early twentieth century. In the later part of the century, historians who emphasized the unnecessary slaughter that characterized the First World War suggested that it was the conjunction of these very forces that made the First World War such a devastating conflict.[24]

During the years of the First World War, Fenwick was still very much in charge of the *BJN*'s content, although some editorials may have been authored by the journal's assistant editor, Margaret Breay. The journal carried different emphases from *The Nursing Times* and *The Nursing Mirror and Midwives Journal*. Not only did it report, in almost every issue, the "progress" of the registration movement and the "advance" of the nursing profession, but it also engaged directly with knowledge production and laid claim to the distinct expertise of nursing as a profession. Fenwick's ideas – as promulgated through the *BJN* – were very firmly rooted in the view that, in addition to their vocational calling and their moral correctness, nurses must possess a thorough grounding in scientific knowledge in order to practise safely and competently.[25] Her choice of material for inclusion in the *BJN* during the war years clearly reflects this emphasis, as will be demonstrated in the remainder of this chapter.

The production of knowledge does not necessarily imply its reception and absorption. Precise circulation figures for the *BJN* are not known, but the journal's contents probably reflect the perspectives only of a small elite within the profession.[26] There are some indications, however, that practices it recommended were adopted by nurses in casualty clearing stations and base hospitals – particularly on the Western Front.[27]

Military medicine during the First World War

Warfare has typically been associated with medical advance.[28] The military medical services were faced with a number of unexpected challenges during the First World War. Significant among these was the need to handle large "rushes" of severely traumatized casualties; an unexpectedly high number of severe life-threatening anaerobic wound infections on the Western Front; and the dilemma posed by infectious diseases such as typhoid fever on all fronts.[29] These challenges were met by an emphasis on the rational organization of medical services, the rapid movement of casualties "down the line" and scientific and technological advance. A number of medical historians have focused on specific medical innovations, such as blood transfusion;[30] surgical advances – particularly in the realm of wound care;[31] the control of infectious diseases;[32] and efforts to rehabilitate disabled veterans.[33] Others have explored the attempts of the military medical services to understand, and provide a coherent response to, the emotional trauma of war.[34]

Although a number of recent studies have focused on the organization of military nursing during the First World War, and on the experiences of the nurses themselves,[35] very few have attempted to place nurses at the centre of debates about clinical practice and innovation.[36] The remainder of this chapter focuses more specifically on the way in which nurses' writings – particularly those published by the *BJN* – offered an opportunity for the journal's readership to familiarize themselves with scientific knowledge and assimilate that knowledge into their practice. It examines, in particular, nurses' written responses to treatments for trauma and wound infection on the Western Front.

Nursing and the reception of medical knowledge

The *BJN* adopted three strategies to facilitate the presentation of medical knowledge: firstly, it presented long excerpts from medical journals, sometimes accompanied by brief editorial comment; secondly, it invited medical authors to contribute pieces giving advice to nurses on how medical innovations might be implemented; and thirdly, it provided opportunities for nurses to write essays and articles on specific medico-scientific topics. An exploration of these approaches can permit insight into how Fenwick and her colleagues chose to present scientific knowledge, though it cannot (and does not claim to) measure its reception.

Medical writings in nursing journals

Mark Harrison has shown that the medical profession had great difficulty in tackling the severe anaerobic wound infections that were encountered on the heavily fertilized fields of France and Flanders during the early months of the war.[37] Articles on the treatment of wounds began to appear frequently in *The Lancet* during the late autumn of 1914.[38] This focus was mirrored by a rapid increase in the number of articles on wounds, extracted from medical writings or medical presentations and published by all three nursing journals during the last four months of 1914.[39]

By December 1914, physicians realized that gas gangrene infections were a much more serious problem than had hitherto been recognized. *The British Journal of Nursing* quoted extracts from a paper by Sir Anthony Bowlby (consulting surgeon with the British Expeditionary Force) and Sir Sidney Rowlands (head of a mobile field laboratory), who had published their work in the *British Medical Journal*.[40] The editors of the *BJN* pointed out that it was important for nurses to familiarize themselves with the appearance of a gangrenous wound, so that they could more rapidly report the onset of gangrene to their medical colleagues and prompt surgical intervention.[41] They clearly anticipated that, by including such material in the pages of the *BJN*, they would ensure that it found its way into practice in military hospitals both in Britain and close to the front lines – particularly on the Western Front.

The frequency with which practising military nurses wrote letters in response to articles in the *BJN* indicates that copies of the journal were mailed and did reach nurses in field hospitals. There are, indeed, some interesting examples of letters to the *BJN* in which writers refer to the dilemmas they experience during their current practice in military hospitals, or to their experiences serving overseas. Many letters to the journal were clearly written by nurses working overseas with the British military medical services.[42] One writer commented directly that "since the war began, I have been working hard in a military hospital".[43]

It was around the time of publication of Bowlby and Rowlands's article that both doctors and nurses began to change their views on the use of antiseptics, which were being rapidly reintroduced into practice. Among the most frequently used antiseptics – which were applied to wounds to kill invading microbes directly – were iodoform, flavin, hydrogen peroxide, perchloride of mercury and hypochlorous acid.[44] In November 1914, Fenwick reproduced a paper that had been read by Sir W. Watson Cheyne to the Medical Society of London and subsequently published in the *British Medical Journal*:

> Some surgeons seem to take a particular pride in emphasizing their contempt for antiseptics and the extreme simplicity of their methods. A surgeon comes to an operation and finds a dish containing some fluid. He asks what that is, and the nurse, who has been carefully trained in real aseptic work, says, in fear and trembling, "That is carbolic lotion for your instruments." It is most instructive to see the look of contempt on the surgeon's face as he says: "Carbolic lotion! Who on earth uses antiseptics nowadays? I thought that no one out of an asylum ever thought of them. Take it away and bring me a bowl of boiled water" . . . The futility and littleness of it all makes me sick![45]

Fenwick's willingness to reproduce an article that hinted at the need for nurses to be independent in their thinking rather than deferential to medical authority could have been a significant item in her repertoire of professionalizing tactics. It made the point that even eminent surgeons could sometimes be wrong. It also suggested that it was useful for nurses to be conversant with medical science, rather than merely blindly following medical orders.

Medical authors

Fenwick introduced medical knowledge into the pages of her journal by inviting medical doctors to write pieces pitched deliberately to the needs and requirements of practising nurses. One of her favourite medical authors was the retired Cambridge-educated doctor A. Knyvett Gordon, who had held a number of important clinical and teaching positions during the early years of the twentieth century: Medical Superintendent of the City of Manchester Fever Hospital; Lecturer on Infectious Diseases in Queen's College, Cambridge; and, later, Lecturer on Infectious Diseases in the University of Manchester. Knyvett Gordon authored pieces for the *BJN* on a range of subjects over a period of about 16 years.[46] Soon after the outbreak of war, Fenwick invited Knyvett Gordon to comment on the significance of the war for nursing work. One of his main foci was wound infection, and he recommended a number of ways in which nurses could influence wound healing by: "washing and dressing the wound, opening up pockets of pus, assisting the patient by such measures as fomentations, which stimulate the leucocytes and relieve pain. Or we can sometimes kill some of the microbes in a wound by the application of disinfectant solutions."[47]

Knyvett Gordon emphasized the role of the nurse in strengthening the general constitution of the patient, to allow the body to produce a better defence against the infective microorganisms. This was achieved by good food and "skilful general nursing", along with tepid sponging to reduce an excessively high temperature. He added that: "*The* most important factor in the later stage is careful, untiring, intelligent nursing in healthy surroundings, and it is most important to keep the patient quiet and to give him plenty of fresh air".[48]

It is easy to see why Fenwick was keen to invite this particular medical author to contribute to her journal. His references to "skilful general nursing" and "careful, untiring, intelligent nursing" indicate that he recognized the significance of (even though he may not have fully understood) those many actions taken by nurses to keep a patient clean, well-nourished, calm and comfortable during a serious illness or infection. His text presented scientific knowledge that could be of use in nursing practice.

In writing of wound shock, Knyvett Gordon advised that:

> The first factor in the treatment of shock is the inversion of the patient, so that the blood may run towards the nerve centres in the head . . . Next comes warmth. In hospital a warm drink (unless this should be contraindicated by the presence of internal haemorrhage) should be given . . . Then we have narcotics, such as morphia . . . Another valuable remedy is the injection of normal saline solution.[49]

Hallett records significant use by nurses in casualty clearing stations on the Western Front of the treatments listed by Knyvett Gordon.[50] Although this does not necessarily prove a causal link between their publication in the *BJN* and their adoption in the field, it nevertheless demonstrates a correlation between what nurses were reading about in the *BJN* and what their personal writings – letters, diaries and memoirs – reveal about their practice.

Nurse-authors

One of the ways in which the *BJN* worked to promote scientific knowledge among nurses was to invite its readers to enter essay-writing competitions. In September 1914, soon after the outbreak of war, the essay question chosen was: "What do you mean by shock and what can you do to combat it?" The winner, C. Phyllis Armitage, offered a detailed description of this very imprecisely understood condition:

> "Shock" has been rather aptly defined as "the result of a bleeding into a man's own vessels." It is the result of paralysis of the vaso-motor system . . . The biggest blood vessels are in the abdomen, and these suck the blood from the blood vessels in the other parts of the body. Then we have most of the blood in the body concentrated in the abdomen, and we get the condition known

as "shock" . . . The signs and symptoms are very much the same as in internal haemorrhage: the skin becomes cold, white and clammy on the withdrawal of blood; the temperature falls; the pulse-beats are quicker and thinner; the respirations are shallow; the face wears an anxious expression; the eyes are half shut, with the pupils distended. The patient is inert, and dislikes to be moved; he sees flashes of light before his eyes, and is conscious of curious tastes and smells and of a ringing in his ears. There may also be nausea and vomiting.[51]

Armitage's remarkable description raises a number of points. It shows a nurse giving an original description of a condition that was not well understood. Her willingness to tackle its intricacies (and, indeed, Fenwick's willingness to invite her readership to do so) indicates that some nurses were not afraid to discuss matters that might well have been seen, until that time, to have been part of a medical domain of knowledge. Armitage's prose is scientifically empirical in its precision, and yet also manages to portray the patient as a suffering human being: precise lists of medical "signs and symptoms" are juxtaposed with descriptions of his physical and mental state. Not only was Armitage showing a nurse's sharp observation for her patient's holistic state of body and mind; she was also stepping comfortably into a medico-scientific domain in confidently describing physiological processes.

In recommending treatments for "shock", Armitage advocated some of the same remedies as Knyvett Gordon in the passage quoted in the previous section. She also, however, departed from his recommendations. Where Knyvett Gordon had advised against the use of stimulants such as strychnine and alcohol,[52] Armitage advocated their careful employment, provided the treatment was not "taken too far" and was accompanied by morphia.[53] These distinctions between the perspectives of Armitage and those of Knyvett Gordon are striking. The journal did not shy away from publishing an essay, part of which was in direct contradiction to a previous article published by a doctor.

A number of other entrants in the same essay competition were each given an "honourable mention" and extracts from their essays were printed. Amy Phipps, for example, had pointed out that "much depends on the intelligent and prompt recognition and treatment of the first symptoms of shock".[54] Fenwick's choice of quotation from this essay suggests that she considered intelligence, combined with good observational skills, as among the most important nursing qualities.

Gladys Tatham won a *BJN* competition in the late summer of 1914 for her paper answering the question: "What precautions may be adopted to minimize the danger to the patient, in the case of a wound which has been exposed to infection?" Tatham recommended that a dressing of hydrogen peroxide should be kept in contact with the wound for about five minutes before re-dressing with an aseptic gauze, wool and a bandage. She went on to describe the battle that takes place within the body of the wounded soldier between infective microorganisms and leucocytes, pointing out that resistance can be lowered by poor general physical and mental health: "To prevent these untoward results we must do everything in our power to increase the resistance of the patient. He must have fresh air, warmth, light, nourishing food, plenty of water to drink, clean surroundings and intelligent nursing."[55] This nurse's recommendations were thus accompanied by a scientific rationale.

One of the most striking features of this piece of writing, and of nurses' writings more generally, was the tendency to focus not only on the treatment of the wound itself, but also on all of those measures that could be adopted to promote the general health and strength of the patient. As in earlier examples, the phenomenon "intelligent nursing" makes an appearance, with the assumption that the readership will know what is meant by this phrase. And yet it leaves the modern reader with unanswered questions. Was "intelligent nursing" something that was acquired through experience of working with numerous individuals, building up expertise, over several years, of how to both strengthen and comfort the patient? Or was it something that could be taught?

The main premise of this chapter is that the *BJN* saw the presentation of scientific knowledge as part of its purpose. The phenomenon "intelligent nursing", as it appears in the pages of the *BJN*, suggests that the journal's editors and authors believed that practice was more effective when it was based on such knowledge.

Nursing textbooks and the development of new knowledge

The documentation of a corpus of knowledge for nurses can be viewed as a slow but steady process, which had begun in the late nineteenth century. Textbooks such as Eva Luckes' *General Nursing*, which entered its ninth edition just before the outbreak of war in 1914,[56] and Isla Stewart's *Practical Nursing*[57] had been used as guides to nursing practice since the 1880s. Alongside these authoritative texts were more specialist outputs such as Emily Stoney's *Bacteriology for Nurses*, one of the earliest attempts to synthesize scientific knowledge with nursing practice.[58]

During the war itself, a number of texts were written by practising nurses to support their colleagues in synthesizing their existing practice with newly emerging scientific knowledge, and to adapt to the conditions of war. Significant among these were the works of M.N. Oxford, a former sister of Guy's Hospital,[59] and Minnie Goodnow, an American nurse, whose textbook was circulated in Britain as well as the USA.[60] The most detailed and comprehensive text was, however, *A Textbook of War Nursing*, authored by London Hospital-trained nurse, Violetta Thurstan.[61] This text contains not only information on the latest treatments for shock and wound sepsis – along with how to implement these – but also advice on how to set up a camp hospital, and how to survive the physical and emotional stresses of war.

Thurstan had spent over two years as County Superintendent of the West Riding District Nursing Association before accepting a position at the new civil hospital in Spezia, Italy in 1913. She was "a strong believer in the need for higher education of nurses, and with other educationalists, a warm supporter of State Registration of Trained Nurses".[62] On the outbreak of war she had led one of the first nursing units to enter Belgium. After being overtaken by the advancing German forces and deported to Denmark, Thurstan had travelled to Russia via Sweden and Finland, to offer her services to the Russian Red Cross.[63] Invalided home with a shrapnel wound and pneumonia, Thurstan had returned to active service at L'Hôpital de L'Océan, La Panne, Belgium after a period of convalescence. Her decision to distil her remarkable knowledge and experience into a textbook resulted in one of the most comprehensive books on war nursing produced during the twentieth century.

One of Thurstan's achievements was to make medico-scientific knowledge relevant to nursing assessment and nursing practice. For example, she advised that, when assessing a patient with wound shock, the nurse should firstly examine his physical condition – skin colour, pulse and respirations – to gain an insight into his physiological state. She then, however, took the assessment further, advising the nurse to understand the person as an individual with a particular age, experience and background: "An inexperienced boy going into battle for the first time, overtired, too excited probably to eat beforehand, deafened by the thunder of heavy guns, terrified by the sights and sounds all round him, his friends perhaps killed at his side, will suffer more from shock with a comparatively small wound than will his more severely wounded comrade who is older and more seasoned".[64]

Nurse-writers such as Thurstan saw it as part of their role to give their fellow nurses a clear insight into the knowledge bases in which their practice was grounded. Not only would this make them safer, more enlightened practitioners, but it would elevate their practice above that of a mere cipher following doctors' orders. This meant that Thurstan, like other nurse-writers, engaged with the prevailing medical controversies of the day.

Nursing knowledge and medical controversy

Since the mid-nineteenth century the professions of nursing and medicine had existed side by side. Medicine had acquired a professional register in Britain in 1858. Nursing, because of its female gendered status, and because its "reform movement" and professionalization had begun later, was by far the weaker of the two.[65] Its relationship with medicine had, at times, been an invidious one. In the first issue of the *BJN* in 1902, Ethel Bedford Fenwick had expressed her wish that the medical profession should "afford to the associated profession of nursing its intelligent moral support – a totally different thing from intolerant personal control".[66] This sense in which nursing had to confront the assumption that it was inferior to medicine had an important influence on the way in which nurse-writers engaged with medical controversy.

As indicated earlier, one of the most controversial areas of medical treatment during the early months of the First World War was the treatment of infected wounds. Drawing on their experience of dealing with clean gunshot wounds during the Second Boer War (1899–1902), surgeons began by advocating conservative treatment: the application of a sterile dressing, which was not removed for several days. Within a few months, it became clear that wounds contracted by heavy artillery fire on the muddy, heavily manured fields of Northern France and Flanders were very different from those encountered on the dry, dusty veldt of South Africa. Bacteriological investigation showed that soil samples from these areas contained large numbers of anaerobic bacteria, causing a range of infectious diseases, among which the most serious were gas gangrene and tetanus. One influential school of thought, led by experts such as William Watson

Cheyne and Sir Anthony Bowlby, advocated the rigorous use of antiseptics. Others continued to advocate the conservative treatment. During the later months of 1914, and throughout 1915, controversy persisted as new treatments were tried by different surgeons. Nurses, in implementing surgical treatments, found themselves a part of this trial-and-error process.

Among the most significant of the prevailing treatments was the excision of massive areas of damaged tissue, recommended by H. M. W. Gray,[67] and the use of hypertonic saline solution, advocated by Sir Almroth Wright.[68] In 1915, the Carrel–Dakin treatment was developed as a result of a partnership between two individuals working in a field hospital in Compiegne supported by the Rockefeller Institute. The British scientist Henry Dakin had discovered that sodium hypochlorite had powerful antiseptic properties, while Frenchman Dr Alexis Carrel invented an ingenious means of delivering this solution so that it continuously flowed through and soaked the tissues of deep penetrating wounds.[69] This innovation offered surgeons yet another option in what was, by now, a complex repertoire of treatments. The ways in which nursing journals and textbooks reported on these methods offer an intriguing insight into the nursing perspective on medical treatment choices, and cast further light on episodes such as the one quoted from the paper by Sir W. Watson Cheyne earlier in this chapter.

A columnist in the *BJN* commented in April 1915 on the work of Drs Carrel and Dakin in Compiegne,[70] and was reporting, in August 1915, that both French and British medical scientists were positive about the use of the Carrel–Dakin technique and that "arrangements [were being] made at the Leeds University for preparing the antiseptic in considerable quantity for use in the military hospitals in this country [Britain]".[71]

The Carrel-Dakin system of treatment soon came to be adopted in a number of casualty clearing stations, hospital trains and base hospitals both on the Western Front and in Britain.[72] The technique was described by Violetta Thurstan in her *A Text Book of War Nursing* as an ingenious solution to the problem of deep, infected wounds. She described how the treatment began with a thorough washing of the wound, followed by its surgical cutting and trimming, to ensure good drainage. Nerves and tendons were sutured, and then the Carrel tubes were put into position and the wound was "irrigated under pressure every two hours".[73] A bottle of Dakin solution was hung by the patient's bedside and valves in the rubber portions of the Carrel tubes were opened, allowing gravity to push the solution into and through the wound cavity. There are numerous examples in the personal writings of nurses to show that the Carrel–Dakin treatment was extensively used on the Western Front, and that British nurses were very experienced in implementing it.[74]

The *BJN* continued to publish articles on the Carrel–Dakin technique throughout the war. One published in March 1917 reproduced verbatim a lecture presented by Dr Depage at the Hôpital de l'Océan, La Panne, Belgium, where Violetta Thurstan was matron.[75] Another *BJN* article reproduced an excerpt from an article in the *British Medical Journal*, offering advice to those implementing the treatment.[76] In December 1917, the journal's prize essay question, "What do you know of the Carrel–Dakin treatment of septic wounds?", yielded the view from winner Margaret Cornock that the treatment "is a thoroughly effective method of dealing with septic wounds, and has proved of enormous value in saving the lives of numbers of soldiers".[77] This comment offers persuasive evidence that Cornock was a practising nurse who was, herself, implementing the treatment. The use of the Carrel–Dakin treatment can be seen as one of the foci for the *BJN's* attention to medical science throughout the war years, demonstrating the journal's emphasis on scientific knowledge transmission.

By 1917, the army medical and nursing services had learned much from their three years' experience of dealing with devastating wound infections such as gas gangrene and tetanus. Thurstan distilled this knowledge into a clear and precise chapter in her *Text Book of War Nursing*, observing that "the treatment of wounds has been revolutionised since the beginning of the war". She commented on the two schools of thought that had existed at the outset of war, one which held that wounds should be left undisturbed, while the general constitution was strengthened by good nutrition and rest; the other – the "more radical school" – believing in "tremendous incisions, horizontal and transverse, making the drainage from the wound as free as possible, so that the toxins or poisons formed by the bacteria might not be absorbed into the system".[78]

By 1917, alongside the use of a range of antiseptics, three other approaches were in use on various war fronts, depending on the preference of certain highly assertive surgeons. First, there was the "plan of no dressings", in which a "loose but ample sterile dressing is put on the wound, the part well mobilised and the whole left severely alone".[79] Second was Sir Almroth Wright's method of "hypertonic saline treatment", still used in a number of British hospitals. Third was "the dry method", which was extensively used on the Eastern Front, where patients might have a long journey following initial treatment at the Front before reaching a base hospital. In this approach, the skin around the wound was cleansed with benzene or alcohol, the wound was painted with iodine, and then the whole was covered with a dry dressing and a large quantity of wool or sphagnum moss and a firm bandage.[80] It is possible to trace the introduction of the treatments referred to by Thurstan through the pages of the *BJN*,[81] suggesting that there is a strong degree of consistency between Thurstan's descriptions and the treatments offered in the journal.

Thurstan offered an intriguing insight into the nurse's position *vis-à-vis* the use of a range of very different treatments. Her first observation was that trained nursing sisters were well aware that the treatment applied often depended heavily on the opinion of the individual surgeon. She added, significantly, that as trained professionals, nurses would have their own opinions on the benefits and disadvantages of particular treatments:

> It is probably unnecessary to remind any trained nurse that she is there to carry out treatment, not to suggest it; very few sisters would openly criticise any treatment offered by the surgeon, but there are some people who *look* their disapproval of methods to which they are not accustomed . . . Loyalty is the first of virtues, and sisters should be very careful never to give the impression that they disagree with the surgeon for whom they are working. The soldier is one of the quickest people in the world to discover any want of harmony, and certainly the feeling that the best possible is not being done for him would

react on his mental condition, retard his recovery and make him anxious and suspicious.[82]

(emphasis in original)

Thurstan's astringent comments illustrate both the acumen of the nurse and her role in medical treatment. The power structure of the British hospital is accepted – and seen as being even more significant in a military environment. Loyalty is the primary virtue. And yet Thurstan's arguments are highly ambiguous. Although overtly asserting the pre-eminence of the doctor in decision-making, she expresses numerous views, hints and opinions that seem to imply that she believes the nurse herself carries a full armoury of judgements, which she may sometimes feel obliged to suppress. In October 1917, the *BJN* published a glowing review of the book, referring to it as "the first [book] which provides the trained nurse on war service with a professional text book dealing with the special branch in which she is engaged, which has developed so much during the present war".[83]

The *BJN*'s strong endorsement of *A Text Book of War Nursing* probably had much to do with the way in which the book emphasized the need for practising nurses to thoroughly understand the scientific principles behind their work. It is interesting that Thurstan also authored articles in the *BJN* that strongly endorsed nurse registration, thus aligning herself with *BJN* editor, Ethel Bedford Fenwick.[84]

Conclusion

This chapter has reviewed some of the material presented during the First World War in *The British Journal of Nursing*. Alongside these materials, it has also considered what is probably the most significant and comprehensive contemporary text on wartime nursing practice: Violetta Thurstan's *A Text Book of War Nursing*. I argue that, while these writings demonstrate deference to medical authority, they also contain a powerful implicit message about the need for the nurse to base her practice on a clear under-standing of science. Hence, the argument is made that nursing knowledge is scientific knowledge.

Medical innovation in the early twentieth century was highly dependent on the individualistic "trial-and-error" efforts of physicians and surgeons. Both *A Text Book of War Nursing* and articles in the *BJN* emphasize the need for both intelligent practice and loyalty to the surgeon. Professional nurses had been taught during their training to offer "intelligent obedience" to the doctor's orders. This concept is an interesting one. Such obedience was a complex phenomenon. One of the most powerful illustrations of this can be found in the way in which controversies between different medical theories were presented in detail in the nursing press. Nurses did not want to simply offer their surgeon-colleagues blind obedience. Rather, they wished to understand thoroughly any treatment they were consenting to carry out. Nursing journals did not, therefore, shy away from reporting on medical controversy. They did so in neutral or overtly positive tones; yet their willingness to engage with medical innovation was part of their own presentation of nursing knowledge as scientific knowledge, as well as an indicator that nurses' perception of their role went well beyond blind obedience to medical authority.

The professional writings of nurses speak eloquently of the intricacy and attention to detail with which their work was infused, and this chapter has interpreted these writings in terms of an emergent understanding of the science behind nursing work. A man with an injury was, for example, much more than a wound to be dressed. Close attention to providing cleanliness, rest and a "strengthening" diet that would enable tissue repair was an essential part of his regime and was recognized by both nurse-authors and medical writers in the *BJN* as "intelligent nursing".

Nurses saw themselves as the guardians of their patients' wellbeing rather than just the executors of doctors' orders. The ways in which a small group of nurses were working to present scientific knowledge are particularly well illustrated by the ways in which they engaged with the treatment controversies of the First World War. Those controversies came at a time when nurses were not only grappling with the horrors of industrial warfare, but also consciously engaging in their own struggle for recognition, by campaigning for a professional register – a campaign that achieved its goal on December 23 1919, with the passing into law of the Nurses Registration Act. Nurses' writings at this time illuminate not only their conscientious attention to the needs of their patients, but also their drive for professional recognition and their confident assertion of the scientific basis of their knowledge.

Notes

1 Quotation taken from the first issue, in July 1902, of *The British Journal of Nursing in which is incorporated The Nursing Record,* vol. XXIX, no. 744, 5 July, p. 3 (previously published as *The Nursing Record* from 1888 onwards).

2 C. Maggs, 1983, *The Origins of General Nursing,* Croom Helm, London; C. Davies, 1995, *Gender and the Professional Predicament in Nursing,* Open University Press, Buckingham; A.M. Rafferty, 1996, *The Politics of Nursing Knowledge,* Routledge, London.

3 C. Hallett, 2009, *Containing Trauma: Nursing Work in the First World War,* Manchester University Press, Manchester; K. Harris, 2011, *More than Bombs and Bandages,* ABC Press, Sydney; K. Harris, 2006, "Not Just 'Routine Nursing': The Roles and Skills of the Australian Army Nursing Service during World War I", unpublished PhD thesis, University of Melbourne.

4 Born Ethel Gordon Manson, Ethel Bedford Fenwick frequently used the name "Mrs Bedford Fenwick" following her marriage to the surgeon, Dr Bedford Fenwick. For ease and clarity, she will be referred to in this chapter by her married surname: "Fenwick". See W. Hector, 1973, *The Work of Mrs Bedford Fenwick and the Rise of Professional Nursing,* Royal College of Nursing, London.

5 V. Thurstan, 1917, *A Text Book of War Nursing,* G.P. Putnam's Sons, London. For examples of reviews in the *BJN* see: Anonymous, 1917, *British Journal of Nursing,* vol. 59, 15 September, pp. 468–493; Anonymous, 1917, "A Professional Review of 'A Text Book of War Nursing'", *British Journal of Nursing,* Vol. 60, 13 October, p. 244.

6 The first journal devoted to nursing issues was *Nursing Notes,* founded by Rosalind Paget in 1887, but this journal came to represent the interests of midwives rather than those of nurses. The *Nurses' Journal* was founded in 1891 to represent the interests of the British Nurses' Association. See L. Brake and M. Demoor, 2009, *Dictionary of Nineteenth-Century Journalism,* Academic Press and the British Library, London. Because of their limited influence, these journals are not discussed in this chapter.

7 B. Abel-Smith, 1960, *A History of the Nursing Profession*, Heinemann, London.

8 A.M. Rafferty, 1996, *The Politics of Nursing Knowledge*, Routledge, London.

9 S. McGann, 1992, *The Battle of the Nurses: A Study of Eight Women Who Influenced the Development of Professional Nursing, 1880–1930*, Scutari Press, London.

10 C. Helmstadter, 2007, "Florence Nightingale's Opposition to the State Registration of Nurses", *Nursing History Review*, vol. 15, pp. 155–165.

11 A. Young, 2008, "Entirely a Woman's Question? Class, Gender and the Victorian Nurse", *Journal of Victorian Culture*, vol. 13, no. 1, pp. 18–41.

12 A. Summers, 2000, *Angels and Citizens: British Women as Military Nurses, 1854–1914*, rev. edn, Threshold Press, Newbury.

13 C. Maggs, 1983, *The Origins of General Nursing*, Croom Helm, London; S. Hawkins, 2010, *Nursing and Women's Labour in the Nineteenth Century: The Quest for Independence*, Routledge, London; S. Hawkins, 2010, "From Maid to Matron: Nursing as a Route to Social Advancement in Nineteenth-century England", *Women's History Review*, vol. 19, no. 1, pp. 125–143.

14 W. Hector, 1973, *The Work of Mrs Bedford Fenwick and the Rise of Professional Nursing*, Royal College of Nursing, London; R. Dingwall, A.M. Rafferty and C. Webster, 1988, *An Introduction to the Social History of Nursing*, Routledge, London; M. Baly, 1995, *Nursing and Social Change*, 3rd edn, Routledge, London.

15 E.R.D. Bendall and E. Raybould, 1969, *A History of the General Nursing Council for England and Wales, 1919–1969*, H.K. Lewis and Co., London.

16 A.M. Rafferty, 1996, *The Politics of Nursing Knowledge*, Routledge, London, pp. 69–73.

17 M. Burr, 1908, "The British Journal of Nursing and the British Nursing Press", *American Journal of Nursing*, vol. 8, no. 5, pp. 372–376. See also K. Waddington, 2000, *Charity and the London Hospitals, 1850–1898*, Royal Historical Society, Boydell Press, Rochester, NY.

18 Select Committee of the House of Commons, 1905, *Report on the State Registration of Nurses*, Her Majesty's Stationery Office, London.

19 M. Burr, 1908, "The British Journal of Nursing and the British Nursing Press", pp. 373–375.

20 L. Brake and M. Demoor, 2009, *Dictionary of Nineteenth-Century Journalism*, Academic Press and the British Library, London, p. 463.

21 S. McGann, A. Crowther and R. Dougall, 2009, *A History of the Royal College of Nursing, 1916–90*, Manchester University Press, Manchester, p. 44.

22 L. Brake and M. Demoor, 2009, *Dictionary of Nineteenth-Century Journalism*, p. 464.

23 M. Burr, 1908, "The British Journal of Nursing and the British Nursing Press", p. 372.

24 M. Ferro, 1973, *The Great War*, Routledge, London; E. Leed, 1979, *No Man's Land: Combat and Identity in World War I*, Cambridge University Press, New York; M. Eckstein, 1989, *Rites of Spring: The Great War and the Birth of the Modern Age*, Houghton Mifflin, Boston; D. Pick, 1993, *War Machine: The Rationalisation of Slaughter in the Modern Age*, Yale University Press, New Haven; N. Ferguson, 1998, *The Pity of War*, Allen Lane, London.

25 A. Bradshaw, 2001, *The Nurse Apprentice, 1860–1977*, Ashgate, Aldershot.

26 Susan McGann and her colleagues have argued that *The Nursing Mirror* remained the journal with the largest readership throughout the war, with, in 1919 a circulation figure of 31,000: S. McGann, A. Crowther and R. Dougall, 2009, *A History of the Royal College of Nursing, 1916–90*, p. 81 fn. 10.

27 C. Hallett, 2009, *Containing Trauma: Nursing Work in the First World War*.

28 R. Cooter, M. Harrison and S. Sturdy, 1999, *Medicine and Modern Warfare*, Rodopi, Amsterdam; J. Lane, 2001, *A Social History of Medicine: Health, Healing and Disease in England, 1750–1950*, Routledge, London; M. Harrison, 2004, *Disease and the Modern World, 1500 to the Present Day*, Polity Press, Cambridge; M. Harrison, 2010, *The Medical War: British Military Medicine in the First World War*, Oxford University Press, Oxford.

29 M. Harrison, 2010, *The Medical War: British Military Medicine in the First World War*.

30 K. Pelis, 2001, "Taking Credit: The Canadian Army Medical Corps and the British Conversion to Blood Transfusion in World War I", *Journal of the History of Medicine and Allied Sciences*, vol. 56, pp. 238–277.

31 D. Simpson, 2005, "Brain wounds in the First World War: Lessons from the Steel Thunderstorms", *War and Society*, vol. 23, pp. 53–57; S. Callister, 2007, "Broken Gargyoles: The Photographic Representation of Severely Wounded New Zealand Soldiers", *Social History of Medicine*, vol. 20, no. 1, pp. 111–130; P. Selcer, 2008, "Standardizing Wounds: Alexis Carrel and the Scientific Management of Life in the First World War", *British Journal of the History of Science*, vol. 41, no. 1, pp. 73–107.

32 D. Linton, 2000, "Was Typhoid Inoculation Safe and Efficient during World War I? Debates within German Military Medicine", *Journal of the History of Medicine and Allied Sciences*, vol. 55, no. 2, pp. 101–133.

33 D. Linton, 2000, "The Obscure Object of Knowledge: German Military Medicine Confronts Gas Gangrene during World War I", *Bulletin of the History of Medicine*, vol. 74, no. 2, pp. 291–316; J. Reznick, 2004, *Healing the Nation: Soldiers and the Culture of Caregiving in Britain during the Great War*, Manchester, Manchester University Press; B. Linker, 2011, *War's Waste: Rehabilitation in World War I America*, University of Chicago Press, Chicago.

34 J.E. Talbott, 1997, "Soldiers, Psychiatrists and Combat Trauma", *Journal of Interdisciplinary History*, vol. 27, no. 3, p. 347; A. Young, 1999, "W.H. Rivers and the War Neuroses", *Journal of the History of Behavioural Sciences*, vol. 35, no. 4, pp. 359–378; B. Shephard, 2002, *A War of Nerves: Soldiers and Psychiatrists, 1914–1994*, Pimlico, London; E. Jones and S. Wessley, 2005, *Shell Shock to PTSD: Military Psychiatry from 1900 to the Gulf War*, Psychology Press, Hove.

35 J. Piggott, 1975, *Queen Alexandra's Royal Army Nursing Corps*, Leo Cooper, London; J. Bassett, 1992, *Guns and Brooches: Australian Army Nursing from the Boer War to the Gulf War*, Oxford University Press, Melbourne; G. Allard, 2005, "Caregiving at the Front: The Experience of Canadian Military Nurses During World War I", in C. Bates, D. Dodd and N. Rousseau (eds) *On All Frontiers: Four Centuries of Canadian Nursing*, Ottawa University Press, Ottawa.

36 C. Hallett, 2009, *Containing Trauma: Nursing Work in the First World War*; K. Harris, *More than Bombs and Bandages*; K. Harris, 2006, 'Not Just "Routine Nursing": The Roles and Skills of the Australian Army Nursing Service during World War I'.

37 Anaerobic wound infections were caused by bacteria that thrived in conditions where oxygen was absent. The most serious were gas gangrene, caused by a range of bacteria, and tetanus, caused by *Clostridium tetani*. See M. Harrison, 2010, *The Medical War: British Military Medicine in the First World War*.

38 G.H. Makins, 1914, "A Note upon the Wounds of the Present Campaign", *The Lancet*, vol. II, 10 October, pp. 905–907; G.H. Makins, 1914, "Note on the Wounds Observed during Three Weeks' Fighting in Flanders", *The Lancet*, vol. II, 21 November, pp. 1210–1212; J. Swan, I. Jones and J.W. McNee, "The Occurrence of Acute Emphysematous Gangrene (Malignant Oedema) in Wounds Received in the War", *The Lancet*, vol. II, 14 November, pp.1161–1162; Sir W. Watson Cheyne, 1914, "An Address on the Treatment of Wounds in War", *The Lancet*, vol. II, 21 November, pp. 1185–1194; Sir A. Bowlby, 1914, "The Treatment of Wounds in War", *The Lancet*, vol. II, 19 December, pp. 1427–1430.

39 Anonymous, 1914, "Gangrene" (notes from a lecture of Mr Max Page), *Nursing Times*, vol. X, 5 September, p. 1111; Anonymous, 1914, "Medical Matters in France", *British Journal of Nursing*, 24 October, p. 318; Anonymous, 1914, "The Nurse's Clinic. Tetanus", *Nursing Mirror and Midwives Journal*, vol. XX, no. 501, 31 October, p. 71; Anonymous, 1915, "Gunshot Wounds", *The Nursing Times*, vol. XI, no. 50, 2 January, p. 15.

40 Sir A. Bowlby and Sir J.S. Rowlands, 1914, "Report on Gas Gangrene", reproduced in *The Lancet*, vol. II, 28 November, pp. 1265–1266.

41 Sir A. Bowlby and Sir J.S. Rowlands, 1914, "Gas Gangrene" [directly quoting "Report on Gas Gangrene"], *British Journal of Nursing*, vol. 53, 5 December, pp. 442–444.

42 Anonymous, 1914, "Letters from the Front: France", *British Journal of Nursing*, vol. 53, 3 October, p. 265; Anonymous, 1914, "Letters from the Front: Belgium", *British Journal of Nursing*, vol. 53, 10 October, p. 286; Anonymous, "Indignant", *British Journal of Nursing*, vol. 55, 13 November, p. 410; Anonymous, 1916, "Nursing a Dead Art: TFN Sister", *British Journal of Nursing*, vol. 56, 11 March, p. 238.

43 Anonymous, 1916, "Mere Merchandise: One Who Has No Right to Communicate With the Press", *British Journal of Nursing*, vol. 57, 7 October, p. 301.

44 C. Hallett, 2009, *Containing Trauma: Nursing Work in the First World War*, p. 54.

45 Sir W. Watson Cheyne, 1914, "The Treatment of Wounds in War" (citing the words of Sir W. Watson Cheyne), *British Journal of Nursing*, vol. 53, 28 November, pp. 419–420.

46 See, for example: A. Knyvett Gordon, 1903, "Some Aspects of the Nursing of Infectious Diseases", *British Journal of Nursing*, 4 July, p. 5; A. Knyvett Gordon, 1906, "A Short Series of Lectures to Ward Sisters: Lecture 8 – Diphtheria", *British Journal of Nursing*, 15 September, p. 203; A. Knyvett Gordon, 1919, "The Examination of the Blood", *British Journal of Nursing*, 26 April, p. 272.

47 A. Knyvett Gordon, 1914, "Some Thoughts on the War (continued)", *British Journal of Nursing*, vol. 53, 29 August, pp. 171–172.

48 A. Knyvett Gordon, 1914, "Some Thoughts on the War (continued)", p. 172.

49 A. Knyvett Gordon, 1914, "Some Thoughts on the War (continued)", p. 171.

50 C. Hallett, 2009, *Containing Trauma: Nursing Work in the First World War*, pp. 28–35.

51 C.P. Armitage, 1914, "What Do You Mean by Shock and What Can You Do to Combat It?", *British Journal of Nursing*, vol. 53, 12 September, p. 202.

52 A. Knyvett Gordon, 1914, "Some Thoughts on the War (continued)", p. 172.

53 C.P. Armitage, 1914, "What Do You Mean by Shock and What Can You Do to Combat It?", p. 202.

54 A. Phipps, 1914, "What Do You Mean by Shock and What Can You Do to Combat It?", *British Journal of Nursing*, vol. 53, 12 September, p. 203.

55 G. Tatham, 1914, "What Precautions may be Adopted to Minimize the Danger to the Patient . . ." *British Journal of Nursing*, vol. 53, 5 September, p. 186.

56 E. Luckes, 1914, *General Nursing*, new and revised (9th) edn, Kegan Paul, Trench, Trubner and Co., London.

57 I. Stewart and H.C. Cuff, 1899–1903, *Practical Nursing*, 4 Volumes, William Blackwood, Edinburgh.

58 E. Stoney, 1900, *Bacteriology and Surgical Technique for Nurses*, W.B. Saunders and Company, London.

59 M.N. Oxford, 1914, *Nursing in War Time: Lessons for the Inexperienced*, Methuen and Co., London.

60 M. Goodnow, 1917, *War Nursing*, W.B. Saunders, Philadelphia.

61 V. Thurstan, 1917, *A Text Book of War Nursing*, G.P. Putnam's Sons, London.

62 Anonymous, 1913, "Nurses of Note: Miss Violetta Thurstan", *British Journal of Nursing*, vol. 50, 15 February, p. 130

63 V. Thurstan, 1915, *Field Hospital and Flying Column: Being the Journal of an English Nursing Sister*, G.P. Putnam's Sons, London.

64 V. Thurstan, 1917, *A Text Book of War Nursing*, p. 137.

65 E. Gamarnikow, 1991, "Nurse or Woman: Gender and Professionalism in Reformed Nursing, 1860–1923", in P. Holden and J. Littlewood, *Nursing and Anthropology*, Routledge, London; C. Davies, 1995, *Gender and the Professional Predicament in Nursing*, Open University Press, Buckingham.

66 Anonymous, 1902, "Editorial. The 'British Journal of Nursing'", *British Journal of Nursing in which is incorporated The Nursing Record*, vol. XXIX, no. 744, p. 1.

67 M. Harrison, 2010, *The Medical War: British Military Medicine in the First World War.*

68 Sir Almroth Wright, 1915, "An Address on Wound Infection: And on Some New Methods for the Study of the Various Factors which come into Consideration in their Treatment", *British Medical Journal*, 24 April, pp. 720–723.

69 C. Hallett, 2009, *Containing Trauma: Nursing Work in the First World War*, pp. 56–58; M. Harrison, 2010, *The Medical War: British Military Medicine in the First World War*, p. 31.

70 Anonymous, 1915, "The Care of the Wounded", *British Journal of Nursing*, vol. 54, 24 April, p. 342.

71 Anonymous, 1915, "A New Antiseptic", *British Journal of Nursing*, vol. 55, 14 August, p. 126.

72 C. Hallett, 2009, *Containing Trauma: Nursing Work in the First World War*, pp. 56–58.

73 V. Thurstan, 1917, *A Text Book of War Nursing*, pp. 118–119.

74 Miss Bickmore, MS essay about life on an ambulance train in France; 3814, 85/51/1; Imperial War Museum, London, UK; Anonymous, 1915, *Diary of a Nursing Sister on the Western Front, 1914–1915*, Blackwood and Sons, Edinburgh; K.E. Luard, 1930, *Unknown Warriors: Extracts from the Letters of K.E. Luard, RRC, Nursing Sister in France, 1914–1918*, Chatto and Windus, London.

75 Anonymous, 1917, "Nursing and the War", *British Journal of Nursing*, vol. 59, 14 July, p. 21; Anonymous, 1917, "Notes on 'Carrel' Treatment", *British Journal of Nursing*, vol. 58, 31 March, p. 219.

76 Anonymous, 1918, "The Technique of the Carrel–Dakin Treatment", *British Journal of Nursing*, vol. 60, 23 February, pp. 127–128.

77 M. Cornock, 1917, "What Do You Know of the Carrel–Dakin Treatment of Septic Wounds? Describe the Method of its Application", *British Journal of Nursing*, vol. 59, 1 December, p. 348.

78 V. Thurstan, 1917, *A Text Book of War Nursing*, p. 110.

79 Ibid., p. 112.

80 Ibid., p. 114.

81 Anonymous, 1916, "The Treatment of Infected Wounds by Physiological Methods", *British Journal of Nursing*, vol. 56, 24 June, p. 538; Anonymous, 1915, "Shell Wounds", *British Journal of Nursing*, vol. 54, 16 January, p. 42; Anonymous, 1916, "On the Salt Pack Treatment of Infected Gunshot Wounds", *British Journal of Nursing*, vol. 57, 2 September, p. 187.

82 V. Thurstan, 1917, *A Text Book of War Nursing*, pp. 114–115.

83 Anonymous, 1917, "Professional Review: A Text-Book of War Nursing", *British Journal of Nursing*, vol. 59, 13 October, p. 244; Anonymous, 1917, "Professional Review: A Text-Book of War Nursing (continued)", *British Journal of Nursing*, vol. 59, 20 October, pp. 260–261.

84 V. Thurstan, 1916, "A B C of State Registration", *British Journal of Nursing*, vol. 56, 6 May, p. 404; Anonymous, 1916, "National Union of Trained Nurses", *British Journal of Nursing*, vol. 56, 17 June, p. 525.

7

ENGENDERING HEALTH

Pronatalist politics and the history of nursing and midwifery in colonial Senegal, 1914–1967

Jonathan Cole

Quand nous amenons un garçon à l'école française, c'est une unité que nous gagnons; quand nous y amenons une fille, c'est une unité multiplié par le nombre d'enfants qu'elle aura.

(*George Hardy,* Une Conquête Morale, *1917*)

In 1964, four years after Senegal's independence, Madame Cissé Lary Seye, a Senegalese *infirmière d'état* and *sage-femme d'état,* relocated from the capital Dakar to the remote eastern town of Bakel. Madame Cissé Lary Seye had begun her education at primary school, continued at secondary school, and received her professional training at nursing school. Assigned to this post with her husband and two children, she and her husband were placed in charge of running the local health post. According to Seye, at the time of her relocation, there was no maternity staff except for the local *matrone* (traditional midwife), who performed almost all the deliveries and care. Without a proper staff or provisions, Seye had to rebuild the maternity[1] from the ground up. She recalled the strain this had placed on her relationship with the *matrone,* who had run the maternity for many years. It was the arrival of Madame Cissé Lary Seye – a women with a Western education and medical training – that disrupted the operation of the maternity by the *matrone,* whose authority, in contrast, rested on her own life experiences as a mother, grandmother and midwife. In the end, the *matrone* would not compromise and Seye sought permission to train several young local girls to serve as her assistants in the maternity.[2]

Madame Cissé Lary Seye's retelling of this story, with both disappointment and pride, reflected the impact of colonial health policy on women's education and professional opportunities. Rather than focus on curing disease, the French administration of Senegal redirected its efforts towards preventive care, particularly concerns over hygiene and health education. As we shall see, this shift reflected the colonial desire to impose a particular vision of health as a tool to control bodies and minds. However, Seye's story reveals the ways that the hegemony of Western medicine in Senegal was only partially achieved. Maternal and infant health policies seized upon the social and biological roles of women as a tool for producing a healthy work force. But through its focus on women, colonial health policy subverted women's traditional roles as wives and mothers while empowering them with new opportunities to define themselves as professionals.

This chapter examines how and why colonial health policies that aimed at remaking the African family in Senegal, and in particular at changing African child-rearing and birthing practices, provided a crucial impetus for the expansion of female education and marked the point of entry for women into medicine in the 1920s and 1930s as nurses and midwives. African women were to play an instrumental role in the French colonial civilizing mission. This role was directly related to their reproductive capacity, in a physical sense, but it extended farther than that. African women would be bearers of a new social and cultural order; they were to be the second front to colonial conquest, "a moral conquest," intended to capture the hearts and minds of the indigenous population. While at first this role was limited to the private sphere of the household, women's function within society as reproducers of the colonial social order gradually extended into the public sphere, transforming them first into good wives and mothers, and later into teachers, nurses, and midwives. To the degree that women embraced these pre-defined roles as a means of social and economic advancement, they also sought to exercise their own influence over their professional identities.

Colonial intermediaries and the construction of colonial rule

Female nurses and midwives were instrumental to the colonial-era health reforms aimed at promoting hygiene and preventive care, particularly around the issue of maternal and infant health. Indeed, in Senegal as in other parts of Africa, indigenous intermediaries – whether interpreters, soldiers, porters, nurses, or clerks – played a critical role in the expansion of empire and the day-to-day operations of colonial rule.[3] In the field of health this was particularly true, as the shortage of European personnel residing in the colonies forced colonial administrators to recruit and train indigenous actors as medical auxiliaries. Recent scholarship has only just begun to illuminate how these previously unknown "colonial middle figures" shaped the workings of the colonial state and left their imprint on the development of the health profession in Africa. John Iliffe, for example, traces the origins of the medical profession in East Africa back to a tiny group of nineteenth-century "pioneers" who received rudimentary medical training from local missionaries.[4] Iliffe goes on to chart these doctors' quest for professional recognition and autonomy, from the opening of the Makrere medical college in 1926, through the disintegration of the profession in the 1970s under Idi Amin, ending with an analysis of their role in combating the AIDS epidemic that ravaged East Africa in the late 1980s and early 1990s. While the context of British and German colonization provided the impetus for the emergence of the profession in East Africa, Iliffe demonstrates that the quest for professional recognition and autonomy was part of a broader, more complicated narrative.

As scholars have begun to pay closer attention to the individual attitudes and motivations of those who pursued careers in the health professions, they have called into question the tendency to read the actions of these African intermediaries and other colonial personnel simply in terms of collaboration with or resistance to colonial rule. Indeed, African health personnel were in some cases despised and in others envied for their close ties to the colonial state. Nevertheless, these health personnel were hardly passive agents of the colonial regime. In fact, professional grievances, such as unequal pay, lack of professional advancement, and political marginalization, often placed African health personnel at odds with the colonial administration. In the end, the deployment of indigenous medical intermediaries in the service of imperial interests came back to haunt colonial regimes, as health professionals rallied around such grievances and marshaled their professional networks and affiliations towards a broader goal: national independence.[5]

Accounts centered on these binaries of domination/resistance and colonized/colonizer obscure the fluidity and complexity of the colonial encounter.[6] As Shula Marks demonstrates in her study on the history of nursing in South Africa, the obstacles South African women faced in their efforts to transform nursing into a "respectable" and autonomous profession could not be explained in terms of tensions between "black" and "white," or even male and female. Rather, the "divided sisterhood" that characterized the development of the nursing profession in South Africa represented the complex articulation of notions of race, class, and gender over the course of this history.[7] As Marks so powerfully demonstrates, the history of the nursing profession in Africa provides a productive lens for understanding the complexities of the colonial encounter and its impact on the everyday lives of African actors, particularly women.

The connection between gender and work reveals how notions of domesticity were fluid and contested. In particular, the introduction of nurses and midwives challenged existing hierarchies of age and sex. As Elizabeth Schmidt points out, the emergence of Western-trained nurses and midwives, culled from the local population, had the effect of eroding the power of traditional female healers and midwives. Nevertheless, such positions also permitted women a newfound autonomy and independence *vis-à-vis* their male relations, i.e. their fathers, husbands, brothers, and uncles.[8] The imposition of colonial rule thus subverted gender roles by replacing and in some instances reinventing relations between the sexes.[9] Along these lines, both Nancy Rose Hunt and Pascale Barthélémy illustrate how the training and employment of female nurses and midwives subverted gender norms and in the process created both opportunities and constraints for women living under colonial rule.[10] This chapter likewise explores the intersection and entanglement of the domains of power held by traditional female healers and midwives and the new professional class of female nurses.

From household to hospital

As the foregoing discussion suggests, nurses and midwives played a critical role in the elaboration of colonial rule, and more particularly the expansion of the colonial health services. Focusing on the case of Senegal, the following sections illustrate how the history of nursing and midwifery care can inform the study of colonialism in Africa. As we see in the first section, critical shifts in policy in the wake of the First World War afforded African women unprecedented opportunities for professional advancement as midwives and nurses. Furthermore, these reforms also placed new emphasis on the importance of female education, both in terms of improving the quality and quantity of female recruits for the nursing school and in regard to promoting a preventive health agenda, particularly around the twin issues of maternal and infant health. However, as the second section will show, colonial efforts to expand girls' education encountered the resistance of local actors, particularly that of parents who feared the destabilizing effects of Western education and culture on family life. These attitudes demonstrate how concerns over girls' education were driven not so much by the politics of the colonial encounter as by the local dynamics of African society and culture. The last section considers how nurses and midwives juggled the competing interests of work, family life, and social identity in their personal and professional lives. Specifically it addresses how "domesticity" redefined female authority for these women professionals.

The professional trajectory of female nurses in Senegal reveals much about the social dynamics at play in Senegal during the nineteenth and twentieth centuries. By the 1930s, the feminization of nursing was already well under way in France, yet in France's West African colonies African women were only just beginning to enter the profession. The absence of female health personnel was a result of the peculiar nature of colonial rule. French wars of conquest of West Africa in the nineteenth century gave rise to the need for medical auxiliaries to assist army surgeons and doctors and to administer care to sick and wounded soldiers. As the ranks of the colonial military mostly comprised African recruits, so too did this early corps of medical assistants. Thus, men formed the core of both the nursing and the medical professions from an early stage. African women's entry into the profession in the wake of the First World War signaled not only a dramatic shift in the evolution of the nursing and medical professions but also a sea change in imperial policy.

The appearance of female midwives and nurses in the 1920s and 1930s was linked to major changes in French colonial health policy. Following the First World War, the priorities of *Assistance Medicale Indigène* (AMI) were redefined to favor preventive health measures. In turn, these reforms not only expanded the range of services offered but extended the scope of these services to include areas outside the reach of existing public health infrastructure. In particular, new emphasis was placed on maternal and infant health.

French concerns over maternal and infant health in the colonies drew inspiration from metropolitan preoccupations. In France as well as in England, declining birth rates coupled with high maternal and infant mortality were seen as a cause for alarm, particularly in the face of the enormous casualties sustained during the First World War.

Fears of racial degeneration, particularly in relation to other imperial powers, prompted calls for the strengthening of the imperial body politic and the elaboration of an ideology of imperial motherhood.[11] These concerns were translated into the colonial context by the application of metropolitan measures to the colonies as well as through the growing emigration of French women into the colonies, particularly in their professional capacities as teachers, nurses, and midwives.[12]

Pro-natalist policies transplanted from France dovetailed well with the political economy of colonial rule. As hostilities drew to a close in Europe, France looked back to the colonies afresh, with an eye to capitalizing on the huge swaths of land that it possessed, straddling the continent from Cap Vert to the Somali coast. Administrators believed in the tremendous potential of their African colonies; they needed only a sufficient labor force to exploit it. Albert Sarraut had expressed this vision more precisely in his elaboration of the notion of *faire du noir*, literally translated as "[re]making of the black." The goal was to augment the population of its African colonies, in quantity as well as in quality. In this way, Sarraut linked the *mise en valeur*, or economic exploitation of the colonies, to the longstanding humanitarian goals of the French civilizing mission.

By virtue of their reproductive capacities, women were the central focus of this new health policy. Annual reports and correspondence from French administrators provided a grim picture of health in the colonies, particularly the high rates of infant mortality. Umbilical tetanus, dysentery, pneumonia, malaria, and hereditary syphilis were the most important contributors to infant mortality. As reports from administrators noted, these conditions were traced back to the fault of the mother, whose ignorance or carelessness endangered her children's health. The key to reducing infant mortality, Governor-General Carde wrote in his circular to the lieutenant governors of *Afrique Occidentale Française* (AOF), was "the education of mothers and the progressive penetration of notions of childrearing into family life."[13]

Initially, European women were asked to spearhead the objectives of the *Protection Maternelle et Infantile* (PMI). Those who possessed formal training served as midwives and nurses in the hospitals and dispensaries of major cities such as Dakar and Saint-Louis. However, even those without formal training also played important roles. For example, administrators cited the important role played by the voluntary organization, Ladies of the Red Cross (*Dames de la Croix Rouge*), who operated a section for infant care three days each week at the *Polyclinique Roume* in Dakar, giving consultations for healthy infants, distributing condensed milk, soap, foodstuffs, and baby clothes to the mothers, and redirecting infants showing any signs of ill-health or malnutrition to the hospital or dispensary for follow-up care.[14] They also ran other charitable activities that concerned maternal and infant health, such as the *Gouttes de Lait* (Drops of Milk) and the *Berceau Africain* (African Cradle).

While reports highlighted the supportive role that the *Croix Rouge* and the *Gouttes de Lait* played in the fight against infant mortality, they also signaled the need to extend these services beyond the confines of the major health centers in cities such as Dakar and Saint Louis. However, the shortage of European personnel and the excessive physical demands of this work required the administration to recruit auxiliaries from the local population. Thus, African female medical personnel such as midwives, nurses, and social workers (*assistantes sociales*) would play an indispensable role spreading the "discourse of the microbe."

A key event in the formation of this corps of female medical auxiliaries was the creation of the medical school in Dakar (*Ecole de Médecine de Dakar*[15]) in 1918. The medical school was intended as a gesture of appreciation for the important sacrifices that the colonies made in support of the war – a symbol of France's investment in the health and well-being of its subjects.[16] More practically, though, the school was a response to the urgent need for trained health personnel in the colonies.

Prior to the First World War, the colonial administration of French West Africa made several fitful attempts at promoting the formation of a professional class of trained assistants. An early effort in this regard was the recruitment of male medical assistants called *aides-médecins*, who were given two years of basic instruction on issues of hygiene, prophylaxis, basic medicine (*médecine usuelle*), and minor surgery. Still, doctors complained that these assistants were "incapable of assimilating the most basic and essential notions of medicine."[17] In order to execute their functions more competently, the assistants required further instruction in the fields of biology, chemistry, and the natural sciences, not to mention more than rudimentary knowledge of French. In response to these complaints, a preparatory section for medical studies was held on the island of Gorée in October 1916, and it was from these first students that the medical school drew its first cohort of (male) medical students: the *médecins-africains*.

The first female students were admitted to the section for *sages-femmes*, or midwives, in 1918. To enter the program, these women needed to be eighteen to twenty years of age, and were required to hold a certificate of graduation from primary school and to pass a four-part entrance exam. In addition to these requirements, students had to submit a dossier that included a letter signaling their intentions to enter the medical school, a signed decennial agreement which stipulated that students would serve in the *Assistance Médicale Indigène* (AMI) for at least ten years, a birth certificate and clean bill of health signed by a doctor, a letter of good conduct from the director of their school of origin, and a letter from their parent or guardian endorsing their entry into school.[18]

In contrast to their male counterparts, who completed four years of study, midwives followed a three-year program. A special section for *infirmières-visiteuses* (visiting nurses) was added in 1930, which provided almost identical training but lasted only two years. After their first year of instruction, students could opt to complete the program in either nursing or midwifery. In both cases, the training provided to nurses and midwives reflected the overarching goals of the health services, particularly as they related to the issues of maternal and infant health.

Administrators stressed the practical as well as ideological importance of nurses and midwives to the colonial public health agenda. In the annual report for the health services of the colony of Senegal for 1936, the education of mothers and young women was put on par with curative measures. Citing the growing number of prenatal and postnatal consultations, officials insisted that the measures aimed at infant and maternal health not only would yield results, but also would provide good propaganda for the

AMI.[19] Midwives and nurses thus provided a critical point of contact between the colonial public health system and the indigenous population. The curriculum for nurses and midwives reflected their key roles as interlocutors for new ideas about health and hygiene, and more importantly as health educators.

The medical school in Dakar thus provided an important springboard for women's entry into the profession of nursing. As Figure 7.1 illustrates, the female students graduating from the medical school significantly outnumbered men. Though women remained a minority in the field of nursing, as demonstrated in Figure 7.2, the numbers reveal a slow but steady stream of entrants to the nursing profession. Nevertheless, many officials lamented both the quantity and the quality of female recruits to the medical school. At the heart of the matter was the issue of girls' education.

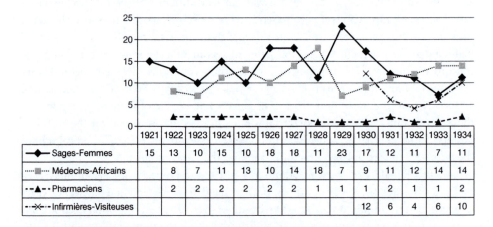

	1921	1922	1923	1924	1925	1926	1927	1928	1929	1930	1931	1932	1933	1934
Sages-Femmes	15	13	10	15	10	18	18	11	23	17	12	11	7	11
Médecins-Africains		8	7	11	13	10	14	18	7	9	11	12	14	14
Pharmaciens		2	2	2	2	2	2	1	1	1	2	1	1	2
Infirmières-Visiteuses										12	6	4	6	10

Figure 7.1 Number of graduates from the Dakar Medical School by section, 1921–1934.

Source: Gouvernement Général de l'Afrique Occidentale Française (1934), *L'Ecole de Médicine de L'Afrique Occidentale Française (de son fondation à l'année 1934).* Séries O: Enseignement de l'AOF 1895–1958, ANS O 161 (31). Dakar, Senegal: Archives Nationale du Sénégal.

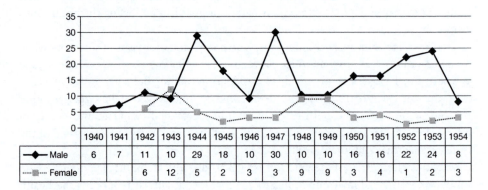

	1940	1941	1942	1943	1944	1945	1946	1947	1948	1949	1950	1951	1952	1953	1954
Male	6	7	11	10	29	18	10	30	10	10	16	16	22	24	8
Female			6	12	5	2	3	3	9	9	3	4	1	2	3

Figure 7.2 Number of male and female nurses accredited at the Hospitals of St Louis and Dakar, 1940–1954.

Source: M'Baye, E.M. (2002), *Etude d'une profession de santé: Les infirmiers au Sénégal de 1889 à 1968.* Mémoire de Maitresse. Dakar, Senegal: Université Cheikh Anta Diop de Dakar.

The state of girls' education in the colony of Senegal prior to the First World War reflected the initial ambivalence of the colonial state to the question of girls' education.[20] While the reorganization of the colonies in 1903 ushered in the development and expansion of government schools, the first few decades of the twentieth century marked a reversal in terms of women's access to education. By the time the Dakar Medical School opened in 1918, only one girl for every 45 boys was enrolled at primary school in French West Africa. Though girls fared better in Senegal, boys still outnumbered girls almost 10 to 1 at government schools, with 448 girls to 4368 boys in 1922. Sex ratios at missionary schools were more balanced, with 349 girls to 308 boys. Only 32 percent of the total female population of Senegal received any sort of primary education.[21]

These persistent inequalities in women's access to education not only compromised the quality of these female health professionals, but also threatened to undermine the long-term goals of reducing infant and maternal mortality and promoting higher standards of hygiene and public health. In order to bridge the gap between male and female students entering the medical school, the *Conseil Supérieure de l'Enseignement* headed by the Inspector General for Education, Albert Charton, proposed the addition of a two-year program to fill the gap between the time girls finished primary school and their entry into nursing school. In line with this recommendation, the administration created the *Ecole Normale de Jeunes Filles de Rufisque* in 1940. The instruction offered to young women at the Ecole Normale in Rufisque differed significantly from that given to their male colleagues at the *Ecole Normale William Ponty*. Specifically, the curriculum of girls' education emphasized women's domestic roles as wives and mothers through lessons in childrearing and homemaking. Thus instruction in French language, math, and science was coupled with the domestic sciences (*économie domestique* and *enseignement ménagère*), which emphasized skills such as sewing, cooking, and cleaning. The aim was to inculcate in these young women an appreciation of their dual role as female functionaries, the "social" as well as the "domestic."[22]

The opening of the *Ecole Normale de Jeunes Filles* solved a key concern over the quality of women's education. However, it did not address a key factor behind lagging rates of female enrollment: parental resistance. According to Papa Gueye Fall, Director of the *Ecole Urbaine de Dakar*, there were many reasons that parents refused to send their girls to the French schools. Above all, parents feared that the French schools would turn their girls into *"desmoiselles"* who were more interested in flirting than fulfilling their religious or household duties.[23] These concerns were echoed in Denise Savineau's report *La Famille en AOF: La condition de la femme*, which stated that Muslim parents often refused to send their girls to school for fear that they would convert to Catholicism, lose their virginity, or simply emancipate themselves.[24] Parents further worried that allowing their girls to pursue their education would endanger their daughters' chances of finding a husband.[25] For these reasons, many parents viewed girls' education as a threat to the social order.

The administration took these concerns seriously. To guard against the potential for impropriety, female students lived a cloistered life at the medical school. They received free room and board, and were subjected to close supervision and strict discipline by the *surveillantes*, whose job it was to protect as well as nurture the moral character of these female students. This not only served to assuage parents' fears of sexual deviance, but also protected the administration's investment in the education of these young female professionals.

Administrators also worked tirelessly to convince parents that the education their children received at the French schools not only would better prepare these young women for fulfilling the duties of the household, making them better wives and mothers, but also would provide opportunities for professional advancement. This potential for professional advancement was an important inducement for reluctant parents. As Mamadou Diouf, a former *infirmier d'état* (state-certified nurse) recounted, many Muslim parents began sending their children to French schools instead of Quranic schools because they worried that their children would not be able to compete in the job market against their Christian counterparts. Furthermore, facing the erosion of their rights as French citizens, parents in the four communes of Rufisque, Dakar, Saint-Louis and Gorée sent their children to French schools in order to meet the fluency requirement for establishing French citizenship.[26]

Women's professional transition from household to hospital, and ensuing debates about girls' education, thus reveal the complexities of life under colonial rule. In particular, attitudes to girls' education changed in relation to the reconstitution of colonial society. As Diane Barthel illustrates in her study of female professionals in Senegal, parents' educational backgrounds influenced attitudes to girls' education. Therefore, women whose parents worked as colonial functionaries enjoyed certain advantages in access to education compared to women whose parents were peasants. Nevertheless, the complexities of class position do not take account of the gendered dimensions of women's professional trajectories. As Barthel has argued, "the delicate balance of sex roles had been upset through colonialism's differential treatment of men and women."[27] The gains that women made in securing access to education and professional status were mitigated by a gendered appreciation of their labor. As we shall see in this final section, the struggle of female professionals to define themselves within a shifting cultural and social landscape elucidates how women confronted the challenges imposed on them by their own profession, but also by the social and cultural norms of their own society.

Prior to the administration's concerted efforts to recruit women into the medical field, women's place in the nursing profession was heavily circumscribed by a gendered appreciation of women's labor value. Those women who did gain entry into the profession, particularly in the period prior to the First World War, were often confined to the hospitals and dispensaries of important urban centers such as Dakar and Saint-Louis. In this capacity, they performed the domestic tasks such cooking, cleaning, and doing laundry. Women were seen as unfit for work in the "bush" where they would often be left alone and unsupervised, in a locale where they most likely did not know anyone and, in certain instances, did not speak the same language. As one retired state nurse (*infirmier d'état*) claimed, the task of running a rural health post was seen as too physically demanding for women.[28]

Even as women began to move on to higher levels of specialization and training, the gendered division of nursing labor persisted. For example, the male *infirmier-sanitaire* (sanitary nurse) and the female *infirmière-visiteuse* (visiting nurse) were intended to serve as key mobile health personnel, ideally suited to fulfill the preventive health agenda of the reorganized AMI.[29] Both were tasked with exerting their influence on African society, notably by educating the populace in matters of proper hygiene and care. Their training also overlapped in terms of identifying and treating diseases such as tuberculosis, syphilis, and leprosy and the collection of demographic data. Still, their respective functions as health auxiliaries, within the structures of health as well as in relation to the communities they served, reflected gendered assumptions about women's labor.

The divergences between the male *infirmier-sanitaire* and the female *infirmière-visiteuse*, in terms of both their duties and their training, revealed a spatial division of labor that constrained the sphere of female action. The female nurse's duties centered on the domestic sphere, specifically aiding and advising mothers during pregnancy and child-birth. They provided mothers with essential information about childcare, instructing them on how to feed, clothe, and care for their children. These tasks confined female nurses to the sphere of the household, and provided them a degree of authority over matters concerning the female domestic sphere. The male nurse's role, on the other hand, engaged him in the public sphere as an agent of hygiene giving practical advice to the general population on matters of propriety, sanitation, and general hygiene. It was hoped that he would become a trusted counselor to the village chiefs, helping to advise and oversee measures taken to promote public health such as the provision of potable water, the disposal of waste, and the destruction of parasites, insects, and vermin linked to diseases such as malaria, plague, and yellow fever. He was also authorized to apply any measures deemed necessary for the preservation of public health, whether following state decree or the instruction of his direct superior. The male nurse thus enjoyed significantly more power and authority than his female counterpart.[30]

The inferior status of female nurses was further evident in their place in the hierarchy of personnel. While both the male nurse and the female nurse answered to a command structure in which the European doctor reigned supreme, the men typically enjoyed a higher position than women in the medical hierarchy, reporting directly to the European doctor or to the *médecin-africain* (the medical assistant). This male-dominated hierarchy further placed female medical personnel, including midwives, below their male counterparts. The female nurses thus reported to the *sage-femme africaine* (the African midwife), the European *sage-femme coloniale* (the colonial midwife) if attached to the maternity, or else to their male superiors, the *médecin-africain* or the European doctor. The irony of this subordination was that while the profession may have opened new doors for women in terms of social advancement, financial autonomy, and professional authority, it came at the price of submitting to a different set of patriarchal norms. The exigencies of colonial rule thus shaped women's entry into the nursing profession in seemingly contradictory ways. While colonial interest in the promotion of maternal and infant health opened up new opportunities for women in terms of education and professional advancement, women simultaneously found their roles within the nursing profession circumscribed by their gender.

Despite the limitations placed on women's role as nurses as well as midwives, administrators continued to signal the importance of these female medical auxiliaries to the goals of the AMI. Colonial administrators hoped that female nurses and midwives would be vehicles for spreading notions of domesticity, hygiene, and cleanliness, among the local population. In certain instances, the authority vested in these roles gave women license to do things that other woman could not, particularly in the face of male authority.[31] However, what authority and standing these women had came from their relationship to the state and not to the society at large. Relocated to remote and sometimes alien communities, these nurses and midwives, educated in French schools and trained in the field of nursing and midwifery care, found themselves in an awkward position *vis-à-vis* the population at large. Teased for their *toubab* (i.e. European) ways, African nurses walked a fine line between their devotion to the profession and their desire to earn the trust and acceptance of the communities they served.

In this battle for hearts and minds, nurses and midwives not only confronted the skepticism of the populace but also bumped up against the entrenched interests of local healers and midwives. Initially, colonial administrators hoped that the introduction of Western-trained midwives and nurses would obviate the need for traditional midwives. This proved difficult for several reasons. First, the lack of personnel made this unfeasible. There were simply not enough nurses and midwives to administer to the entire population of the colonies, particularly those living outside of the major and secondary centers. Second, there was the issue of demand. Many women either preferred to give birth at home or were convinced to do so by their husbands or their families; thus traditional midwives remained relevant even in the face of the introduction of this new corps of female nurse and midwives. Finally, as women decided to forsake the help of the *matrone* and give birth at the colonial maternity or dispensary in increasing numbers, there were often not enough beds to accommodate them.[32] Expediency therefore dictated that traditional midwives be integrated into the ranks of health personnel, provided that they complete a short training course dealing specifically with infant and maternal health and hygiene, and submit to the supervision of colonial-trained nurses and midwives.[33] While some *matrones* accepted this bargain, and the material bonuses it entailed,[34] their subordinate position to colonial nurses and midwives clearly created tensions.

The introduction of Western-trained nurses and midwives challenged the autonomy and authority that traditional midwives had long enjoyed over matters of birth and women's health. In Senegal, as elsewhere in West Africa, women's authority traditionally rested on their social status as married, post-menopausal women. Furthermore, traditional midwives drew their expertise from their training as well as their personal experience with childbirth. The subordination to younger and more inexperienced women thus challenged not simply their autonomy but also their authority. The tensions that Madame Seye recalled between her and the *matrone* in Bakel echoed the experiences of other African nurses and midwives who served during the colonial period. Even as there existed mutual recognition, and in some cases respect of each other's craft, there remained an insuperable gap between the world of the modern midwife and that of the *matrone*.[35] The experiences of Seye, in this respect, challenge the narrow perception of these female professionals as pawns in a battle against native superstition and ignorance. Instead, their roles as intermediaries, or more aptly interlocutors for a Western model of health care and medicine, reflect a more complicated story about the evolution of nursing and midwifery in the colonial period.

Conclusion

The politics of maternal and infant health left an indelible imprint on the development of nursing and midwifery in Senegal. Colonial health policies aimed at remaking the African family marked the point of entry for women into the health professions. These policies shaped the trajectories of female professionals in colonial Senegal and the colonial Federation of French West Africa as a whole. Nevertheless, the imposition of these measures was not a one-way street. Rather, the translation of these metropolitan concerns into the colonial setting marked a process of negotiation and dialogue between the interests of imperial policymakers and those of local actors. The history of nursing thus provides fertile ground for grappling with the complexities of the colonial encounter and exploring how aspects of race, class, and gender shaped the evolution of the profession as it was transplanted into France's overseas colonies.

Notes

1 In this chapter I use the word "maternity" to refer to the location where women receive their birthing care. In the context of colonial French West Africa, maternities could be attached to hospitals, but more often than not they were connected to rural dispensary posts. To call them "maternity centers," as the term is used in the context of US and UK history, would be misleading as it would overstate their autonomy in relation to the existing health infrastructure.

2 L.C. Seye, 2011. Interview with Madame Lary Cissé Seye, *ancienne infirmière d'état et sage-femme d'état*. This chapter draws on extensive archival research in France and Senegal and interviews with current and former health personnel conducted in 2010 and 2011. This was made possible thanks to the support of the Sigmund Martin Heller Traveling Fellowship provided by the Department of History and a grant from the Center for African Studies at the University of California at Berkeley. The sources consulted in Senegal were primarily from Series O and Series H in the Archives Nationales du Sénégal, dealing with education and health respectively. I conducted the interviews cited in this chapter with the assistance of William Carvallo and Badara Sissokho.

3 B.N. Lawrance, E.L. Osborn, and R.L. Roberts (eds), 2006, *Intermediaries, Interpreters, and Clerks: African Employees in the Making of Colonial Africa*, Madison: University of Wisconsin Press.

4 J. Iliffe, 1998, *East African Doctors: A History of the Modern Profession*, Cambridge: Cambridge University Press.

5 M. Lyons, 1994, "The Power to Heal: African Auxiliaries in Colonial Belgian Congo and Uganda," in D. Engels and S. Marks, eds, *Contesting Colonial Hegemony: State and Society in Africa and India*, London: British Academic Press, pp. 202–223.

6 F. Cooper, 1994, "Conflict and Connection: Rethinking Colonial African History," *American Historical Review*, vol. 99, no. 5, pp. 1516–1545.

7 S. Marks, 1994, *Divided Sisterhood: Race, Class, and Gender in the South African Nursing Profession*, New York: St Martin's Press.

8 E. Schmidt, 1992, *Peasants, Traders, and Wives: Shona Women in the History of Zimbabwe, 1870–1939*, Portsmouth, NH: Heinemann.

9   Schmidt, *Peasants, Traders, and Wives*; T. Kanogo, 2005, *African Womanhood in Colonial Kenya, 1900–50*, Athens, OH: Ohio University Press.

10 P. Barthélémy, 2010, *Africaines et Diplômées à L'époque Coloniale (1918–1957)*, Rennes: Presses Universitaires de Rennes; N.R. Hunt, 1999, *A Colonial Lexicon of Birth Ritual, Medicalization, and Mobility in the Congo*, Durham, NC: Duke University Press.

11 A. Conklin, 1998, "Redefining 'Frenchness': Citizenship, Race Regeneration, and Imperial Motherhood in France and West Africa, 1914–1940," in J.A. Clancy-Smith and F. Gouda (eds), *Domesticating the Empire: Race, Gender, and Family Life in French and Dutch Colonialism*, Charlottesville, VA: University Press of Virginia; A. Davin, 1997, "Imperialism and Motherhood," in F. Cooper and A.L. Stoler (eds), *Tensions of Empire: Colonial Cultures in a Bourgeois World*, Berkeley: University of California Press.

12 Conklin, "Redefining Frenchness," p. 71.

13 Gouvernement Général de l'Afrique Occidentale Française (GGAOF), 1926, *Instructions relatives à l'orientation et au developpement des services de l'Assistance Medicale Indigène, 15 fevrier 1926*, Series H (AOF), Archives Nationales du Sénégal.

14 GGAOF, 1935, *AOF – Inspection Générale Des Services Sanitaires Et Medicaux. Rapport Annuel: Partie Administrative Et Partie Medicale*. Series 2G. Dakar, Sénégal. Archives Nationales du Sénégal.

15 The medical school was later renamed *Ecole de Médecine Jules Carde* in honor of the former governor-general who had dedicated so much of his attention to the twin issues of education and public health.

16 J. Turritin, 2002, "Colonial Midwives and Modernizing Childbirth in French West Africa," in S. Geiger, N. Musisi, and J.M. Allman (eds), *Women in African Colonial Histories*, Bloomington, IN: Indiana University Press.

17 GGAOF, 1930a, *A.O.F. École de Médecine. L'école de médecine indigène par L. COUVY*. Séries 2G: Rapports périodiques, Première Tranche, 1895–1940, ANS 2G 30-58. Dakar, Sénégal. Archives Nationales du Sénégal.

18 Barthélémy, *Africaines et Diplômées*, 53–61.

19 GGAOF, 1936, *Sénégal. Service de santé. Rapport annuel: Partie Administrative et Partie Médicale*. Séries 2G: Rapports périodiques, Première Tranche, 1895–1940, ANS 2G 36-22. Dakar, Sénégal. Archives Nationales du Sénégal.

20 Quaranic schools had been the primary venue by which both girls and boys were educated.

21 Barthélémy, *Africaines et Diplômées*, p. 36; P.M. Diop, 1997, "L'enseignement de la fille indigène en AOF, 1903-1958," in *AOF, réalités et héritages, Sociétés ouest-africaines et ordre colonial, 1895–1960*, Dakar: Direction des Archives du Sénégal, pp. 1081–1096.

22 A. Charton, 1935a, *Conseil Supérieure de l'Enseignement, 1935: L'Education des filles et la formation des elèves-sages-femmes*. Séries O: Enseignement de l'AOF 1895–1958, ANS O 161 (31). Dakar, Sénégal. Archives Nationales du Sénégal; 1935b *La préparation des Elèves Sages-Femmes et l'enseignement des filles*. 1935. Séries O: Enseignement de l'AOF 1895–1958, ANS O 161 (31). Dakar, Sénégal. Archives Nationales du Sénégal. The instruction offered at the *Ecole Normale des Jeunes Filles* is described in detail in Barthélémy, *Africaines et Diplômées*. See also dossiers in the Archives Nationales du Sénégal relating to girls' education and the training of midwives and nurses, specifically ANS O 454 (31), O 212 (31), O 307 (31).

23 P.G. Fall, 1934, "La Vie Scolaire: L'Enseignement des Filles au Sénégal et dans la Circonscription de Dakar," *L'Education Africaine: Bulletin de l'enseignement de l'Afrique occidentale française*, vol. 23, no. 87.

24 D. Savineau, 1938, *Rapport de Madame Savineau sur la famille en AOF: les conditions de la femme. 1937–1938*. Séries 1G: Études Générales Thèses, Mémoires et Monographies, 1903–1978, ANS 1G 00021. Dakar, Sénégal. Archives Nationales du Sénégal, pp. 146, 183.

25 N. Guèye, 2003, *Etude d'une profession médicale?: Les sages-femmes du Sénégal de 1918 à 1968*. Mémoire de Maitresse, Université Cheikh Anta Diop de Dakar.

26 M. Diouf, 2011. Interview with Mamadou Diouf, *ancien infirmier d'état*.

27 D.L. Barthel, 1975, "The Rise of a Female Professional Elite: The Case of Senegal," *African Studies Review*, vol. 18, no. 3, p. 17.
28 Diouf, 2011. Interview.
29 The *infirmier-sanitaire* and the *infirmière-visiteuse* were rather specialized in their training and job duties. They were distinguished then from other health personnel who also wore the title of nurse (*infirmier/infirmière*).
30 GGAOF, n.d., *Programme de l'Enseignement à Donner aux Infirmiers sanitaires, aux Infirmières Visiteuses et aux Matrones Traditionnelles*. Séries H: Santé, Fonds de l'AOF, 1920–1959, ANS 1 H 102. Dakar, Sénégal. Archives Nationales du Sénégal.
31 P. Barthélémy, 2004, "Sages-femmes africaines diplômées en AOF des années 1920 aux années 1960: Une redéfinition des rapports sociaux de sexe en contexte colonial," in A. Hugon, ed., *Histoire des femmes en situation coloniale: Afrique et Asie, XXe siècle*. Paris: Éditions Karthala, pp. 119–171.
32 To remedy the problem of capacity and encourage women from more rural and remote areas to give birth at the clinics, the administration created *centres d'hebergement*, shelters for those who came to have their babies but had no other place to stay ANS 2 H 14.
33 GGAOF, 1940, *Instructions sur la lutte contre La Mortalité Infantile et Les Maladies Endémo-Epidémiques*. Séries H: Santé, Fonds de l'AOF, 1920–1959, ANS 1 H 102. Dakar, Sénégal. Archives Nationales du Sénégal; 1949, *Rapport sur la protection maternelle et infantile en A.O.F. 1949*. Séries H: Santé, Fonds de l'AOF, 1920–1959, ANS 2 H 14. Dakar, Sénégal. Archives Nationales du Sénégal.
34 Upon completing their training, these state-sanctioned *matrones* received a special kit that included some basic supplies such as scissors, tongs, gauze, and eye drops. They also received cash bonuses for the pregnant women they referred to the maternities. GGAOF, 1933, *Dakar. Hôpital Central Indigène. Rapport annuel (partie administrative et partie médicale)*. Séries 2G: Rapports périodiques, Première Tranche, 1895–1940, ANS 2G 33-20. Dakar, Sénégal. Archives Nationales du Sénégal; GGAOF, 1940, *Instructions sur la lutte contre La Mortalité Infantile*; GGAOF, 1949, *Rapport sur la protection maternelle et infantile*.
35 Turritin, "Colonial Midwives and Modernizing Childbirth"; Barthélémy, *Africaines et Diplômées*, pp. 195, 206.

Bibliography

Primary sources

Interviews

Diao, S., 2011. Interview with Samba Diao, *ancien infirmier d'état*.
Diouf, M., 2011. Interview with Mamadou Diouf, *ancien infirmier d'état*.
Seye, L.C., 2011. Interview with Madame Lary Cissé Seye, *ancienne infirmière d'état et sage-femme d'état*.

Archival documentation

Charton, A. (1935a) *Conseil Supérieure de l'Enseignement, 1935: L'Education des filles et la formation des elèves-sages-femmes*. Séries O: Enseignement de l'AOF 1895–1958, ANS O 161 (31). Dakar, Sénégal. Archives Nationales du Sénégal.
—— (1935b) *La préparation des Elèves Sages-Femmes et l'enseignement des filles*. 1935. Séries O: Enseignement de l'AOF 1895–1958, ANS O 161 (31). Dakar, Sénégal. Archives Nationales du Sénégal.

Fall, P.G. (1934) "La Vie Scolaire: L'Enseignement des Filles au Sénégal et dans la Circonscription de Dakar," *L'Education Africaine: Bulletin de l'enseignement de l'Afrique occidentale française*, 23(87).

Gouvernement Général de l'Afrique Occidentale Française (GGAOF) (1939) *Organisation de l'enseignement et l'education de jeunes filles d'AOF: 1934–1939*. Séries O: Enseignement de l'AOF 1895–1958, ANS O 212 (31). Dakar, Sénégal. Archives Nationales du Sénégal.

—— (1926) *Instructions relatives à l'orientation et au developpement des services de l'Assistance Medicale Indigène, 15 fevrier 1926*. Séries H: Santé, Fonds de l'AOF, 1920–1959, ANS 1 H 102. Dakar, Sénégal. Archives Nationales du Sénégal.

—— (1930a) *A.O.F. École de Médecine. L'école de médecine indigène par L. COUVY*. Séries 2G: Rapports périodiques, Première Tranche, 1895–1940, ANS 2G 30-58. Dakar, Sénégal. Archives Nationales du Sénégal.

—— (1930b) *Sénégal. Service de santé. Rapport annuel (partie administrative et partie médicale)*. Séries 2G: Rapports périodiques, Première Tranche, 1895–1940, ANS 2G 36-22. Dakar, Sénégal. Archives Nationales du Sénégal.

—— (1933) *Dakar. Hôpital Central Indigène. Rapport annuel (partie administrative et partie médicale)*. Séries 2G: Rapports périodiques, Première Tranche, 1895–1940, ANS 2G 33-20. Dakar, Sénégal. Archives Nationales du Sénégal.

—— (1934) *L'Ecole de Médecine de L'Afrique Occidentale Française (de sa fondation à l'année 1934)*. Séries O: Enseignement de l'AOF 1895–1958, ANS O 161 (31). Dakar, Sénégal. Archives Nationales du Sénégal.

—— (1935) *A.O.F. Inspection générale des services sanitaires et médicaux. Rapport annuel: Partie Administrative et Partie Médicale*. Séries 2G: Rapports périodiques, Première Tranche, 1895–1940, ANS 2G 30-58. Dakar, Sénégal. Archives Nationales du Sénégal.

—— (1936) *Sénégal. Service de santé. Rapport annuel: Partie Administrative et Partie Médicale*. Séries 2G: Rapports périodiques, Première Tranche, 1895–1940, ANS 2G 36-22. Dakar, Sénégal. Archives Nationales du Sénégal.

—— (1940) *Instructions sur la lutte contre La Mortalité Infantile et Les Maladies Endémo-Epidémiques*. Séries H: Santé, Fonds de l'AOF, 1920–1959, ANS 1 H 102. Dakar, Sénégal. Archives Nationales du Sénégal.

—— (1941) *Dakar Et Dépendances. Hôpital central indigène. Rapport Annuel*. Séries 2G: Rapports périodiques, Deuxième Tranche, 1895–1940, ANS 2G 41-9. Dakar, Sénégal. Archives Nationales du Sénégal.

—— (1946) *Correspondance échangée entre la Direction générale et les Directeurs locaux de la Santé publique, 1946–1951*. Séries H: Santé, Fonds de l'AOF, 1920–1959, ANS 1 H 44. Dakar, Sénégal. Archives Nationales du Sénégal.

—— (1949) *Rapport sur la protection maternelle et infantile en A.O.F. 1949*. Séries H: Santé, Fonds de l'AOF, 1920–1959, ANS 2 H 14. Dakar, Sénégal. Archives Nationales du Sénégal.

—— (n.d.) *Programme de l'Enseignement à Donner aux Infirmiers sanitaires, aux Infirmières Visiteuses et aux Matrones Traditionnelles*. Séries H: Santé, Fonds de l'AOF, 1920–1959, ANS 1 H 102. Dakar, Sénégal. Archives Nationales du Sénégal.

Hardy, G. (1917) *Une Conquête Morale, L'enseignement En A.O.F*, Paris: A. Colin.

Savineau, D. (1938) *Rapport de Madame Savineau sur la famille en AOF: les conditions de la femme. 1937–1938*. Séries 1G: Études Générales Thèses, Mémoires et Monographies, 1903–1978, ANS 1G 00021. Dakar, Sénégal. Archives Nationales du Sénégal.

Secondary sources

Allman, J. (1994) "Making Mothers: Missionaries, Medical Officers and Women's Work in Colonial Asante, 1924–1945." *History Workshop*, 38, pp. 23–47.

Barthel, D.L. (1975) "The Rise of a Female Professional Elite: The Case of Senegal." *African Studies Review*, 18(3), pp. 1–17.

Barthélémy, P. (2002) "La professionnalisation des africaines en AOF (1920-1960)." *Vingtième Siècle. Revue d'histoire*, 75, pp. 35–46.

—— (2004) "Sages-femmes africaines diplomées en AOF des années 1920 aux années 1960: Une redéfinition des rapports sociaux de sexe en contexte colonial." In A. Hugon (ed.) *Histoire des femmes en situation coloniale: Afrique et Asie, XXe siècle*. Paris: Éditions Karthala, pp. 119–171.

—— (2010) *Africaines et diplômées à l'époque coloniale, 1918–1957*, Rennes: Presses universitaires de Rennes.

Clancy-Smith, J.A. and Gouda, F. (eds) (1998) *Domesticating the Empire: Race, Gender, and Family Life in French and Dutch Colonialism*. Charlottesville, VA: University Press of Virginia.

Conklin, A. (1998) "Redefining 'Frenchness': Citizenship, Race Regeneration, and Imperial Motherhood in France and West Africa, 1914–1940." In J.A. Clancy-Smith and F. Gouda, (eds), *Domesticating the Empire: Race, Gender, and Family Life in French and Dutch Colonialism*. Charlottesville, VA: University Press of Virginia.

Cooper, F. (1994) "Conflict and Connection: Rethinking Colonial African History." *American Historical Review*, 99(5), pp. 1516–1545.

Davin, A. (1997) "Imperialism and Motherhood." In F. Cooper and A. L. Stoler (eds), *Tensions of Empire: Colonial Cultures in a Bourgeois World*. Berkeley: University of California Press.

Dieng, I. (1974) "Evolution of the nursing profession in Senegal." *International Nursing Review*, 21(6), pp. 172–173.

Diop, P.M. (1997) "L'enseignement de la fille indigène en AOF, 1903-1958." In *AOF, réalités et héritages, Sociétés ouest-africaines et ordre colonial, 1895–1960*. Dakar: Direction des Archives du Sénégal, pp. 1081–1096.

Engels, D. and Marks, S. (eds) (1994) *Contesting Colonial Hegemony: State and Society in Africa and India*. London: British Academic Press.

Frieson, K. (2000) "Sentimental Education: Les Sages Femmes and Colonial Cambodia. *Journal of Colonialism and Colonial History*, 1(1).

Gaye, P. (1998) "La diffusion institutionnelle du discours sur le microbe au Sénégal au cours de la Troisième République française (1870–1940)". Doctoral Thesis, Université Paris VII-Denis Diderot.

Guèye, N. (2003) *Etude d'une profession médicale?: Les sages-femmes du Sénégal de 1918 à 1968*. Mémoire de Maitresse, Université Cheikh Anta Diop de Dakar.

Hansen, K.T. (ed.) (1992) *African Encounters with Domesticity*, New Brunswick, NJ: Rutgers University Press.

Hodgson, D.L. and McCurdy, S. (1996) "Wayward Wives, Misfit Mothers, and Disobedient Daughters: 'Wicked' Women and the Reconfiguration of Gender in Africa." *Canadian Journal of African Studies/Revue Canadienne des Études Africaines*, 30(1), pp. 1–9.

Horwitz, S. (2007) "'Black Nurses in White': Exploring Young Women's Entry into the Nursing Profession at Baragwanath Hospital, Soweto, 1948–1980." *Social History of Medicine*, 20(1), pp. 131–146.

Hunt, N.R. (1990) "Domesticity and Colonialism in Belgian Africa: Usumbura's Foyer Social, 1946–1960." *Signs*, 15(3), pp. 447–474.

—— (1999) *A Colonial Lexicon of Birth Ritual, Medicalization, and Mobility in the Congo*. Durham, NC: Duke University Press.

Iliffe, J. (1998) *East African Doctors: A History of the Modern Profession*, Cambridge: Cambridge University Press.

Kanogo, T. (2005) *African Womanhood in Colonial Kenya, 1900–50*. Athens, GA: Ohio University Press.

Knibiehler, Y. and Goutalier, R. (eds) (1985) *La Femme Au Temps Des Colonies*. Paris: Stock.

Lawrance, B.N., Osborn, E.L. and Roberts, R.L. (eds) (2006) *Intermediaries, Interpreters, and Clerks: African Employees in the Making of Colonial Africa*. Madison, WI: University of Wisconsin Press.

Lyons, M. (1994) "The Power to Heal: African Auxiliaries in Colonial Belgian Congo and Uganda." In D. Engels and S. Marks (eds), *Contesting Colonial Hegemony: State and Society in Africa and India*. A Publication of the German Historical Institute. London: British Academic Press, pp. 202–223.

M'Baye, E.M. (2002) *Etude d'une profession de santé: Les infirmiers au Sénégal de 1889 à 1968*. Mémoire de Maitresse. Dakar, Sénégal: Université Cheikh Anta Diop de Dakar.

Marks, S. (1994) *Divided Sisterhood: Race, Class, and Gender in the South African Nursing Profession*. New York: St Martin's Press.

Summers, C. (1991) "Intimate Colonialism: The Imperial Production of Reproduction in Uganda, 1907–1925." *Signs*, 16(4), pp. 787–807.

Turritin, J. (2002) "Colonial Midwives and Modernizing Childbirth in French West Africa." In S. Geiger, N. Musisi, and J.M. Allman (eds), *Women in African Colonial Histories*. Bloomington, IN: Indiana University Press.

8

WINDSOR'S METROPOLITAN DEMONSTRATION SCHOOL AND THE REFORM OF NURSING EDUCATION IN CANADA, 1944–1970

Steven Palmer

A 1948 feature in Toronto's *Star Weekly* invited readers to contemplate a "quiet street in Windsor [where there] stands a dignified old stone house that could well become as symbolic to the nursing profession of Canada as Florence Nightingale." The house in question was the first home of the Metropolitan School of Nursing, an experimental academy operated by the Canadian Nurses Association (CNA) between 1948 and 1952.[1] With core funding from the Canadian Red Cross, and a partnership with the Metropolitan Hospital of Windsor, Ontario, the CNA "demonstration school" was designed to show that an autonomous academic institution run by nurses could attract better candidates to the field than existing hospital-controlled schools, provide superior training, and produce professional nurses in less time. The CNA was confident that, if judged pedagogically successful, the experiment would entrench the legitimacy of academic instruction for nursing students, introduce elements of the university nursing curriculum into the standard model of nurse education, and fatally expose the administrative and pedagogical irrationality of the exploitative hospital schools that still monopolized registered nurse training in Canada. Along the way, it was hoped, permanent sources of funding would be found (most likely from government) to allow the school to carry on as a model and beacon for reform after its five-year experimental phase came to an end.

A shortage of registered nurses and the reticence to enter nursing among educated, middle-class women threatened the planned expansion of qualitatively distinct hospital care in the post-war era. This context, and the enhanced influence of Canadian nurses stemming from their participation in the war effort, made it possible for leaders of the profession to launch an experimental project in nurse education whose ultimate objective was to improve the professional standing of nursing.[2] The demonstration school was overseen by leading figures in Canadian nursing, principal among them faculty associated with the University of Toronto (U of T) School of Nursing. As an internationally recognized pioneer in nursing education, U of T Nursing received significant funding from the Rockefeller Foundation (RF), a philanthropic organization promoting reforms in medicine and public health.[3] Because it was an experiment designed to advance the agenda of these important institutional actors, the Metropolitan School of Nursing became a national and international showcase for the reform of nurse training over its five years of operation.

The mayor of Windsor and administrators at the hospital, which had no in-house nurse training program of its own, were initially enthusiastic about the school at a time when increasing amounts of government money were becoming available for innovative expansion of hospital services. The hospital board agreed to build a dedicated school and residence building, and to pay the school $200 per year per student for the work they would perform on the wards. Despite this promising start, a number of problems compromised the experimental school's budget model and eroded its local political support. Most serious was a 1949 "sex scandal" involving Metropolitan Hospital nurses and the hospital administrators and municipal politicians with whom the CNA had entered into agreement. Though neither its personnel nor the students were implicated in the scandal, the demonstration school found itself engulfed in a fog of community skepticism and fiscal woes stemming from conflict with a new and more conservative post-scandal hospital regime.

Though never explicitly framed as a feminist project, the CNA demonstration school did embrace a rhetoric of radical reform – a "New Deal for nurses in training," in the words of one reporter in attendance at the first graduation ceremony in 1950.[4] Moreover, the manner in which its authority and continuity were damaged by the 1949 scandal – for which neither the school nor its students bore any responsibility – revealed the challenge that the CNA experiment posed not only to patriarchal hospital institutions, but also to gendered community expectations that tax dollars invested in nurse training would buy bedside care from women trainees. The Metropolitan School of Nursing may have been backed by powerful national and international forces of reform (the U of T, the CNA, the Red Cross, and the RF), but it rose and fell at the intersection of strong personalities, gendered domains of authority, and community politics. Though discontinued in 1952, the CNA demonstration school did succeed in completing its five-year mission to show that competent nurses could be trained in two years. Moreover, the template, rationale, and findings of the school experiment would be key reference points for the new standard nursing education model that took shape in Ontario in the 1950s and 1960s, one that embraced a twenty-four month general nurse training of a largely academic character, though still within the institutional confines of hospitals.

"Can nurses train in 25 months?" Mid-century innovation in North American nursing education

The Metropolitan School of Nursing was one of a cluster of carefully designed and monitored experiments in North American nursing education conducted around 1950. Many of them sought to establish the legitimacy of a two-year period of instruction with greater academic content for nurse trainees, objectives formally articulated in North American nursing as early as the Goldmark Report of 1923, and on the CNA's agenda since the late 1920s.[5] The headline of a national magazine report on the Windsor demonstration school asked the bold question, "Can nurses train in 25 months?"[6] Researchers in nursing education used the critical shortage of hospital nurses in the post-Second World War era to answer that question, in the process prying open and transforming what Susan Reverby has identified as the "political economy of the hospital–nursing school relationship" that had previously undermined the autonomy and professionalizing ambition of nurse educators.[7]

The CNA Windsor demonstration school was an early and influential project in this experimental wave, its progress closely watched by nurse educators in both Canada and the United States.[8] It was soon followed by others. For example, in 1950, deciding to "follow the example of the Demonstration School in Windsor," Toronto Western Hospital's Atkinson School of Nursing implemented an experimental "2 + 1" nurse training program. The school remained under hospital control, but was administered autonomously, with two years of academic instruction followed by one year of clinical work on the wards that would repay the cost of the education.[9] In the US, Mildred Montag at Teacher's College, Columbia University, directed an important study of a two-year "associate degree nurse" training model. Carried out between 1952 and 1957 with a grant from the Kellogg Foundation, the objective was to create "nursing technicians" or "semi-professional" nurses in community colleges.[10]

These experiments have received very little attention from historians. The dramatic changes in nursing education after mid-century are sometimes explained through reference to criticism of the hospital training model made by influential academic leaders in nursing or in landmark reports by the American Nurses Association or the CNA; other times they are simply understood in terms of the general spread of colleges and universities in the post-Second World War era.[11] While class-related differentiation in the nursing ranks and its relationship to professional identity has been a strong theme in the social history of nursing, the effect of pedagogical projects on stratification has been largely overlooked, and outcomes tend to be ascribed to long-term structural transformations in educational and labor markets.[12] One exception to this is Julie Fairman's recent study of the evolution of nursing in modern healthcare. She points to the importance of Montag's study in this reform conjuncture in legitimizing the expansion of associate degree programs in community colleges over the 1960s. The result was the "development of a new level of worker . . . that compounded an already hierarchical workforce" – a "new type of nurse, the associate degree nurse, to perform technical tasks," leaving the registered nurse at the top of a "nursing pyramid."[13]

The central role played by U of T faculty in the Windsor school, and the close connection between that faculty and the health reform initiatives of the RF, suggest that the Canadian experiment was comparable in nature to Montag's. In both instances, university-based educators and a major philanthropic foundation came together in a highly self-conscious effort to design the post-war nursing work force. In the case of the CNA demonstration school, however, rather than producing elite nurses as the university schools were doing, or associate technical nurses, its stated purpose was "to give basic education for professional nursing, and a recognized background for post-graduate study in public health or nursing education" to "the great intermediary group of nurses giving bedside care in hospitals and homes – the original nurses, coming from the traditional three-year hospital schools."[14]

The attempt to bring to life a single-discipline, stand-alone school of nursing as a model for the training of registered nurses, and to nurture in the students a strong professional ethos wrapped in a "new deal" discourse, made the CNA demonstration school an audaciously nurse-autonomist and professionalizing experiment. The history of the Windsor school contributes to an appreciation of the spectrum of reform initiatives undertaken at this time, revealing different approaches by professional associations, university-based researchers and major philanthropic organizations, and underlining the need for more case studies to allow for greater comparative analysis. At the same time, the consequences of the Windsor experience for the future of nursing reform in Canada remind us of the importance of local history and case studies of "failed reforms" for understanding the dynamics at play in the evolution of nursing education.[15]

A New Deal for nurses

After the First World War, nursing leaders had convinced the Canadian Red Cross to use funds accumulated from public donations during the conflict to sponsor programs in public health nursing education. This initiative gave rise to the country's first university-based nursing programs, including that of the University of Toronto. U of T Nursing, then, also began as a short-term "demonstration" and, with the help of a series of major grants from the RF, was transformed over the 1920s and 1930s into Canada's first administratively autonomous, degree-granting School of Nursing. As the Second World War drew to a close the CNA again petitioned the Red Cross to fund a pedagogical experiment. Showing "statesmanlike leadership," Kathleen Russell, Honorary Advisor in Nursing of the Canadian Red Cross, persuaded the organization to sponsor a demonstration school with a grant of one hundred and fifty thousand dollars.[16] The preeminent figure in Canadian nursing at this time, Russell was also Dean of Nursing at U of T and one of the RF's most respected collaborators.[17] Russell's two main allies in the demonstration school project were Agnes McLeod, Chief Nurse in the federal government's Department of Veterans' Affairs, and Nettie Fidler, a U of T faculty member and President of the Ontario Registered Nurses' Association who would be appointed to set up and direct the experiment.

Over her career, Fidler worked and studied in virtually every major reformist domain of Canadian nursing practice, pedagogy, and politics. She graduated from the Toronto General Hospital training program in 1919 and almost immediately became Head Nurse

(1920–23, 1925–27), a tenure punctuated by two years as a Red Cross Outpost Nurse in Northern Ontario.[18] After a year studying at McGill's School for Graduate Nurses, Fidler returned to Toronto General as an instructor before taking on directorial nursing roles at Ontario Hospital in Whitby and at the Toronto Psychiatric Hospital. In 1936 she became an instructor at U of T Nursing and began preparing for an academic future by completing requirements to enter undergraduate studies. She received her BA in 1943 and was promoted to Assistant Professor.[19]

In the late 1930s Mary Tennant, a senior RF advisor on nursing, described Fidler as an "unusually interesting person" after observing her teach at U of T and speaking with her students. Kathleen Russell told the RF that Fidler was the "strongest person in the School, in fact . . . outstanding in Canada, and within five years will be one of the ablest nurses on the North American Continent." Russell promoted the idea of a fellowship for Fidler, very much her protégée (they had trained together at Toronto General, Russell one year ahead of Fidler), explaining to Tennant that she wanted Fidler to "get the same stimulus that she (Miss R [Russell]) got some years ago when visiting European nursing activities as a guest of the RF – says it opened her mind and started her thinking in entirely new channels."[20] In 1939 the RF awarded Fidler a grant to study in London and visit a number of nursing schools in Europe. Fidler's appointment in 1947 to direct the CNA's Metropolitan demonstration school made the experiment itself an expression of RF nurse education reform. It also consolidated her stature as a leader of Canadian nursing: in 1946 she had been elected President of the Ontario Registered Nurses Association, and her book *Law and the Practice of Nursing*, co-authored with Kenneth Gray, a lecturer in medical jurisprudence and forensic psychiatry at U of T, was set to appear in 1948.[21]

As Fidler wrote in the *Nursing Mirror's* "Experiments in Nurse Training" section, the Canadian system of nursing education had been established on a Nightingale model but its "essential principles were imperfectly understood and interpreted." The system did not prepare students equally for public health and hospital nursing. The response had been to create postgraduate certificate courses in universities to prepare a nursing elite, and on the other hand to train nursing assistants. But the education of the core group of bedside care nurses, who would now require greater skills to operate in a more technologically demanding hospital environment, had languished in a traditional, pedagogically inefficient hospital training school model.[22] The objective of the CNA demonstration school, according to an internal report, was to "establish a nursing school as an educational institution; a separate entity in its own right" in order to demonstrate that a "skilled clinical nurse can be prepared in a shorter period than three years, *once the school is given control of its students' time*" (emphasis in original). Financial and administrative independence would provide "the necessary freedom for research on the curriculum," reveal the real cost of a nursing school, and allow the training of "nurses who are in good health, who are developing personalities, and who like nursing and want to nurse."[23]

Nurse educators perceived a precipitous decline in the academic and social standing of young women entering the nursing ranks, and blamed it largely on what they felt was an unjust and outmoded model of hospital training schools (Fidler skewered them as "money-saving devices" and "not . . . educational institutions").[24] Marjorie Earl, writer of the 1948 *Star Weekly* feature, noted "the fishy eye with which young women choosing a career view the nursing profession."[25] One contemporary calculation argued that a nursing student in an Ontario hospital training school spent a minimum of 121 forty-eight-hour weeks of ward service, which if calculated at the sweatshop wage of fifty cents meant she paid $2,000 in labor for her education. Given that stenographers could make $1.50 an hour with virtually no training, the increasing numbers of young women entering the work force eschewed nurse training. The CNA estimated that in many hospitals student nurses were performing eighty percent of the ward service.

Echoing long-standing criticisms by proponents of nursing reform, the CNA felt that such programs damaged the health of the students. Demanding twelve-hour days and six-day weeks doing foul work in pathogen-rich hospital environments further slowed their education or ended it through illness, while demoralizing others into dropping out of school or exiting the profession quickly.[26] The Metropolitan School of Nursing was designed as a counter-model to the hospital training school. A report in the *Montreal Standard* called it "a revolutionary new type of nursing school . . . where the student is Queen, where her education and training is the sole paramount concern . . . where she does NOT donate time and work during her training period free of charge, often at the expense of health and study." The demonstration school added up to nothing less than "a new deal for nurses in training on the North American continent."[27]

The Windsor connection

The CNA wanted to set up the demonstration school in partnership with an established, mid-sized hospital in a centrally located area, preferably non-sectarian and without its own in-house nurse-training program. Finding one proved difficult. Ontario legislation permitted a twenty-four month minimum period of training for nurses, and its Department of Health approved the demonstration school curriculum for RN certification eligibility, making that province the most likely option.[28] At one point the CNA tried to convince the federal and provincial governments to provide a subsidy that would have allowed them to locate the demonstration school in St Catherine's through a kind of buy-out of the existing in-house school at the General Hospital (a sentimental favorite because it was the site of the first formal nurse training program in Canada, established in 1873). This did not happen, and Fidler began to promote the Windsor option after two site visits to Windsor's Metropolitan General Hospital and a meeting with the superintendent of nursing, Mildred Maybee, the hospital superintendent, Horace Atkin, and the mayor, Arthur Reaume (a key figure since it was a municipal hospital). Partnering with the Metropolitan became irresistible when Reaume and Atkin assured her that a dedicated school and residence building would be constructed adjacent the hospital.[29]

Metropolitan Hospital was adequate for the purposes of the demonstration school plan, with 150 beds, fifty nurses on general staff with five supervisors and a head nurse, and a medical staff of twelve physicians.[30] The city's Catholic Hotel Dieu Hospital and the Salvation Army's Grace Hospital both had nurse training programs, and Metropolitan Hospital initially had reasonable access to graduates of those programs and did not create its own school.[31] The growing demand for nurses in the post-war period, however, put pressure on nurse recruitment. More immediately, the end of wartime restrictions on cross-border employment led to an increased flow of Canadian nurses to the United States – nationally, 246 left for US jobs in 1946, while by 1948 the figure was 779 – and the proximity to Detroit, with its rapidly growing medical complex, accelerated competition for nurses and drove up salaries in Windsor. Graduates from Hotel Dieu and the Grace could easily find employment in Detroit and reported better wages and more respectful treatment.[32] The Metropolitan Hospital board hoped that the CNA school would alleviate staff shortages; students would perform some clinical work and graduates might develop a loyalty to the institution and become staff rather than simply seek higher-paying jobs across the border.

Fidler reported to the Demonstration School Administration Committee that the Metropolitan Hospital "is quite new, with a progressive medical staff and very fine laboratory."[33] The hospital's origins in the late 1920s were connected to an experimental tradition of local public health collaboration with province-wide initiatives in vaccination and school and community nursing. The "progressive" medical staff Fidler referred to were among those involved in the promotion of Windsor Medical Services, a physician-run, pre-paid full service medical and hospital insurance program pioneered by the Essex County Medical Society in the late 1930s with the help of an RF grant. Nathan Sinai, a leading economist at the University of Michigan School of Public Health who advised state and federal governments on progressive health insurance reform, used Windsor Medical Services as a "field laboratory" to accumulate data designed to show the viability of similar health insurance schemes being proposed in the US.[34] The Windsor area Member of Parliament, Paul Martin, was Minister of Health and Welfare in the federal Liberal government, and he guaranteed fifty thousand dollars of federal health research funding to help with construction of the new school build-ing (which would be matched by the province). Given the enthusiastic welcome, the progressive and innovative history of local health institutions, and the larger social context of a unionized work force expanding in an era of prosperous collective bargaining based on automobile manufacturing, Windsor likely seemed an ideal place to pilot the future of nursing education and perhaps find synergies that would promote a successful outcome for the experiment.[35]

The New Deal demonstrated

The School of Nursing opened in January 1948 with twelve students from five Canadian provinces, three of them from the Windsor area. Until the new building became available in the fall of 1949 the school established its headquarters, classrooms and residence in the "dignified old stone house" acquired for the CNA by the city. Eleanor Martin, an instructor at the highly regarded Calgary General Hospital School of Nursing, was brought in as Fidler's assistant and the main clinical teacher; she spent her time at the hospital while Fidler dealt with administrative matters and oversaw classroom instruction in the temporary school building. The senior staff would be complemented later by Nancy McPhedran, another U of T professor, while nurses at the Metropolitan Hospital were to cooperate in providing opportunities for clinical instruction.[36]

In her 1950 article in the *Nursing Mirror*, Fidler described the Windsor course as a "Streamlined Nursing" program, "similar in many ways to the one at U of T." First year included anatomy, physiology, bacteriology, chemistry, psychology, materia medica, nutrition and diet, therapy, medicine, and surgery; second year covered psychology, obstetrics, pediatrics, communicable disease, public health and community nursing, and ward administration. A pre-clinical science and nursing term lasted three months; medical nursing (including nutrition) four months; surgery (including operating room) four or five months; psychiatry three months; obstetrics and pediatrics four or five months; TB and communicable disease a month and a half; public health nursing half a month; ward administration one month; and two months were spent on vacation. The various experiences were "not rigidly segregated" and the "social aspects of nursing" were emphasized throughout the course of study.[37] The curriculum met the requirements for nurse registration in Ontario, and thereafter through reciprocity in all Canadian provinces. In character and scope it roughly corresponded to the curriculum classification of a "good school of nursing" as defined in a major 1949 US report on nursing education.[38]

Prospective students had to meet academic requirements equivalent to university entrance. They had to be at least eighteen years of age, of "good background" and in good health.[39] The first dozen would be joined by twenty-four more in September 1948, a further twenty-four in September 1949, and a final class of thirty-five in September 1950. School directors felt that the quality of applicants was high; the dropout rate was certainly very low, and the numbers of applicants from across the country, mostly recruited through provincial nursing associations, constantly outstripped capacity. The regional background of the students in the final graduating class was representative of the previous cohorts: nine came from Windsor and Southwestern Ontario, nine from other parts of Ontario, four each from British Columbia and Saskatchewan, two from Manitoba, and three from Quebec and the Maritimes (one student was from Massachusetts in the US, while three others did not complete the program).[40] After a debate among board members during the establishment of the school it was decided that Black students would be eligible for admission (south-western Ontario was an important area of Afro-Canadian settlement) and, while none were accepted during the life of the school, graduates included three Japanese-Canadians and possibly at least one aboriginal woman.[41]

A concerted effort was made to humanize the school. The director insisted on an eight-hour day with "relaxed discipline," a limit of four to five hours' practice on wards and the rest spent in class. A good deal of attention was paid to nutrition, and the students were given significant vacation and "community" time.[42] A spread in the local newspaper to celebrate the inauguration featured a charming photograph of students Huguette Quenneville and Corinne Anderson reading *Gray's Anatomy*, and emphasized that these "pioneer girls in nursing experiment" enjoyed "modern sectional furniture and appointments" in their living and study quarters that avoided "all touches of an institutional life."[43] When the school was able to occupy the new building in November 1949 the students' situation improved considerably. They had access to "bright study halls and modern laboratories," a library, and classroom facilities, while the school and residence building had direct access via a tunnel to the hospital wards.[44] Because the school had not reached full capacity most students had their own room with "combined desk and dresser with built-in cosmetic tray, roomy closets and comfortable, modern beds."[45] As the total complement of students rose, traditions and structures of nursing school life began to take shape and, internally, the school appears to have developed harmoniously.[46]

The inauguration of the CNA demonstration school received considerable local and national press coverage.[47] Fidler also promoted the project in Canadian and US nursing and medical periodicals.[48] Among the school's notable features was the stream of international visitor-observers. As Fidler testified in 1949, the demonstration school had welcomed "hundreds of visitors so far, coming from pretty well everywhere," including Europe and Asia.[49] Many of them were RF fellows from around the world doing a one-year graduate nursing program at U of T (by far the most popular destination for Rockefeller nursing fellows).[50] Visiting nurse educators from Canada, Great Britain, France, Switzerland, and elsewhere gave the school favorable reviews, and it also received two endorsements in high-profile medical periodicals.[51] A leading researcher in nursing education from Great Britain, Gladys Beaumont Carter, having studied the school during a visiting instructor stint at U of T, extolled the Windsor experiment in *The Lancet* by way of excoriating the lack of innovation in nurse training in England.[52] A report in the *Canadian Medical Association Journal* summarized a favorable independent review conducted for the Canadian Education Association and the CNA by a panel of senior public servants in education, medical policymakers, and nursing educators who compared the demonstration project with three control hospital schools.[53]

The first graduation took place in February 1950, exactly twenty-five months from the start date of the pedagogical experiment, thus answering in the affirmative the question posed in the headlines at the time of the school's inauguration. The ceremony in the new school building was attended by a distinguished list of nurses from Canada, Great Britain, and the United States. Fidler "greeted the visitors in a smart navy crepe dress, the skirt knife-pleated," and Kathleen Russell gave the address to the graduating class of eleven who had finished their "'No Drudgery' Course."[54] But even as these "leading women" of Canadian nursing celebrated a mission accomplished in the presence of the federal minister of health, things were badly awry in the school's relationship with the Metropolitan Hospital and the Windsor public.

The school and the scandal: Transgressions of nursing's New Deal

As became evident in the course of the 1949 royal inquiry, the mayor, Arthur Reaume, and the hospital superintendent, Horace Atkin, used Metropolitan Hospital as a kind of municipal harem. Atkin systematically approached nurses to invite them to a variety of public and private social events involving the mayor and associates, and oversaw a system of rewards for nurses who responded favorably. In February 1949 Reaume and Atkin arranged to have four single nurses from the hospital attend, "unchaperoned," a party thrown in a suite of rooms rented by the mayor for the Press Photographers Ball at Detroit's glamorous Book-Cadillac Hotel.[55] The Metropolitan Hospital's Superintendent of Nursing, Mildred Maybee, resigned when she discovered that nurses under her charge – including one who missed a shift under false pretenses – had attended the ball as guests of the mayor and hospital superintendent. The incident became public due to rampant rumors about sexual antics at the party, and because a woman physician on the board insisted, against the mayor's wishes, that Maybee should be called to explain the reasons for her resignation. Political opponents forced Reaume to ask the provincial government to create a royal inquiry into the administration of Metropolitan Hospital. Eric Cross, the judge who presided, while finding no evidence of sexual improprieties, dismissed Atkin for unprofessional conduct, dissolved the old board and restructured hospital governance to eliminate any direct representation on the new board from the mayor and city council.[56]

While the students and faculty of the Metropolitan demonstration school had no direct role in the Book-Cadillac affair, testimony at the inquiry revealed dynamics that likely consolidated resentment against Fidler and the CNA experiment in the context of the scandal. For one thing, in her testimony Fidler reiterated her strong support for the progressive healthcare vision of both the mayor and the hospital superintendent even in the face of the sordid details that were emerging about their treatment and use of hospital nurses. This showed considerable courage of conviction, but it underlined the degree to which she and the school were aligned with the hospital's now disgraced leadership. Fidler also confirmed that she had been centrally involved in the design and construction of the new nursing school building.[57] Among a medical staff that had seen its petition for a new hospital wing sidelined in favor of the nursing school construction, Fidler's project management role would have accentuated a feeling that she wielded illegitimate power and authority within the hospital due to her special relationship with a board controlled by the mayor and the superintendent.

At a 1949 emergency joint meeting of the board of the Metropolitan School of Nursing and the Demonstration School Administration Committee of the CNA, called to address the implications of the scandal, there was some surprise that after two years Fidler had still not met with the Metropolitan Hospital physicians' group. Whether symptomatic of autonomist hubris or of hostility from the physicians, Fidler's inability to cultivate any working relationship with the hospital medical staff now left the school in a weak position. She was urged to send a formal request to the hospital board for payment of the outstanding sum for student services (which surprisingly, and no doubt to Fidler's embarrassment, had yet to be billed), and to write to the President of the Medical Staff "suggesting that as the School has now been in operation for over a year, it would now be an opportune time to permit the Director of the School to meet with the Medical Staff to discuss the School."[58]

It also became clear during the inquiry that Maybee's resignation over the Book-Cadillac affair coincided with a breakdown in her relations with Fidler and Martin. At the outset of the CNA demonstration school program she had been an enthusiastic ally, perhaps hoping to realize earlier academic aspirations through involvement with the school.[59] Her relations with Fidler and Martin did not prosper, however; due, it seems, to the demonstration school faculty's criticism of the quality of instruction the students received from the Metropolitan nursing staff. Martin suggested a series of changes that were not well received by Maybee, and Fidler and Martin took to resolving disputes by appealing to their ally, hospital superintendent Atkin. This unfortunately duplicated the pattern of nurses going to Atkin above Maybee's authority that was at the heart of her motives for resigning after the Book-Cadillac affair.[60]

The school, in short, had been living in a vulnerable bubble of proud self-reliance, sustained by the goodwill of one faction of the local elite, but not securely anchored in its host institution or community and indeed facing the strong resentment of many, including the hospital's medical staff. The Metropolitan School of Nursing was now re-evaluated by the public according to gendered notions of legitimate domains of moral and institutional authority that had been clarified and deployed in the Metropolitan Hospital inquiry, and condemned as excessive and transgressive in analogous ways. In her testimony at the inquiry, Maybee showed she was bound still to a code of hospital nursing in which the moral reputation of the nursing staff was integral to the character of the institution. "I know it is their (the nurses who attended the ball) business when they are off duty, until such time as it affects the name of the hospital where they work."[61] Given that the Metropolitan was a municipal hospital and therefore a civic symbol, in bringing the "name of the hospital" into disrepute through their improper conduct (appearing "unchaperoned" in public festivities and private hotel rooms with "married men" who were high civic officers) the young nurses of Metropolitan Hospital had brought dishonor onto the city of Windsor itself. The nurses of the Metropolitan (and by extension the students in the school), then, were daughters of the city – in some way the property of the city – and the municipal public had the right and duty to control and restrict their conduct in order to preserve the moral character of the community.

Maybee's traditional authority had been eroded by the young nurses' overly modern notions of acceptable conduct displayed on the other side of the border in connivance with the hospital administrator and mayor; modern transborder medical economies had eroded her disciplinary power by giving nurses alternative employment options. When it came to the nurse trainees of the Metropolitan School of Nursing, who were pushing at the borders of female nursing autonomy, Maybee had no authority whatsoever. With its implicitly feminist ethos and leadership, its basis in a quest for full nurse autonomy, its reconception of the political economy of healthcare, and its construction of a female nurse-governed domain of scientific authority, the Metropolitan School of Nursing also violated traditional lines of hospital authority and jurisdiction.[62] The demonstration school's connection with the Atkin and Reaume board, the conflicts of its directors with the hospital matriarch who was keeper of the civic nursing honor, its women directors' insistence on autonomy and control over knowledge and use of students' time, the cosmopolitan nature of the school, the "outsider" character of its faculty and the majority of the students – all were held against it. In the context of the Book-Cadillac scandal, Atkin and Reaume's decision to build a gynoecium to house young single nurse trainees who would come from across the country was reinterpreted as part of the same pattern of improper hospital administration.

The demonstration school was an early attempt by nursing elites to attract students of "good social standing" back to the fold. To do so, as Kathryn McPherson points out, they capitalized "on the powerful youth culture of the postwar era" which allowed for innocent sexual encounters between the sexes, considered healthy, and in which "women's sexual possibility was highly visible."[63] The demonstration school's promotional material, for example, focused on the contemporary cut of the school's uniforms and the dorms with their sectional furniture, comfortable beds, and vanities. A feature in the Toronto *Globe and Mail* celebrating the first graduation ran with a picture of "three attractive girls [students] . . . seen during leisure time in one of the attractively furnished rooms."[64]

The official opening of the school and residence building in November 1949 in the immediate wake of the scandal involved an ill-advised "open house" that gave a guided tour of the school and residence to 700 members of the public. They were treated to an inside look at an underutilized facility in which young women enjoyed spacious, private, and independent accommodation while having their education subsidized by the taxpayers of Windsor even though they provided limited ward care. From the perspective of the late 1940s, with an early Cold War moral conservatism emboldening those looking to roll back the relaxation of gender norms that had taken place during the war years, the conduct of the young Metropolitan Hospital nurses who attended the party at the Book-Cadillac Hotel was evidence of the danger and dishonor that could come of these new feminine lifestyles and freedoms.

In retrospect, as Fidler herself came to realize, the school had started prematurely in rushing to begin in January 1948 (perhaps due to timeline strictures for spending the Red Cross grant). Because the new building was not finished, and due to the size of the "old stone house" that had been made available as a temporary building, the school had to restrict the first cohort to twelve students. The subsequent two entering classes were limited to twenty-four for the same reason, with half housed in private lodging; only the final cohort of thirty-five, admitted in 1950 after the school and residence building were inaugurated, matched initial expectations for class size. This not only introduced unexpected costs for additional lodging and reduced potential enrolment revenues, it limited the number of students available for work on the wards and early on established a sense among Metropolitan Hospital staff that students were not shouldering a workload of any significance.

When details of the arrangement between the former board and the school were brought to the attention of the city council and the public through reportage on the Metropolitan debacle, the payment of two hundred dollars per student per year was portrayed in language that had overtones of payment to mistresses and prostitutes. In December 1949, just after the inauguration of the new school building and with the first graduation ceremony less than two months away, the *Windsor Star* published a story headlined "Hospital Problems." The report explained that the "problem of the nurses in the new training school" was to be taken up by city council in the context of their discussion of "the Metropolitan Hospital question." Following the revelation that the city, through the hospital, was said to have "to pay for the services of these young women . . . a keen debate can be started concerning whether these girls are more trouble than they are worth at the hospital."[65]

Indeed, the new Metropolitan Hospital board quickly reneged on the earlier memorandum of agreement signed between the Reaume-controlled board and the school, arguing that it did not constitute a contract (again to the likely embarrassment of Fidler, author of a book on nursing and the law).[66] Crucially, they refused to pay for student services – a sum that had been counted on for a significant portion of the school's budget ($34,000 dollars over the five years, or roughly 15 percent). Though the school was allowed to occupy the new building in the fall of 1949, some hospital departments began poaching on the unused capacity and demanding use of other space in the school building. Lawyers became involved, with the CNA demonstration school threatening to withhold certain payments and services to the hospital, and using its contacts to exert national and provincial political pressure on the city behind the scenes. In the end it was an astute lawyer for the city, Lorne Cumming, who negotiated an entente that allowed the school to ride out its five-year experimental lifespan with dignity and without suffering further major affronts from the hospital or the city.[67] After the Red Cross refused to increase its original grant, the budget shortfall was met by a special grant from the provincial and federal governments that allowed the school to graduate its final class of thirty-two in May 1952.[68] The autonomous CNA School of Nursing, however, would not carry on in post-experimental guise as originally hoped. In 1952 the Metropolitan Hospital reclaimed the building and began to make plans for its own in-house nurse training school.

Ultimately, in the context of the Book-Cadillac scandal, the demonstration school fell victim to the same gendered notions of institutional honor relying on traditional lines of authority and labor discipline that it had been set up to challenge. It also suffered from a gendered mid-century political economy of healthcare in which nursing education remained, in the words of historian Celia Davies, a "constant casualty."[69] Fidler herself was not hurt professionally by the Windsor experience, and her mentors evidently forgave her political and administrative mistakes. She left the Metropolitan School of Nursing in 1951 to finish her distinguished career as Russell's successor in the Dean's chair at U of T. That same year she was named to the Dominion Council of Health, a senior national planning body that included all provincial deputy ministers of health and Chief Medical Officers, and from 1952 to 1955 served as Chair of the Red Cross Outpost Nursing Committee.[70]

The CNA Demonstration School and educational innovation after 1952

The final report of the Demonstration School Administration Committee outlined the "numerous problems" faced by the experimental school and "generally regret[ted] the necessity for its discontinuance."[71] Despite the bittersweet aftertaste, Canada's nursing elite was determined to hold onto and hold up the experience of the demonstration school. Academically, the promoters of the school felt comfortable making the case that the school had proved that an autonomous nurse-run program focusing on the learning and human needs of the students trained a better nurse in two-thirds the time of the traditional hospital school. Its approach to assessing the value of students' clinical work also became a standard point of reference – accepted without discussion as reliable, for example, in the proceedings of a conference of directors of Ontario nursing schools convened by Fidler at U of T in 1958.[72]

As an institutional model, the research results were less promising. In her February 1950 article in the *Nursing Mirror*, written as the first class graduated from the Metropolitan School of Nursing, but also with the Book-Cadillac scandal still fresh and the school's fight with the hospital board ongoing, Fidler claimed that among the project's goals was research "to find the form of contract which is feasible in such a situation." One of the major findings in this regard was "the possibility that the whole arrangement is transitional and that a nursing school should not be tied up financially in any way to a hospital."[73] Fidler already felt that the only reasonable source of financing for nursing schools was the State: "The source of this for other schools is the State, and this appears to be the only source for the nursing school. The task of obtaining this would seem to be the next task of the Association."[74]

In the short run, however, the Windsor demonstration school became the reference point for a compromise Canadian solution in which "2 + 1" schools of nursing would be established, still under the control of hospitals, but as independent academic units.[75] Students would "pay back" roughly half the expense of their two-year education with a third year of internship in the hospital (though still under the supervision of the school), while the state would cover the other half through special grants to the hospitals who were willing to innovate along these lines. In 1963 ninety-five percent of nursing students in Canada were still enrolled in the country's 171 hospital schools, all of which were three-year programs, but these were increasingly of the new "2 + 1" type.[76] Fittingly, the second school to adopt this model (after Toronto Western, discussed above) was the hospital-run Metropolitan School of Nursing in Windsor, inaugurated in 1954.[77] Dorothy Colquhoun, hired to develop and direct the new in-house school of nursing and perhaps aware of the "2 + 1" program at Western, insisted that Metropolitan Hospital "use the findings" of the original demonstration school and create the new Metropolitan School of Nursing as an independent academic unit.[78]

Between 1955 and 1965, the majority of hospital schools of nursing in Ontario changed from the traditional three-year apprenticeship system to "2 + 1" programs, and the Metropolitan school's second director, Kate Moderwell, who took over from Colquhoun in 1958, repeatedly declared that this shift was primarily due to the success of the school and its basis in the findings from the CNA demonstration school that preceded it. In 1970, again in the face of nursing shortages in an era of further institutional expansion, the Ontario government moved to two-year programs under the auspices of community colleges – according to Moderwell, still with the Metropolitan demonstration school's experiment of 1948 to 1952 as a point of reference. In doing so, the government finally did two of the things the CNA had advocated since the 1940s: training nurses in two-year academic programs and using general public expenditure on post-secondary education to pay for it. Because the "2 + 1" and then the community college system were implemented in relatively uniform fashion, however, the transition also may have conserved the original school's homogenizing thrust. In any case, until further research is done it should not be taken for granted that the shift to the community college model in Canada reproduced the earlier US experience in its effects on professional identity and stratification in the ranks of registered nurses.

The way that the international, the national, the provincial, and the local aligned, and then misaligned, underlines the importance of place in determining the course of Windsor's Metropolitan demonstration school. If the CNA experiment might not have been conducted at all had it not been for the politics of health in the Windsor area, its demise was also the result of fallout from local political affairs. Nevertheless, because it was the product of powerful institutional interests, it would have lasting significance due to its ability to demonstrate success in building professional nurse education and identity through progressive innovation, pedagogical autonomy, and academic rigor. Though formally under the CNA and the Red Cross, the central role played by RF fellows Russell and Fidler in its creation, design, and direction shows that the Metropolitan School of Nursing has to be understood in pedagogical terms as primarily the offspring of the RF-supported U of T Faculty of Nursing, and its academic, research-oriented, and professional agenda for all nurse education. Indeed, in a real sense, we can see Windsor's Metropolitan Demonstration School as an effort to make a stripped-down version of the U of T School of Nursing the prototype for the Canadian nursing school of the future – not oriented to producing the university-trained elite nurse, but not mutually exclusive of university education either. It was designed to provide two years of post-secondary academic schooling that would be the basis for nursing certification and professional identity, while also dovetailing in all essential ways with later studies at university. In this sense, the CNA Metropolitan School of Nursing both promoted and anticipated a university-based model of mass, professional nursing education in North America that was still decades away.

Notes

1 Marjorie Earl, "A new plan for nurse training," *The Star Weekly* (Toronto), February 7, 1948, n.p., in "Metropolitan Demonstration School of Nursing (Windsor, ON), Scrapbook," Papers of the Canadian Nurses' Association (hereafter CNA Papers), MG 28, I 248, 163, Library and Archives Canada (hereafter LAC), Ottawa. The author would like to thank Ron Foster of Windsor Regional Hospital's Public Relations Department, Loryl Macdonald of the University of Toronto Archives and Records Management Services, and Michele Hiltzik of the Rockefeller Archive Center for access to materials; the Essex County Historical Society and the Barbara Bates Center for the Study of the History of Nursing at the University of Pennsylvania for opportunities to present this work at an earlier stage; and Steve Malone, Larry Kulisek, Marty Gervais, Jayne Elliott, Dominique Tobbell, Miriam Wright, Christina Simmons, Barbara Melosh, and the editors for critical feedback on the manuscript.

2 On the enhanced authority of nurses following the war, see Toman, C. 2007, *An Officer and a lady: Canadian military nurses and the Second World War*, Vancouver: UBC Press.

3 On the RF "infatuation" with the U of T program, which it saw as "the model nursing institution against which all others were measured," not just in North America but internationally, see Farley, J. 2003, *"To cast out disease": a history of the International Health Division of the Rockefeller Foundation (1913–1951),* London: Oxford University Press, pp. 216, 230–5; quote from p. 230.

4 M.W. Bowman, "New Deal for nurses in training," *Montreal Standard,* April 1950, typescript copy, p. 1, "Scrapbook." In the international arena, stripped of its contentious US domestic political and ideological baggage, Roosevelt's New Deal became synonymous with fundamental reform in the interest of social justice. Probably not coincidentally, *A new deal for nurses* was also the title of a 1939 book by Great Britain's Gladys B Carter, a visiting lecturer at the U of T in 1950 who attended the graduation.

5 Josephine Goldmark's landmark report, *Nursing and nursing education in the United States* (1923) had proposed reducing the fundamental period of nurse training to 28 months "by eliminating unessential, non-educational routine," and proposed greater fiscal and curricular independence for nursing schools as a way to attract "capable young women"; West, M. & Hawkins, C. 1950, *Nursing schools at the mid-century. A report prepared under the auspices of the Subcommittee on School Data Analysis for the National Committee for the Improvement of Nursing Services,* New York: National Committee for the Improvement of Nursing Services, p. xiii. A 1929 survey, the basis of Weir, G. 1932, *Survey of nursing education in Canada,* Toronto, led to the formation of the CNA's committee for curricular reform.

6 "Can nurses train in 25 months?" *Home Magazine. The Farmer's Advocate* [1948], n.d., "Scrapbook."

7 Reverby, S.A. 1987, *Ordered to care: the dilemma of American nursing, 1850–1945,* Cambridge: Cambridge University Press, p. 60.

8 Allen, M. & Reidy, M. 1971, *Learning to nurse: the first five years of the Ryerson nursing program,* Toronto: Registered Nurses Association of Ontario, pp. 14–15.

9 Wallace, W.S. 1955, *Report on the experiment in nursing education of the Atkinson School of Nursing, the Toronto Western Hospital, 1950–1955,* Toronto: University of Toronto Press, pp. 5–6; and Duncanson, B. 1970, "The development of nursing education at the diploma level," in Mary Innis, ed., *Nursing education in a changing society,* Toronto: University of Toronto Press, pp. 118–19.

10 Montag, M.L. 1951, *The education of nursing technicians,* New York: GP Putnam; and Montag, M.L., 1959, *Community college education for nursing,* New York: McGraw-Hill.

11 See, for example, McPherson, K. 2003, *Bedside matters: the transformation of Canadian nursing, 1900–1990,* Toronto: University of Toronto Press, pp. 159–60; 209–10, 221; Lynaugh, J.E. 2008, "Nursing the Great Society: the impact of the Nurse Training Act of 1964," *Nursing History Review,* vol. 16, pp. 14–15, 20; and Lynaugh, J.E. 2006, "Mildred Tuttle: private initiative and public response in nursing education after World War II," *Nursing History Review,* vol. 14, pp. 203–11.

12 Melosh, B. 1982, *"The physician's hand": work culture and conflict in American nursing,* Philadelphia: Temple University Press, esp. Chapter 2; and Fairman, J. 2008, *Making room in the clinic: nurse practitioners and the evolution of modern health care,* New Brunswick, NJ: Rutgers University Press, pp. 42–3. For Canada, McPherson, *Bedside matters,* esp. Chapter 6.

13 Fairman, *Making room in the clinic,* p. 42. Kalisch, P.A. & Kalisch, B.J. 2004, *American nursing: a history,* 4th ed., New York: Lippincott Wilkins and Williams, p. 383, briefly discusses the Montag experiment, but emphasizes its importance in moving "nursing education into the overall system of American higher education."

14 The first quote is from Nettie Fidler, "Demonstration School of Nursing in Ontario, Canada," *Nursing Mirror,* 17 February 1950, pp. i–iii; the second quote is from "Canadian Nursing Association – The Metropolitan Demonstration School of Nursing," n.p.; Faculty of Nursing, 1893–1964, A73011/4, University of Toronto Archives and Records Management Services (hereafter UTARMS).

15 I am indebted to Tobbell, D. 2012, "'Coming to grips with the nursing question': the politics of nursing education reform in 1960s and 1970s America," American Association for History of Medicine conference, Baltimore, for drawing out these issues in her comparison of struggles over nursing education autonomy at UCLA and the University of Minnesota.

16 Emory, F.H.M. "Edith Kathleen Russell: an appreciation of her professional life and work," p. 4; ms., Helen Maude Carpenter Speeches, 1958–1964, A1973-0011/1 (2), UTARMS. The CNA decision to create the demonstration school dated from 1944 and by December 1945 Russell reported to the CNA executive that the Red Cross grant had been secured. Canadian Nurses' Association Executive Committee Papers, Demonstrator School Administrative Committee, Papers of the Canadian Nurses' Association, MG 28, I 248, 163, LAC.

17 Kirkwood, R. 1994, "Blending vigorous leadership and womanly virtues: Edith Kathleen Russell at the University of Toronto, 1920–52," *Canadian Bulletin of Medical History / Bulletin canadien d'histoire de la médecine*, vol. 11, pp. 175–205.

18 Jardine, P.O. 1989, "An urban middle-class calling: women and the emergence of modern nursing education at the Toronto General Hospital, 1881–1914," *Urban History Review / Revue d'histoire urbaine*, vol. 17, no. 3, pp. 177–90. On Red Cross Outpost nursing as a space for creating innovative professional identities, see Elliott, J. 2008, "(Re)constructing the identity of a Red Cross outpost nurse: the letters of Louise de Kiriline," in Elliott, J., Stuart M. & Toman, C., eds., *Place and practice in Canadian nursing history*, Vancouver: UBC Press, pp. 136–52.

19 "Personal history record and application for travel grant," RG 10.1 Fellowship; Series 427L; Box 3, Folder Nettie Fidler, Rockefeller Foundation Archives (hereafter RFA); "Miss Nettie Fidler heads U of T School of Nursing," *Globe and Mail*, 17 March 1952; and "School of Nursing head retires," *Globe and Mail*, 30 March 1962, Nettie Fidler, UTARMS clippings, University of Toronto official file card, UTARMS A2003-0025/054; Nettie Fidler, Application for Admission to Faculty of Arts, "Pass course for teachers," 1939, UTARMS A1969-0008/220; Nettie Fidler, academic record for BA Teachers Course, 1939–1943; UTARMS A1989-0011/025.

20 Diary of Miss Tennant, RG 6.1, Series 1.1, Box 19, Folder 196, RFA. On Russell's training, Farley, "To cast out disease," p. 233.

21 Fidler, N & Gray, KG 1948, *Law and the practice of nursing*, Toronto: Ryerson Press.

22 "CNA – The Metropolitan Demonstration School of Nursing," n.p.

23 "CNA – The Metropolitan Demonstration School of Nursing," n.p.

24 Fidler, "Demonstration School of Nursing," pp. i–iii.

25 Earl, "A new plan for nurse training," n.p.

26 Earl, "A new plan for nurse training," n.p.

27 Bowman, "New Deal for nurses in training."

28 Provincial nurses' associations were asked for suggestions and in 1947 Fidler visited 11 hospitals in Manitoba, Quebec, and Ontario.

29 Fidler's testimony on the early meetings she held in July and August 1947 with Atkin and Reaume and discussion about the building are in "Proceedings of a Royal Commission appointed to enquire into the finances, administration and personnel of the Windsor Metropolitan General Hospital, held in the city of Windsor, Ontario, April 25th [1949] et seq.," pp. 850–1, in "Records of the inquiry into the Windsor Metropolitan General Hospital," Record Group 18-129, Archives of Ontario (hereafter AO).

30 "Appendix A, Report of survey of Nursing Department of the Metropolitan Hospital, Windsor, Ontario, during period of May 18–20 inc., 1949," and "Royal Commission on Windsor Metropolitan General Hospital," p. 13, AO.

31 On the history of these two hospitals and their nurse training programs, see www.hdgh.org/en/historymission

32 "Reduce training period of nurses to 2 years hospital head's view," *Toronto Daily Star*, October 1949, "Scrapbook," n.p.

33 Minutes of Meeting of CNA Committee on Educational Policy – Sub-Committee: the Demonstration School Administration Committee, August 12 1947, p. 4, ARC 19, M4B File 1, CNA Papers.

34 Darsky, B.J., Sinai, N. & Axelrod, S.J. 1958, *Comprehensive medical services under voluntary health insurance: a study of Windsor Medical Services*, Cambridge, MA: Harvard University Press; and Muma, J.K. 1995, "Developing comprehensive medical insurance: Windsor Medical Services as an example of a pre-OHIP non-profit scheme," MA thesis, University of Windsor.

35 An overview is Price, T. & Kulisek, L. 1992, *Windsor 1892–1992: a centennial celebration*, Windsor: Chamber Publications.

36 Richardson, S. 2001, "Stand up and be counted: nursing at the Calgary General Hospital after the Second World War, *Canadian Bulletin of Medical History*, vol. 18, no. 2, pp. 297–323. McPhedran would go on to pioneer nursing education at the University of New Brunswick.

37 Fidler, "Demonstration School of Nursing in Ontario, Canada," p. iii.

38 West and Hawkins, *Nursing schools at the mid-century*, p. 4. It was also oriented by a 1936 proposal by the Curriculum Committee of the CNA Nursing Education Section under Marion Lindburgh of McGill University's School for Graduate Nurses; CNA, *Proposed curriculum for schools of Nursing in Canada*, cit. in Emory, "Edith Kathleen Russell," pp. 4, 12–13.

39 Fidler, "Demonstration School of Nursing in Ontario, Canada," p. ii.

40 "32 Metropolitan nurses graduate," *Windsor Daily Star*, 12 Sept, 1952; Scrapbook, CNA Papers.

41 Minutes of Meeting of Board of Directors, 15 January 1948, ARC 19, M4B File 1, CNA Papers. Applications are not part of the archive. The Japanese-Canadians, who had almost certainly spent the war in internment camps, were Hideko Dorothy Yamashita and Nori Arikado, both of Toronto, and Alice Tanaka of Wymark, Saskatchewan; Dorothy Martin was from Oka, Quebec; Metropolitan School of Nursing, Graduation Exercises brochure, 12 October 1950; Metropolitan School of Nursing, Graduation Exercises brochure, 13 Sept. 1952, CNA Papers. On race and nursing in Canada at this time, with details on the experience of Black nurse trainees in Windsor's Hotel Dieu program, see Flynn, K. 2009, "Beyond the glass wall: Black Canadian nurses, 1940–1970," *Nursing History Review*, vol. 17, pp. 129–52.

42 Earl, "A new plan for nurse training," n.p.

43 "These girls pioneers in nursing experiment," *Windsor Star*, 27 January 1948; Scrapbook, CNA Papers.

44 "Nurses' home opens Saturday," *Windsor Star*, n.d.; Scrapbook, CNA Papers.

45 "'Met' nurses' home is officially opened," *Windsor Star*, 26 November 1949, p. 5; Scrapbook, CNA Papers.

46 A house committee was formed to bring students and faculty together to discuss policy and disciplinary matters, organize extra-curricular activities and award prizes, and a student council was formed.

47 Besides the extensive reportage in the *Windsor Star* and the Toronto *Globe and Mail*, and other instances cited here, examples found in the Scrapbook include M.W. Bowman, "Plan new type nursing school," *Canadian Hotel Review and Restaurant*, 15 September 1947; Dorothy Sangster, "New deal for nurses," *Saturday Night* (Toronto); and "Can nurses train in 25 months?" *Home Magazine*; all from Scrapbook, CNA Papers.

48 Fidler, N.D. 1949, "The Canadian Nurses' Association's Demonstration School of Nursing," *Canadian Medical Association Journal*, vol. 60, pp. 514–16; Fidler, ND 1948, "Canada's Demonstration School," *American Journal of Nursing*, vol. 48, no. 4, April, p. 221.

49 "Royal inquiry into the Windsor Metropolitan General Hospital," p. 855.

50 Farley, *"To cast out disease,"* p. 233.

51 A list of international observers would include: Miss Katherine Favell, director of the College of Nursing, Wayne University, Detroit; Lucy Germaine, director of nursing, Harper Hospital, Detroit; Lilli Petschnigg, assistant director of nursing and social welfare bureau of the League of Red Cross Societies in Geneva, whose "first thought" when she knew she was visiting Canada was "I simply must see the new nurses' training school in Windsor, Ontario," "Red Cross nurses from France visit Metropolitan School," *Windsor Star*, 5 July 1950; Scrapbook, CNA Papers.

52 Carter, G.B. 1953, "Experimental training for nurses," *The Lancet*, vol. 111, p. 707.

53 Lord, A.R. 1953, "The nurse training experiment," *Canadian Medical Association Journal*, vol. 69, pp. 629–32.

54 "Leading women attend nursing school exercises," *Windsor Star*, 17 February 1950; Scrapbook, CAN Papers.

55 The Book-Cadillac was featured as a principal setting in a Robert Capra film of 1948, *State of the Union*, starring Spencer Tracy and Katherine Hepburn – a typical comedy of the noir era that involved the transgressions of a powerful, independent woman being overcome by a restoration of proper gender hierarchies re-contained within a loving marriage.

56 "Introduction" to the Eric W. Cross Papers, Eric William Cross Fonds, F-1025, AO. Cross was a provincial magistrate, former chairman of the Ontario Municipal Board (1935–37), and provincial cabinet minister.

57 "Royal inquiry into the Windsor Metropolitan Hospital," pp. 858–9.

58 Minutes of Special Meeting of the Board of the Metropolitan School of Nursing, 5 April 1949; see also Minutes of Joint Meeting of the Demonstration School Administration Committee and the Board of the Metropolitan School of Nursing, 5 April 1949; both in ARC 19, M4B File 1, CNA Papers.

59 A graduate of the Winnipeg General Hospital, Maybee had taken graduate courses at Columbia University while working at Yonkers Hospital in New York from 1937 to 1940; "Royal inquiry into the Windsor Metropolitan Hospital," pp. 65–7.

60 "Royal inquiry into the Windsor Metropolitan Hospital," p. 872.

61 "Royal inquiry into the Windsor Metropolitan Hospital," p. 69.

62 On gendered domains of institutional and professional authority, see Fairman, J. 2004, "Not all nurses are good, not all doctors are bad," *Bulletin of the History of Medicine*, vol. 78, no. 2, pp. 451–60.

63 McPherson, *Bedside matters*, pp. 166–8.

64 "Pioneering nursing school first graduation," *Globe and Mail*, 15 February 1950, Scrapbook, CNA Papers.

65 "Hospital problems," *Windsor Star*, 9 December 1949, n.p.; scrapbook, CNA Papers.

66 Fidler and Gray's *Law and the practice of nursing* has sections on the patient, the doctor, the hospital, drug control, mental illness, public health, nursing legislation, the organized nursing profession, and labor unions, but nothing on institutional contracts.

67 Cumming was an agile negotiator who would go on to be Chairman of the Ontario Municipal Board in the 1950s, presiding over an innovative period of provincial–municipal relations centering on the amalgamation of Toronto. See Kulisek, L. & Price, T. 1988, "Ontario municipal policy affecting local autonomy: a case study involving Windsor and Toronto," *Urban History Review/Revue d'histoire urbaine*, vol. 16, no. 3, p. 265.

68 Helen Anderson Wood, "A new director, a new building," [University of Toronto Varsity magazine?], 1952, Clippings, Nettie Fidler, UTARMS, pp. 18–19.

69 Davies, C. 1980, "A constant casualty: nurse education in Britain and the USA to 1939," in C. Davies, ed., *Rewriting nursing history*, London: Croom Helm, pp. 102–21.

70 "Miss Nettie Fidler heads U of T School of Nursing," *Globe and Mail*, 17 March 1952; and "School of Nursing head retires," *Globe and Mail*, 30 March 1962; Nettie Fidler, clippings, UTARMS; on the Red Cross appointment, Jayne Elliott, personal communication.

71 Agnes J. Macleod, Canadian Nurses' Association, "Demonstration School Administration Committee," Final Report, MG 28, I-248, vol 163, LAC.

72 "Proceedings: Conference Directors of Schools of Nursing," Nov. 1958, Faculty of Nursing, 1893–1966, A73-011/2, UTARMS.

73 Fidler, "Demonstration School of Nursing in Ontario, Canada," p. iii.

74 Fidler, "Demonstration School of Nursing in Ontario, Canada," p. iii.

75 The influence of the demonstration school on the development of this model is noted in Emory, "Edith Kathleen Russell," p. 4; and in a summary of Fidler's career, "School of Nursing head retires," *Globe and Mail*, 30 March 1962.

76 David Spurgeon, "Wanted: A new system for training nurses," *The (Woman's) Globe and Mail*, 23 May 1963; see also Mussallem, H.K. 1960, *Spotlight on nursing education*, Montreal: Canadian Nursing Association.

77 This is the strong and repeated motif of the annotations on the school's origins made by second director, Kate Moderwell, who prior to her retirement prepared a well-organized and precisely annotated archive of the school. Archives of the School of Nursing, Metropolitan Hospital (SNMH), donated by Kate Moderwell (Instructor and Director of School of Nursing, 1958–1973), Windsor Regional Hospital, Windsor, Ontario. Another school that was modeled on the CNA's Windsor demonstration school was Toronto's Nightingale School of Nursing, established as an independent, two-year school in 1960.

78 On Colquhoun, RNAO News, September/October 1967; clipping in Vol. 2, Box 1, SNMH. References to the second Metropolitan School of Nursing modeling itself on the CNA demonstration school were made repeatedly, most along the lines of the following 1964 convocation address by the school's director, Kate Moderwell: "The School began in 1954, and established its philosophy upon research findings of a Demonstration School . . . It was proved that if responsibility for the control of students' time and experience was delegated to teachers, rather than Head Nurses, the quality of student-learning could improve [and] her course of study could be shortened." Kate Moderwell, "Address to Class of 1964," Vol. 2, Box 1, SNMH.

9

CONFLICTING CHRISTIAN AND SCIENTIFIC NURSING CONCEPTS IN WEST GERMANY, 1945–1970

Susanne Kreutzer

The "scientification of the social sphere"[1] is a key aspect in the development of twentieth-century Western societies. Experts in human sciences – representatives of disciplines as diverse as medicine, law, economics, psychology and social sciences – gained interpretive power with regard to social reality, interpersonal relationships and personal wellbeing. For nursing in West Germany this process began comparatively late. While scientification and rationalization were included in the socio-political agenda for private households as early as the 1920s, the field of nursing did not follow suit until the 1950s.[2]

This noticeable resistance to the scientification of nursing had its roots in the motherhouse-bound organizations of Catholic sisters and Protestant deaconesses. In Germany, the motherhouse principle became the dominant form of organized nursing in the nineteenth century. It was based on a simple exchange principle: women who entered committed to devote their lives to the sisterhood and to the sick and needy. In return they received an education and the assurance of lifelong provision. Up until the early 1950s in West Germany it was understood that nurses would be single and be prepared to work out of a sense of charity. A "good" nurse possessed a wealth of practical experience rather than a sound theoretical education.

The picture changed dramatically in the second half of the 1950s. With the growing medicalization, mechanization and specialization of healthcare, the tasks expected of a "good" nurse took on a different character. Practical experience and Christian ethos, highly valued until then, rapidly lost their legitimacy, with nursing turning into an activity that had to be planned and organized to conform to scientific principles. Such reforms were part of the 1960s' *Zeitgeist* with its firm belief in planning, progress and technical feasibility.[3] At the time the hope of being able to control social processes with the help of a scientific planning system informed the history of West Germany as much as that of its European neighbors.[4]

In the 1950s radical changes in the life plans of younger women also considerably affected the field of nursing. The traditional image of the devoted "act of charity" was no longer congenial to an emerging consumer society. The celibate state of the Christian sisters grew less acceptable too, since a woman's lifestyle that was not defined by marriage had lost its social legitimacy.[5] "Being just a sister" was no longer attractive. The development away from celibacy for nurses went hand in hand with the departure from being "just a housewife." Women were no longer expected – nor were they willing – to pursue the ideal of a single vocation, whether it concerned the needs of patients or those of a family. A modern woman's life plan encompassed the possibility of having a job, a husband and children.[6]

Driven by the shortage of nurses and its dramatic exacerbation around the year 1960 – mostly due to the expansion of the hospital system – nursing grew to be a legally regulated woman's profession with union-agreed salary scales and regulated working hours. The tremendous rate at which the professional image of nurses changed within just a few years reflects the development of West German society as a whole at the time. The period of postwar reconstruction was followed in the second half of the 1950s by a phase of unprecedented prosperity. At the same time a fundamental change occurred, impacting on almost all areas of society; a change that is referred to with terms such as detraditionalization, liberalization, democratization, individualization and secularization.[7]

This chapter investigates the reconceptualization of nursing, with an emphasis on the conflicting implementation of scientific principles in a context dominated by Christian nursing traditions.[8] Christian and scientific concepts were, however, not *per se* incompatible. The denominational sisterhoods also conveyed theoretical knowledge in line with the regulations of the nursing law.[9] But the sisters and deaconesses had considerable reservations when it came to enforced scientification since they prioritized other forms of knowledge, including nursing ethics and practical knowhow. The general training schedule for deaconesses illustrates this clearly: students first received practical training on the wards for a year, followed by religious instruction. The theory of nursing was concentrated in one teaching block with examination at the end of the training.[10]

The present chapter demonstrates that a dramatic shift occurred in the 1960s with regard to the conception of authoritative nursing knowledge. According to Brigitte Jordan, authoritative knowledge is the knowledge that is seen as dominant in a field and that has the power to define "facts." In healthcare, that could include the question of whether a person is sick or healthy, competent or incompetent. Authoritative knowledge is recognized by the majority of agents in a particular field as the natural, only sensible form of knowledge. Authoritative knowledge is powerful not because it is correct but because it counts.[11]

This chapter explores the shift in how authoritative knowledge was conceived, using the example of a group of sisters located at the interface between traditional and modern nursing values: The Agnes Karll Association. The Association, re-formed and re-funded after 1945, has a history of being the first "independent" sisterhood, the Professional Organization for German Nurses (*Berufsorganisation der Krankenpflegerinnen Deutschlands*), initiated by Agnes Karll in 1903.[12] The Professional Organization for German Nurses gained international acclaim because of Karll's active involvement in founding the International Council of Nurses with nurses from the United States and United Kingdom.[13] The organization was dissolved in 1938. After World War II, former members reorganized as the Agnes Karll Association and it went on to be instrumental in the professionalization of nursing after 1945.

This chapter throws light on the nursing concept of the Agnes Karll Association. How did traditional Christian, experience-based views of nursing relate to those founded on scientific standards? To which related sciences did the women refer and how did the logic of scientifically planned and organized nursing establish itself? And what does this say about the role of women in West German society?

The dominance of the sisterhood principle

The dominance of the motherhouse-bound sisterhoods had considerable impact on the organization of "independent" nursing professionals, defined as those who had no motherhouse affiliation. The Agnes Karll Association's forerunner, the Professional Organization for German Nurses, did not completely abandon the sisterhood principle when it was founded in 1903. Like the motherhouses, the organization provided a uniform for its members, instituted an employment agency and ensured adequate sickness and retirement provision for its nurses. The image of a sisterhood was seen as an essential means of gaining recognition along with the religious sisterhoods. Being addressed as "sister," a privilege that had so far been reserved for members of denominational sisterhoods, was considered particularly important. By forming associations the independent nurses were able to call themselves "sister," a form of address that, to this day, is used as a synonym for female nurses.[14]

After 1945 the Agnes Karll Association held on to this organizational tradition, re-founding itself as a sisterhood. Just like the motherhouse organizations, it entered into contracts with hospitals to regulate the deployment of its nurses. These contracts also allowed the association to take charge of the nursing school that was attached to the hospital and to have a say in the training of new nurses. The nurses were employed either by the Agnes Karll Association or by the hospital operators. Unlike deaconesses and denominational sisters, who were sent out by their motherhouses, the Association's nurses could choose where they wanted to work.[15]

There were other independent sisterhoods apart from the Agnes Karll Association. They were usually smaller and regionally organized. The only organization that was comparable to the Agnes Karll Association in size and reputation was the Association of Independent Sisters (*Bund freier Schwestern*), a sisterhood that formed part of the German public service and transport workers' union (*Gewerkschaft Öffentliche Dienste, Transport und Verkehr*). While the members of the Agnes Karll Association usually came from Protestant middle- or upper-middle-class families, the Association of Independent Sisters recruited its members primarily from a social-democratic, unionist, often atheist, working-class milieu. While the organization advocated a union-regulated wage system for nurses, it was skeptical about the professionalization of nursing. But among the independent sisterhoods it was the Agnes Karll Association that assumed a pioneering role in the professionalization of nursing.[16]

Starting point: The Agnes Karll Association and the conception of "good" nursing

Given the influence of Protestant deaconesses and Catholic sisters in post-war Germany, "independent" nurses, who were not associated with a motherhouse, were under pressure in Germany to prove that they also were "good" nurses who were concerned primarily with the patients' wellbeing. After the war the situation of independent nurses grew even more sensitive since the Western occupying powers suspected them of having actively supported the Nazis' extermination policies; they saw the denominational motherhouse sisterhoods of Caritas and Inner Mission as less complicit.[17] Although the Professional Organization of German Nurses was dissolved in 1938, many of its members transferred to its Nazi-controlled successor organization (*Reichsbund deutscher Schwestern und Pflegerinnen*) that merged with the national socialist "brown sisterhood" in 1942 (*NS-Reichsbund Deutscher Schwestern*). It was therefore not possible to distinguish at the end of World War II between former members of the Professional Organization and "brown sisters."[18] The Agnes Karll Association especially had the reputation of having accepted formerly devoted Nazis.[19] Thus, the association's direction strove to emphasize Christian principles because a Christian ethos was considered to guarantee "good" caring nursing practice.[20]

The leadership of the Agnes Karll Association shared one of the central tenets of Christian nursing: caring for both body and soul. While physicians were concerned with the symptoms, diagnosis and treatment of illness, the nurses, according to the tenet, devoted themselves wholeheartedly to the patients' entire personality. Conveying a sense of comfort and security to patients was seen as an essential healing factor.[21] The relationship between physicians and nurses was therefore not hierarchical but complementary. This applied particularly to Christian hospitals where, up until the second half of the twentieth century, physicians had to fight to establish their scientifically based biomedical understanding of health and illness.[22] "Love for the sisterhood," that is, the ability to treat nurses with respect, was one of the main criteria of employment for physicians in these hospitals, a fact that did much for the recognition of the nursing profession.[23]

The publications of the Agnes Karll Association tended to emphasize that the reputation of a hospital depended equally on the head physician's expertise and the atmosphere in the house that the nurses created.[24] In order to be able to do justice to that responsibility for the atmosphere, the nurses also needed to feel comfortable in their place of work. Like other sisterhoods, the Agnes Karll Association therefore aimed at staffing hospitals exclusively with its own nurses.[25] This was meant to facilitate the establishment of a community of nurses who supported each other and were able to convey to both sisters and patients the feeling that they were in good hands.

It was consequently an important aspect of the Agnes Karll Association's training concept for nurses that it valued not only the acquisition of technical knowledge but especially the development of a nurse's "personality." A "good" nurse had to be a nurse "at heart." This "heart" – and in this respect the association shared the fundamental precepts of the conventional, experience-based training concept – was best developed if nurses lived and worked together in a community, learning from the example of more experienced sisters and benefiting from the general atmosphere in the hospital and nursing school.[26] Far into the 1960s, women considered it natural to leave nursing once they were married.

Because nurses carried so much responsibility for the patients' physical and mental needs, they had to be in close contact with the patients and highly committed to their work. Even though the Agnes Karll Association insisted that nurses had time to themselves outside working hours, it refused to bring their working hours into alignment with those of other salaried professions. Eight-hour work days were not considered feasible in nursing because the continuous contact with patients was seen as essential to the process of recovery.[27] The close contact between nurses and patients was enhanced by the longer periods that patients spent in hospital: 25 days on average in the early 1950s.[28] In the mid-1960s patients still remained hospitalized for an average of 21 days, which was longer that the comparable 14 days in the United States and Sweden.[29]

It would, however, not do justice to the Christian nursing concept to discuss only its emphasis on devoted care. Beyond the care aspect, the continuity of contact was essential so that nurses could gain competence in patient observation including the monitoring of moods, appearance, sleep and appetite as well as changes to a patient's weight, temperature, respiration and elimination. From the nineteenth century up to the 1950s the close observation of patients had, across sisterhoods, become the specific domain of the nursing staff and the essence of its independence. In 1952, for example, the Federation of German Nurses' Associations (*Arbeitsgemeinschaft deutscher Schwesternverbände*), as the umbrella organization of all German sisterhoods including the Agnes Karll Association, firmly refused to consider leaving the distribution of food to assistant staff, arguing that it was most important for nurses to be aware of what their patients ingested.[30] As long as the provision of care was based on the personal needs of patients, with their exact and continuous observation being its distinguishing feature, the assistant staff should only perform tasks outside the patient room.[31]

Neither the ability to make patients feel comfortable and secure nor the experience-based and often intuitive observation of patients was easily definable according to criteria of scientific rationality. The importance of these aspects for the healing process was even less measurable. That did not pose a problem in the Christian view of nursing; on the contrary, the particular proficiency of nursing lay in the fact that it was based on a – specifically feminine – "mystery" that eluded penetration and imitation.[32] It was that mysteriousness surrounding the nurses' activities that accounted for the profession's specialness and independence in the Christian view.

The radical changes of the 1960s: The scientification of nursing

Postwar medical history in West Germany was not marked by "major" inventions but by growing specialization and mechanization.[33] The logic of a biomedical view of illness that was based on natural scientific concepts established itself also in Christian hospitals in the 1960s. Nursing was transformed into a process based on planning and on the criteria of scientific rationality.

The scientification process in nursing started in the mid-1950s with the labor sciences, a discipline that could justify its importance with the growing shortage of nurses. The labor sciences, which had a long tradition in Germany at the time, strove for the "optimization" of work processes.[34] In the field of nursing they could, however, only be established once the denominational sisterhoods with their views of what nursing should be like lost ground.

The denominational motherhouse sisterhoods had been suffering from recruitment problems since the early 1950s as the social norms for women changed and the labor sciences promised to provide solutions through more effective deployment of the nursing staff available. They introduced new concepts into the field of nursing that were derived from economic cost–benefit calculations. Efficiency was one of their key factors.

The rationalization of workflow in nursing was seen as the key to solving staffing problems. Frederick Winslow Taylor's concept of improving the productivity of work through a division of labor according to tasks and the standardization of process steps had reached the healthcare sector. When new hospitals were built it was seen as important to keep walking distances to a minimum and centralize routine functions such as the sterilizing of instruments in order to reduce labor on the ward. Nurses were to be relieved from non-nursing tasks, especially housekeeping jobs. But the envisaged differentiation between non-nursing and nursing-specific activities called the very foundations of traditional Christian nursing into question. Still in the early 1950s the Agnes Karll Association objected to the deployment of nursing assistants, a concept that had long become established in other countries, including the United States. There was to be no hierarchy of activities as superior or inferior in the immediate delivery of care.[35]

Yet the critical attitude about nursing assistants changed by the end of the 1950s. The rebuilding of hospitals was largely completed and with the growing prosperity of West German society the healthcare system expanded.[36] But the opening of modern hospitals was seriously jeopardized by the shortage of nurses. Hospitals that wanted to attract and keep new nursing staff had to adjust working conditions to the life plans of the next generation of women. The reduction of weekly working hours, introduced in 1956 and 1957, proved particularly effective. It paved the way for comprehensive rationalization in nursing because working hours became a valuable asset that had to be used efficiently. By 1959, even the Agnes Karll Association began to favor the introduction and regulation of nursing assistants.[37]

The successive introduction of functional care and the division of labor into specialized tasks facilitated the fundamental transformation of the nurse–patient relationship. Patients were no longer looked after by one nurse but by a number of nursing professionals who were each allocated one specific task. The demands on staff nurses also changed profoundly. The hallmarks of a "good" staff nurse were no longer her motherly, caring qualities, but increasingly her ability to set up efficient duty schedules and organize the care rather than provide it.[38] The workflow rationalization and the restriction of duties led to a significant reduction in the amount of time available for traditional notions of nursing work that was not directly task-oriented. The concept of motherly, caring devotion rapidly lost importance in the 1960s. Critics, sociologists in particular, found that too much value was attached in the self-image of nurses to "mothering patients," and the role of the nurse was reduced to "a vague 'tending' to the healing process."[39] While bedside attendance and the ability to make patients comfortable made nursing so special in the older model, these activities were not really definable and certainly not divisible into functional work stages. Nurses seemed now in danger of losing their status as caregivers in the modern, mechanized and highly specialized healthcare system.

Psychology eventually offered a way out of this situation since it provided the possibility of restructuring the relationship between nurses and patients along scientific principles. In the 1950s, psychological concepts of different personality types were successively introduced into the realm of nursing. Nurses were expected to learn how to divide patients into scientifically defined types in order to be better able to judge their behavior and adapt care interventions to their particular personality type. It was recommended, for instance, that they separate patients according to the scheme of Carl Gustav Jung, the founder of analytical psychology, into introvert and extrovert types; or that they differentiate between the pyknic, gregarious type and the leptosomic, reserved type, based on the theories of psychiatrist Ernst Kretschmer.[40]

By introducing psychological interpretive patterns into nursing, the Agnes Karll Association followed the general trend at a time when other fields of Christian (mostly Protestant) social work also opened up to psychological theories.[41] Unlike in the United States, however, it was not psychiatric nursing that drove the psychologization process here, since psychiatric nursing appeared rather late in the German professionalization process.[42] In the 1960s psychology evolved as a key factor in the scientification of the nurse–patient relationship in Germany. The provision of care seemed no longer possible without basic psychological knowledge.[43] Knowing something about developmental psychology became an essential prerequisite for gaining an understanding of the patients' age-specific life themes and problems. Nurses were now expected to acquire basic counseling skills so that they were able to control and direct conversations rather then let them evolve "randomly" as they used to do.[44] The direct interaction with patients thus also became subject to efficiency considerations.

Psychology clearly came into its own as the conditions of the older, need-oriented nursing began to deteriorate so dramatically with the introduction of functional nursing. Psychology can therefore be seen as the vehicle that ensured that the patient as a person was not entirely lost from view in the modern hospital. In 1966, psychology began to be included in the training curriculum and examination regulations for nurses.[45] Psychological concepts were probably not put into practice in everyday nursing until the 1970s, the "therapeutic decade,"[46] when the number of therapies offered to persons in need soared in all areas of psycho-social healthcare.

The growing adoption of psychological concepts from the 1960s onward gave rise to new demands in the field of nursing: sisters were now expected to learn to reflect on their own actions by developing awareness of their own feelings of fear, insecurity, aversion or affection. Following Sigmund Freud, the founder of psychoanalysis, nurses were now asked to gain clarity in their dealings with patients about possible transference and countertransference mechanisms in order to be able to control them.[47] This step toward self-reflection was important in that, by the 1960s, the traditional Christian care provision was increasingly suspected of encroaching on and abusing patients' private space.[48] Such criticism was characteristic of the general democratization of the society, whereby established authorities and hierarchical structures were increasingly called into question.[49] In the Christian care concept, patients were indeed highly dependent on the nurses assigned to them. That such a constellation did not have to result in the patient being made comfortable, but could also produce conflicts – for example, if the patients didn't get along with the nurse allocated to them – was a significant taboo in Christian nursing traditions. The introduction of psychological–therapeutic concepts therefore certainly filled a void in the traditional Christian nursing concept.

The character of care delivery changed dramatically with the psychologization and therapeutization of the patient–nurse relationship. Psychological concepts relied on the spoken word and prioritized cognitive awareness. Ritual, more sense-based ways of expression characteristic of Christian nursing traditions – such as songs, prayers, non-verbal religious practices, but also moments of quiet – were forced out of the nursing routine.[50] Since "knowledge of mental experience mechanisms" was declared to be the key skill in dealing with patients, the forms of devotion that had previously been practically acquired and were without scientific foundation were no longer valid or legitimate.

The scientification of the patient–nurse relationship and the arrival of the concepts of efficiency and targeted actions gave rise to a new view of nursing as an organized, well-planned process in the late 1960s. In 1969, *Die Agnes Karll-Schwester*, the journal published by the Agnes Karll Association, first presented the nursing process as a four-phase model consisting of data collection, planning, implementation of nursing interventions and evaluation.[51] The notion of the nursing process first appeared in the United States in the 1950s and, in the 1960s, it was further developed on the basis of the cybernetic model. Cybernetics was introduced in the 1940s and 1950s as an interdisciplinary science connecting technology, natural and human sciences and the humanities.[52] It saw human beings as complex functional mechanisms that were not fundamentally different from machines. With its key concepts of regulation, control, information and feedback, cybernetics restructured the field of nursing to conform to the logic of technology and mathematics. Feedback was its central aspect as it allowed for the success or failure of the nursing activity to be regulated and, if necessary, corrected.[53] The logic of the nursing process made it possible to speak about nursing like an engineer who aims at optimizing production processes with planned interventions. In the 1970s the nursing process found its way into the nursing text books as a model; in 1985 it became statutory in West German nursing training.[54]

The nursing process has been widely criticized by some nursing scholars for its mechanical approach to problem solving, because it promotes an instrumental access to patients as "information and problem carriers," and ignores the importance of intuitive, experiential forms of knowledge.[55] It nevertheless became established in nursing as a "global concept" that is now being taught, discussed and implemented worldwide.[56] The nursing process is another example of the extent to which the scientification of nursing followed the logic of sciences that were alien to it, a logic that is unable to do justice to the specific qualities of nursing and to the special situation of sick, frightened and suffering human beings.

Nursing reform and the scientification of the social sphere

The scientification of nursing needs to be seen as part of a wider "scientification of the social sphere"[57] that was characteristic of the twentieth century. In nursing this led to a dramatic shift in the conception of authoritative knowledge. In Germany in the early 1950s, the knowledge nurses had of the close relationship between the body and the soul, the capacity for personal, caring devotion that was especially ascribed to women, and the competence in patient observation that nurses acquired in dealing with patients were seen as important curative knowledge. The legitimacy of this knowledge was not affected by the fact that it was largely based on intuition rather than objectifiable observations. The nurses' activities were special because of this "mysterious" aspect.

The fact that this concept was considered hopelessly antiquated by the end of the 1960s illustrates how rapidly the fundamentals of nursing were transformed. With the decline of the sisterhood principle, the old Christian nursing concept lost its organizational basis. The reformation of nursing from a Christian "act of charity" to a salaried profession undoubtedly opened up new perspectives for women, such as the possibility of a private life and the chance of getting away from work. But the reduction of working hours led to an overall workflow rationalization in nursing. The introduction of the labor sciences and their logic to the management of hospitals and nursing was the beginning of a paradigm shift in the healthcare system because the labor sciences were about efficiency, not "good" nursing or the wellbeing of patients. Economic efficiency is aimed at relating the deployment of means, such as labor, time or money, to the outcome in a way that is rationally calculable and profitable. It has no place for non-measurable, "mysterious" aspects.

With the arrival of functional nursing it was no longer possible for patients to receive continuous care from one nurse. For nurses it became increasingly difficult to acquire competence in patient observation and security in patient handling. From the point of view of the 1950s this meant that nurses had lost their key competence. With the establishment of a natural scientific understanding of medicine and the growing importance of laboratory tests and imaging techniques in the 1960s, the nurses' observations were reduced to the level of unscientific and therefore irrelevant pronouncements.[58] Compared to the collected "hard" patient data the intimate, personal awareness of patients lost its validity.

The introduction of cybernetics to nursing, in the form of the nursing process, shows that the mechanization of nursing was not restricted to the increasing use of technical equipment. The workflow in nursing was also restructured according to technical production processes and the language of nursing was adapted to the scientific terminology of engineering. Psychology might have provided new, science-based concepts that made space for a personal nurse–patient relationship in the highly technologized hospitals, and the demand for self-reflection might have filled a real void in the conventional nursing concept. But the prioritization of the spoken word in psychology meant that the ear was trained while the eye – the observation of the patient's physical condition – became secondary.

All in all, the scientification of nursing created a new field of conflict that is referred to by German nursing scholars as *doppelte Handlungslogik* (dual "rationale of action"). How can the theoretical, science-based mainstream knowledge with its claim to universality be united with the hermeneutic approach that validates the specialness of individual patients and their subjective experience of illness? This contradiction, which underlies all actions in person-related service professions, is particularly problematic in nursing. Because of their focus on the patients' body, nursing professionals rely on implicit forms of knowledge that cannot be cognitively and rationally explained and that lost their significance with the scientification of healthcare. The two sides of the "rationale of action" – mainstream scientific knowledge and the specialness of the individual patient – are indeed not equivalent. Since mainstream scientific knowledge grew to be *the* authoritative knowledge in the second half of the twentieth century, the subjective knowledge of the patient no longer carried as much weight as it had in the past.

Up to now historical research on nursing, just like the history of science, has dealt primarily with what is new and modern in the process of social development. Phases of forced modernization in society are, however, always phases of forced obsolescence. The fact that non-objectifiable forms of knowledge lost their validity will be highly relevant for the history of nursing but also for the twentieth-century history of gender as a whole: scientification affected women and men in very different ways since women work primarily in person-related, caring fields where intuitive forms of knowledge that cannot be formalized play an important part. Research into the significance, ambivalences and conflicts of scientification processes and the various ways of entering science-based society in the world would be a worthwhile enterprise. A research perspective that challenges the establishment of a hierarchy between scientific and experience-based, intuitive forms of knowledge would lead to a significant reevaluation of progress and backwardness in nursing history, and would throw new light on the "scientification" process.

Notes

1 Raphael, L. 1996, "Die Verwissenschaftlichung des Sozialen als methodische und konzeptionelle Herausforderung für eine Sozialgeschichte des 20. Jahrhunderts," *Geschichte und Gesellschaft*, vol. 22, pp. 165–193.

2 See Wildt, M. 1994, *Vom kleinen Wohlstand: Eine Konsumgeschichte der fünfziger Jahre*, Fischer Verlag, Frankfurt/Main, pp. 116–123.

3 See Schildt, A. 2000, "Materieller Wohlstand – pragmatische Politik – kulturelle Umbrüche: Die 60er Jahre in der Bundesrepublik," Schildt, A., Siegfried, D. & Lammers, K.C. (eds.) *Dynamische Zeiten: Die 60er Jahre in den beiden deutschen Gesellschaften*, Hans Christians Verlag, Hamburg, pp. 21–53, here p. 48.

4 See Haupt, H.G. & Requate, J. 2004, "Einleitung," Haupt, H.G. & Requate, J. (eds.) *Aufbruch in die Zukunft: Die 1960er Jahre zwischen Planungseuphorie und kulturellem Wandel. DDR, ČSSR und Bundesrepublik Deutschland im Vergleich*, Velbrück Wissenschaft, Weilerswist, pp. 7–28.

5 See Heineman, E. 1996, "Complete Families, Half Families, No Families at All: Female-Headed Households and the Reconstruction of the Family in the Early Federal Republic," *Central European History*, vol. 29, pp. 19–60.

6 See Oertzen, C. von 2001, "Fräulein auf Lebenszeit? Gesellschaft, Berufung und Weiblichkeit im 20. Jahrhundert," *WerkstattGeschichte*, no. 27, pp. 5–28, here pp. 16–28.

7 See Frese, M., Paulus, J. & Teppe, K. (eds.) 2002, *Demokratisierung und gesellschaftlicher Aufbruch: Die sechziger Jahre als Wendezeit der Bundesrepublik*, Schöningh, Paderborn; Herbert, U. (ed.) 2007, *Wandlungsprozesse in Westdeutschland: Belastung, Integration, Liberalisierung, 1945–1980*, Wallstein-Verlag, Göttingen; Schildt, A., 2007, *Die Sozialgeschichte der Bundesrepublik Deutschland bis 1989/90*, Oldenbourg Verlag, Munich, pp. 30–53.

8 The chapter is based on the research project "Rationalization of Nursing in Western Germany and the United States. A Comparative History of the Exchanges of Ideas and Practices, 1945 to 1975," sponsored by the German Research Foundation.

9 In the early 1950s training took a year and a half and included 200 hours of theory.

10 See Kreutzer, S. 2008, "'Before, We Were Always There – Now, Everything Is Separate.' On Nursing Reforms in Western Germany," *Nursing History Review*, vol. 16, pp. 180–200, here p. 186.

11 See Jordan, B. 1997, "Authoritative Knowledge and Its Construction," Davis-Floyd, R. & Sargent, C.F. (eds.) *Childbirth and Authoritative Knowledge: Cross-Cultural Perspectives*, University of California Press, Berkeley, pp. 55–79, here pp. 56–61.

12 See Boschma, G. 1996, "Agnes Karll and the Creation of an Independent German Nursing Association, 1900–1927," *Nursing History Review*, vol. 4, pp. 151–168; Hummel, E. 1986, *Krankenpflege im Umbruch (1876–1914): Ein Beitrag zum Problem der Berufsfindung „Krankenpflege"*, Hans Ferdinand Schulz Verlag, Freiburg i. Br., pp. 101–170; Schmidbaur, M. 2002, *Vom „Lazaruskreuz" zu „Pflege aktuell": Professionalisierungsdiskurse in der deutschen Krankenpflege 1903–2000*, Ulrike Helmer Verlag, Königstein/Taunus.

13 See Tomes, N.J. & Boschma, G. 1999, "Above All Other Things – Unity," Brush, B. & Lynaugh, J. (eds.) *Nurses of All Nations: A History of the International Council of Nurses, 1899–1999*, Lippincott, Philadelphia, pp. 1–38, here pp. 26–30.

14 See Hummel, *Krankenpflege*, pp. 101–118; Schmidbaur, *Lazaruskreuz*, pp. 58–78.

15 See Kreutzer, S. 2005, *Vom „Liebesdienst" zum modernen Frauenberuf: Die Reform der Krankenpflege nach 1945*, Campus, Frankfurt/Main, pp. 37–39.

16 See Kreutzer, *Liebesdienst*, pp. 46–50 and 164–273.

17 However, the motherhouses subscribed to the basic assumptions of National Socialist policy regarding race and population policy. For example, forced sterilizations were carried out in deaconess motherhouses. See Lauterer, H.M. 1994, *Liebestätigkeit für die Volksgemeinschaft:*

Der Kaiserswerther Verband deutscher Diakonissenmutterhäuser in den ersten Jahren des NS-Regimes, Vandenhoeck & Ruprecht, Göttingen.

18 See Steppe, H. 1996, "Krankenpflege ab 1933," Steppe, H. (ed.) *Krankenpflege im Nationalsozialismus,* Mabuse, Frankfurt/Main, pp. 61–85, here 65–66.

19 See Kreutzer, *Liebesdienst,* p. 38; Schmidbaur, *Lazaruskreuz,* p. 150.

20 See Elster, R. 1956, "Bericht über eine Studienreise durch die Schweiz, England, Schottland, Schweden und Finnland," *Die Agnes Karll-Schwester,* vol. 10, pp. 96–99, here p. 99.

21 See Elster, R. 1951, "Ein Wort an unsere Examensschwestern," *Die Agnes Karll-Schwester,* vol. 5, pp. 213–214, here p. 213.

22 See Schmuhl, H.W. 2003, "Ärzte in konfessionellen Kranken- und Pflegeanstalten 1908–1957," Kuhlemann, F.K. & Schmuhl, H.W. (eds.) *Beruf und Religion im 19. und 20. Jahrhundert,* Kohlhammer Verlag, Stuttgart, pp. 176–194.

23 See Kreutzer, S. 2010, "Arbeits- und Lebensalltag evangelischer Krankenpflege. Organisation, soziale Praxis und biographische Erfahrungen", *1945–1980* (unpublished postdoctoral thesis, *Habilitationsschrift*).

24 See Rudolph, H. 1956, "Die Stellung des Krankenhauses in unserer Zeit," *Die Agnes Karll-Schwester,* vol. 10, pp. 326–329, here p. 328.

25 See Klitzing, A. von 1953, "Eröffnung der Vor- und Fortbildungsschule des Agnes Karll-Verbandes," *Die Agnes Karll-Schwester,* vol. 7, pp. 285–288, here p. 287.

26 See Plieninger, M. 1950, "Die erzieherische Bedeutung der Krankenpflegeschule: Vortrag auf dem Kurzlehrgang für Lehr-, Operations- und Stationsschwestern an Krankenpflegeschulen vom 27.–29.10.1949 in Stuttgart-Berg," *Die Agnes Karll-Schwester,* vol. 4, pp. 6–11.

27 See Schmidt, G. 1954, "Schwesternprobleme der Gegenwart," *Die Agnes Karll-Schwester,* vol. 8, pp. 7–9, here p. 7.

28 See Spree, R. 1996, "Quantitative Aspekte der Entwicklung des Krankenhauswesens im 19. und 20. Jahrhundert: ,Ein Bild innerer und äußerer Verhältnisse'," Labisch, A. & Spree, R. (eds.) *„Einem jeden Kranken im Hospitale sein eigenes Bett": Zur Sozialgeschichte des Allgemeinen Krankenhauses in Deutschland im 19. Jahrhundert,* Campus, Frankfurt/Main, pp. 51–88, here p. 65.

29 See Anon 1965, "Verkürzte ,Krankenhaus-Verweildauer' – ein Weg?," *Die Agnes Karll-Schwester,* vol. 19, p. 387.

30 See Kreutzer, *Liebesdienst,* pp. 256–257.

31 See Kreutzer, "Before," pp. 183–187.

32 See Rudolph, H. 1956, "Die Stellung des Krankenhauses in unserer Zeit," *Die Agnes Karll-Schwester,* vol. 10, pp. 326–329, here p. 328. At 6.6 percent the proportion of male nurses was relatively low in 1950. Male nurses worked primarily on psychiatric wards or all-male wards, mostly in urology departments. See Kreutzer, *Liebesdienst,* p. 20.

33 See Seidler, E. 1993, *Geschichte der Medizin und der Krankenpflege,* 6th edn., Kohlhammer, Stuttgart, pp. 240–242.

34 When, after World War I, North American nursing scientist Isabel M. Stuart proposed to standardize nursing practice in line with the labor-scientific principles, she was criticized in the United States for attempting to introduce the German model of heartlessness and brutal efficiency into nursing. See Reverby, S. 1989, "A Legitimate Relationship: Nursing, Hospitals, and Science in the Twentieth Century," Long, D. & Golden, J. (eds.) *The American General Hospital: Communities and Social Contexts,* Cornell University Press, Ithaca, NY, pp. 135–156, here p. 143.

35 See Cauer, M. 1950, "Von den menschlichen Anforderungen an die Schwester: Auszug aus dem Hand- und Lehrbuch der Krankenpflege von Fischer-Groß-Krick, Part 2," *Die Agnes Karll-Schwester,* vol. 4, pp. 5–7, here p. 5.

36 See Krukemeyer, H. 1998, *Entwicklung des Krankenhauswesens und seiner Strukturen in der Bundesrepublik Deutschland: Analyse und Bewertung unter Berücksichtigung der gesamtwirtschaftlichen*

Rahmenbedingungen und der gesundheitlichen Interventionen, Hauschild, Bremen, pp. 85 and 98–99.

37 See Elster, R. 1960, "Bericht über die 17. Hauptvorstandssitzung des Agnes Karll-Verbandes und die Delegiertenversammlung," *Die Agnes Karll Schwester*, vol. 14, pp. 342–344, here p. 344.

38 See Günzel, M. 1961, "Ist eine Ausbildung zur Stationsschwester notwendig?," *Die Agnes Karll-Schwester*, vol. 15, pp. 268–269, here p. 268.

39 Leich, H. 1962, "Aufgaben, Pflichten und Rechte der Oberin bei der Betriebsführung im Krankenhaus," *Die Agnes Karll-Schwester*, vol. 16, pp. 12–18, here p. 17.

40 See Höhn, E. 1952, "Die Bedeutung psychologischer Typen für den mitmenschlichen Kontakt," *Die Agnes Karll-Schwester*, vol. 6, pp. 10–11.

41 Kaminsky, U. & Henkelmann, A. 2011, "Die Beratungsarbeit als Beispiel für die Transformation von Diakonie und Caritas," Damberg, W. (ed.) *Soziale Strukturen und Semantiken des Religiösen im Wandel: Transformationen in der Bundesrepublik Deutschland 1949–1989*, Klartext Verlag, Essen, pp. 89–104.

42 It was not until 1957 that psychiatric nursing training became legally regulated in Germany. Until then psychiatric nurses had passed so-called house exams that were conducted and regulated by the respective mental hospitals. See Kreutzer, *Liebesdienst*, p. 244.

43 See Elster, R. 1961, "Das heutige Berufsbild in der Krankenpflege," *Die Agnes Karll-Schwester*, vol. 15, pp. 297–301, here p. 298.

44 See Kelber, M. 1964, "Die Kunst der Gesprächsführung im Einzelgespräch," *Die Agnes Karll-Schwester*, vol. 18, pp. 136–137.

45 "Ausbildungs- und Prüfungsordnung für Krankenschwestern, Krankenpfleger und Kinderkrankenschwestern," 2 August 1966, § 1, section 2, Bundesministerium für Justiz (ed.) 1966, *Bundesgesetzblatt*, Part I, Bundesanzeiger, Bonn, pp. 462–365, here p. 462.

46 See Ziemann, B. 2006, "The Gospel of Psychology: Therapeutic Concepts and the Scientification of Pastoral Care in the West German Catholic Church (1950–1980)," *Central European History*, vol. 39, pp. 79–106.

47 See Baumann, W. 1967, "Gruppenarbeit und Gruppendynamik in der Krankenpflege," *Die Agnes Karll-Schwester*, vol. 21, pp. 4–5, here p. 4; Kelber, M. 1964, "Die Kunst der Gesprächsführung im Einzelgespräch," *Die Agnes Karll-Schwester*, vol. 18, pp. 136–137.

48 See Dörrie, K. 1964, "Zur ,sozialen Rolle' des Patienten," *Die Agnes Karll-Schwester*, vol. 18, pp. 132–135, here 135.

49 See Schildt, A. 1999, *Ankunft im Westen. Ein Essay zur Erfolgsgeschichte der Bundesrepublik*, S. Fischer Verlag, Frankfurt/Main, pp. 181–189.

50 See Ziemann, "Gospel," pp. 98–104.

51 See Hölzel-Seipp, L. 1969, "Der praktische Krankenpflegeprozess," *Die Agnes Karll-Schwester*, vol. 23, pp. 201–203.

52 See Hörl, E. & Hagner, M. 2008, "Überlegungen zur kybernetischen Transformation des Humanen," Hörl, E. & Hagner, M. (eds.) *Die Transformation des Humanen: Beiträge zur Kulturgeschichte der Kybernetik*, Suhrkamp, Frankfurt/Main, pp. 7–37, here pp. 11–12.

53 See Hörl/Hagner, "Überlegungen," p. 11; Friesacher, H. 2011, "Macht durch Steuerung: Zur Kybernetisierung von Pflege und Gesundheit," Remmers, H. (ed.) *Pflegewissenschaft im interdisziplinären Dialog: Eine Forschungsbilanz*, V&R unipress, Göttingen, pp. 343–367, here pp. 347–348.

54 See Juchli, L. 1979, *Allgemeine und spezielle Krankenpflege: Ein Lehr- und Lernbuch*, 3rd edn., Thieme Verlag, Stuttgart, pp. 19–23.

55 See Friesacher, "Macht," p. 348; Henderson, V. 1982, "The Nursing Process – Is the Title Right?," *Journal of Advanced Nursing*, vol. 7, pp. 103–109, here pp. 107–109; Hülsken-Giesler, M. 2008, *Der Zugang zum Anderen. Zur theoretischen Rekonstruktion von Professionalisierungsstrategien pflegerischen Handelns im Spannungsfeld von Mimesis und Maschinenlogik*, V&R unipress, Göttingen, pp. 313–331.

56 See Habermann, M. & Uys, L.R. (eds.) 2005, *The Nursing Process: A Global Concept*, Elsevier Churchill-Livingstone, Edinburgh, p. 3.

57 Raphael, "Verwissenschaftlichung," pp. 165–193.

58 See Eckart, W.U. 2005, *Geschichte der Medizin*, Springer, Heidelberg, pp. 270–277.

PART 4

Nursing and the "practice turn"

10

PROTESTANT NURSING CARE IN GERMANY IN THE 19TH CENTURY

Concepts and social practice[1]

Karen Nolte

With the recent "practice turn" in the field of history, the main focus is again the daily life and the activities of ordinary people.[2] At the center of scholarly interest are people's daily activities and individual practices, but the historians analyze them in close relation to discourses and structures of which these agents were a part. The starting point for this "practice turn"[3] is Pierre Bourdieu's concept of social practice.[4] Bourdieu regards the practices that social agents perform as an implicit knowledge but at the same time assumes that discourses and norms are performatively created through such practices. Utilizing this praxeological point of view, this chapter brings a new perspective to the German history of nursing care in the 19th century and focuses in particular on the nurses' actions and spheres of influence while also investigating the relationship between the practices, discourses and structures in this context. It concentrates on Protestant nursing care which, due to its type of training and community style of living and working, became very influential for German nursing care in the 19th century.

Protestant nurses were mainly deaconesses who lived and worked in a strictly regulated community. While the founder of the first German deaconess motherhouse in Kaiserswerth, Theodor Fliedner (1800–1864), had originally planned to train daughters from the better circles of the educated middle class for this vocation, the actual deaconesses were mainly women from the lower middle class with either an urban or a rural background. Since Fliedner led the community in a family-like and paternalistic way, both the male and the female principals considered themselves as superiors and "parents" of their deaconesses. In return for subordinating their life to the requirements of the motherhouse, the sisters received care when they fell ill and in old age.

Historian Claudia Bischoff[5] emphasizes the normative restrictions and patriarchal structure of the community of deaconesses. Similarly, theologian Jutta Schmidt, in her nuanced study of the social composition of deaconess communities in the 19th century, argues that the community of deaconesses was not very appealing to women from the educated middle class.[6] Both studies emphasize the repressive patriarchic character of the deaconess communities. The notion of suppression that these scholars stress, however, adheres to a one-dimensional notion of power and does not explain why so many young women joined the community of deaconesses. Theologian Silke Köser, by contrast, argues that, following Max Weber, a power relationship needs to be borne by both parties: the rulers and the ruled. She establishes how the principal pastor at the institution for deaconesses in Kaiserswerth managed to create a hierarchical structure (and thus the power of the principals at the motherhouse) by forming this particular mother-house culture and by building an identity of the deaconesses that rested on the community. The deaconesses accepted their (inferior) status in this hierarchical order because their superiors provided the security of belonging that formed the basis of deaconesses' identity. According to Köser, central to this establishment of a "collective identity" were the distinct dresses of the deaconesses, the deaconesses' initiation with a festive confirmation, the maintaining of the community through regular letter exchanges with the deaconesses on site, and finally the regular return of those deaconesses "in the field" to the motherhouse.[7]

My arguments build on Köser's research while also drawing on studies on female religiosity in the 19th century which point out that women were crucial as facilitators of the Christian faith within the context of a bourgeois culture of piety (*Frömmigkeits-kultur*).[8] Thus I will show how the deaconesses appropriated the "collective identities" in their everyday practices and what spheres of action this process opened. I argue that the thorough training the nurses received, to become both missionaries to the unfaithful in their homeland and professionals in physical nursing care, strengthened their position with respect to physicians.

This argument is based on the extensive collection of detailed letters sent by the nurses whom the motherhouse had placed in hospitals as well as in community and private care, held in the archive of the Fliedner foundation in Kaiserwerth near Düsseldorf. The deaconesses reported to the motherhouse not only about their work, their experiences and newly gained knowledge, but also about their daily conflicts with the patients, other deaconesses and, more rarely, the physicians and pastors. Since the letters were addressed to the principal couple of the motherhouse – in the first years Theodor Fliedner and his wife Caroline – the Sisters tried to fulfill their expectations of a deaconess. The principals of the motherhouse, in turn, chose individual letters to present as examples in the in-house journal "The Friend of the Poor and the Sick," published for the community of Sisters and the supporters of the institution for deaconesses. This circumstance may also have influenced the Sisters' writing behavior. The journal appeared six times a year and had between 30 and 40 pages. Keeping this background in mind, these letters are nonetheless foremost self-testimonials shaped by a normative pressure and revealing ruptures – especially when the nurses described conflicts with the social surroundings.[9] These ruptures and the descriptions of the daily routines form the starting point of a history of social practice.[10]

Nursing care in 19th-century Germany

Around 1800 organizations were founded in Germany that dedicated themselves to the nursing care of poor people. These were women's associations that were dedicated to caring for the sick and poor, or Catholic orders for nursing care,[11] or motherhouses of deaconesses. Those working within these organizations of care reacted to the dramatic changes in society at the time. When industrialization began in Germany at the beginning of the 19th century, German cities transformed into metropolises into which the impoverished population from rural areas flocked to search for opportunities to earn a living. In large cities people who became sick could no longer be cared for at home, because all family members had to work for their livelihood. Hence, poor patients received either poor care or none at all. Disease posed a significant risk of impoverishment for the workers, artisans and servants who already lived just above the poverty level. Women earned only half of what men received for working in the factory or service professions. When the male breadwinner of the family either fell ill for a long period of time or died, the family or the widow could only exist with the aid of poor relief. Bourgeois society discussed the impoverishment occurring on a huge scale under the tagline "the social question." Due to the close relation between disease and poverty, care for the sick was understood as a measure against poverty.[12]

In 1836, the young pastor Theodor Fliedner founded a training institution for Protestant nurses in the impoverished community of Kaiserswerth near Düsseldorf which, by happenstance, was a Catholic region. As a model, he drew on the Catholic Sisters of Mercy and referred to the first deaconesses described in the communities of the New Testament. For Fliedner, referring to the occupation of those first deaconesses was not an attempt to be historically precise; rather he was looking for grounds to justify a professional life for women in the community.[13] Fliedner sympathized with a revival movement that, since the end of the 18th century, had been causing a religious awakening. These revivalists had been putting the practical Christian lifestyle of the individual at the center of their Christian self-understanding. Due to the inter-denominational features of this religious awakening movement, Fliedner had no fundamental reservations about Catholicism, which explains the mixture of Catholic and Protestant elements in the community of deaconesses.[14]

After the founding of the deaconate at Kaiserswerth, additional motherhouses were established throughout the German Reich. The institution for deaconesses in Kaiserswerth became a model for all subsequent communities of deaconesses founded within Germany, and also in the rest of Europe and the United States.

The Protestant philanthropists and the deaconesses regarded poverty as a result of a "spiritual poverty," i.e. a lack of piety. For that reason they considered the re-Christianization of the faithless, which was also called "inner mission," to be the central measure against poverty in their homeland. The concept of the "inner mission" must be understood within the context of the colonial history of the 19th century: Numerous associations were founded to convert the so-called heathens – unbelieving Christians – in the home country, a notion that was derived from the missions in the German colonies in Africa. These associations were dedicated to religious social work that focused on fighting alcoholism, prostitution and other manifestations of a sinful life to which the lower classes had succumbed due to their lack of faith.[15] The bourgeois Protestant notion of the "inner mission" was thus a reaction to the pauperization that had been perceived as a problem, especially in larger cities. Fliedner and other protagonists of the "inner mission" shared the opinion that disease and material and spiritual impoverishment were causally linked. For that reason the sisters, in addition to caring for the body, also concerned themselves with the patients' salvation.[16]

Norms and regulations

Theodor Fliedner's concept of a community of deaconesses followed the contemporary model of the bourgeois family according to which the husband was his wife's guardian.[17] Hence, according to bourgeois norms, it was unsuitable for unmarried women to move about in public on their own, and it was likewise inappropriate for reputable bourgeois ladies to have an occupation. Honorable bourgeois women were allowed to pursue very few occupations outside the house. While bourgeois ladies worked as teachers, they straddled the fine line between acceptance and rejection.[18] Taking care of the poor was one of the few tasks that a bourgeois woman could take up in the public sphere without suffering damage to her reputation. Offering unmarried women a community in which the principal couple adopted the position of parents and ensured legal security and respect in society, Fliedner wanted to create a model for a life beyond marriage or the pitiful existence of an unmarried woman who had to live and depend on her parents or siblings until she was old.[19] The pastor introduced a uniform for the nurses that corresponded to the garments of a married woman to provide a visible sign that deaconesses were honorable: Their floor-length dresses in dark blue were made from expensive cloth (Figure 10.1). The deaconesses also wore white lace bonnets which up to then had only been worn by married women when in public to signal that they were literally "under the bonnet," which even entered the German language as an idiom for being married. As Jutta Schmidt has pointed out, it was not the daughters of pastors or other educated women that came to Kaiserswerth to become part of the community of deaconesses, but rather women with very little education from a petty rural or petty bourgeois background.[20]

In the paternally "ruled" family that was the community of deaconesses, the principal's strict role as a patriarch was crucial to earn the respect of society for this cohabitation and collaboration with unmarried women.[21] One expression of the patriarchal structure was the concept of sending the deaconesses to work where they were needed: The principal couple of the deaconesses' motherhouse decided where the nurses were to work and how long they had to stay at their post. The deaconesses from Kaiserswerth were sent to both denominational and municipal hospitals.[22] The municipal hospitals appreciated Protestant nurses since they had received a thorough training in physical care. The hospitals and the deaconesses' motherhouse signed a contract that determined the working conditions according to the "House Order and Rules of Service" in Kaiserswerth and also decided how much the directors of the hospital had to pay the motherhouse for the deaconess' work. In addition to room and

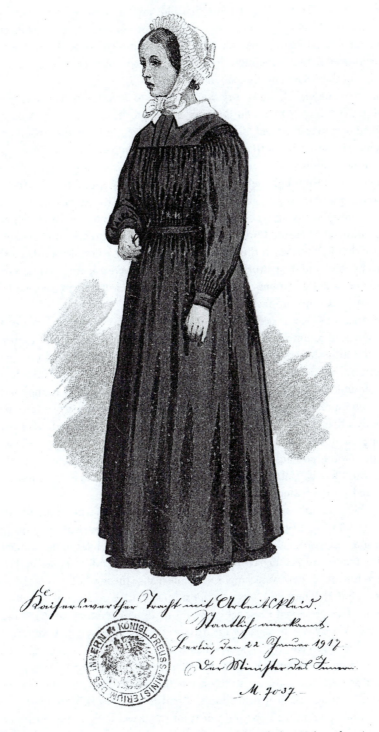

Figure 10.1 A deaconess in her dress. Archive of the *Fliedner Kulturstiftung* in Kaiserswerth. Reproduced with permission.

board, the deaconesses received a financial allowance and everyday necessities from the motherhouse. Deaconesses ended up in private or community care when the church communities hired them to care for members in their own homes. In this case, a contract was negotiated between the motherhouse and the community or, in the case of private care, the motherhouse and the patient.[23]

The deaconesses' life and work were subject to strict rules that had been written down in the "House Order and Rules of Service for Deaconesses."[24] A deaconess was supposed to perceive herself as a servant not only of God but also of her patients and her fellow nurses. It was strongly expected that the nurses were to display an attitude marked by humility and self-denial. The deaconesses were supposed to subject themselves to a thorough "self-examination" with duty, humility and self-denial at its core and, if possible, to do so on a daily basis. Thus they were supposed not only to live a pious lifestyle but also to internalize the central rules of the motherhouse.[25] Furthermore, the "House Order and Rules of Service" also served to secure the social order of the deaconesses in the hospital, in which they had to subordinate themselves to the physician and the pastor. Simultaneously they were asked to assume a dominating position towards the patients and male and female paid untrained care workers, and to keep a social distance from them.

Applying the idea of performative changes of norms to the example of Protestant nursing care, through the deaconesses' everyday dealings and actions, their normative frame of action shifted. The "House Order and Rules of Service" of the first German institution for deaconesses in Kaiserswerth illustrates this well. As Silke Köser points out, its founder had to adapt his orders and instructions constantly to the social practice in the community of deaconesses; between 1837 and 1864 there were five revisions of this body of rules which was meant as a guideline for the attitude and work of the deaconesses. In the second version, created in 1850, a fund for the nurses was initiated since the prohibition against accepting gifts, which had been included in the rules in 1839, could not be upheld because, in reality, when the nurses had been successful in caring for their patients they received such gifts.[26]

Another example of an individual's appropriation of and resultant revision of Fliedner's set of regulations can be seen in a deaconess' personal copy of the "House Order and Rules of Service." The official rules did not only refer to the concrete nursing practice and the Sisters' behavior within the community of deaconesses. Rather, they spoke to how the Sisters were supposed to internalize the ideal of self-denial, willingness to serve and the required religious position using a catalogue of self-examining questions. This preserved personal copy of one deaconess' copy of the "House Order and Rules of Service" shows how she had thoroughly reviewed these questions, replacing the printed passages with her own handwritten expressions, and even deleted whole questions from the catalogue without replacing them. Thus this deaconess obviously regarded as superfluous the question on whether she had always been diligent to learn practices such as "surgical procedures," "female handiwork" or "gardening work." Furthermore, it seems that she did not want to answer daily the question of whether she had sufficiently sought to please and cheer up her patients, the children and other wards. The deaconess even deleted the whole paragraph that discusses whether and how she should conduct devotions with her patients. We cannot know from this source whether she regarded herself as impeccable in these areas or whether she thought these questions unnecessary for other reasons. Most of the small adaptations in the text apparently served the purpose of formulating the self-examining questions so that they corresponded to her own way of expressing herself and giving the catalogue her own touch.[27]

Training

After their arrival in Kaiserswerth the young women who would be deaconesses began their thorough training in matters of physical and spiritual care. The training usually lasted six months but could take much longer depending on the needs and ability of the individual nurse. The "parents" of the motherhouse decided when a nurse on probation was ready to be sent to a hospital or into private care in different communities. After her apprenticeship the nurse on probation was "handed over" to an older, more experienced deaconess, the so-called probation mistress. At first the nurse on probation had to work in the kitchen, the household or the laundry and was taught "female" needle works. Only at the hospital of the institution for deaconesses in Kaiserswerth (Figure 10.2) could a young nurse get practical experience in caring for patients with mild diseases from a mentoring nurse.[28]

Together with a physician, Fliedner lectured on theory in the motherhouse, the so-called "Medical Course" (*Medicinischer Cursus*). The female principal, Caroline Fliedner (1811–1892), taught practical courses on physical care for the nurses on probation.[29] Both the theoretical and the practical courses were based on the manuals on attending to patients that the Berlin physicians Johann Friedrich Dieffenbach (1792–1847) and Carl Emil Gedike (1787–1867) had written. These two doctors worked and taught nursing at the Berlin *Charité*.[30] Handwritten resources on the training of deaconesses illustrate that, contrary to Bischoff's argument,[31] the deaconesses were indeed meticulously trained in physical care and even learned skills that were otherwise executed by non-academic surgeons[32] upon the order of an academic physician.

The transcripts of the lessons from around 1850 by Theodor Fliedner paint a detailed picture of the training. The curriculum demanded the following central qualities of a nurse: "Attention both to the symptoms of the disease but also to what is going on within the patient," "presence of mind," "cold-bloodedness without toughness and indifference," "leniency when dealing with the patients but without sentimentality," "cheerfulness in the right sense," "discretion," "truthfulness," "punctuality" and "agreeableness." Furthermore a nurse had to have "physical strength" and had to get used to practicing "neatness and cleanliness."[33] The transcript further reveals that nurses received a basic knowledge of anatomy, and detailed explanations of all practical activities involved in physical care. Apart from washing the bedding and the patients, wound care and the correct administration of medications, the following practical skills were part of the curriculum: blood-letting, cupping, application of leeches and of fontanelles. This last procedure involved opening the skin and inserting a hair-rope to achieve "good purulence" through which substances of the disease were supposed to be drained

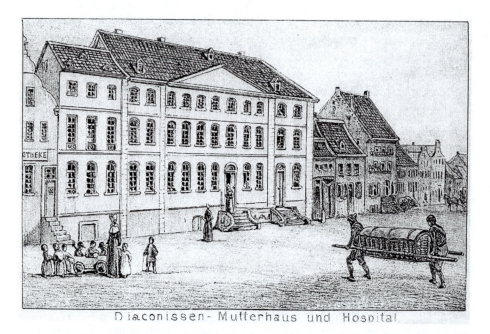

Figure 10.2 Deaconess motherhourse and hospital in Kaiserwerth around 1859, Archive of the *Fliedner Kulturstiftung* in Kaiserwerth. Reproduced with permission.

out. During the first half of the 19th century these surgical procedures were performed by barbers and non-academic surgeons. However, deaconesses were supposed to take on therapeutic tasks when no surgeon was available.[34] Due to their surgical skills, the nurses were in principle capable of crossing the line between the functions of the nurse and of the physician. Letters from community nurses in Kleve who reported to the motherhouse reveal that deaconesses indeed performed these procedures. Cupping and applying leeches were self-evident parts of their daily tasks with the patients.[35]

Theodor Fliedner also instructed "his" deaconesses thoroughly in the care of the patient's soul. While the nurse was required to pay attention to the patient's physical suffering, she also had to silently watch the behavior of her patient to gain an understanding about the condition of his or her soul. It was crucial that these observations occurred right after taking on the patient. After only a few days of observation the deaconesses were to ask the patient about their confirmation and check how well they knew the Ten Commandments. She also had to probe to what extent the patient was willing to reflect on his violations of the Commandments. For the care of the soul the following basic idea applied: The more a patient's character was like that of a child, the more promising the efforts for his or her soul would be. According to contemporary notions of the educated middle class, uneducated people were supposedly more open to the care of the soul than educated patients; young patients were thought to be more willing than older patients and women were assumed to be more open than men.[36] From the deaconesses' point of view the care for their patients' salvation was an act of caring without which the healing from a severe disease was impossible. After all, the

Christian caretakers interpreted disease either as the result of a sinful lifestyle or, when the patients were pious, as a touchstone of God.

Daily nursing routine

Physical care was a significant part of the daily practice, yet the letters the nurses wrote to the motherhouse focused mainly on the care of the soul. A crucial reason for this was that care of the soul was central to the self-understanding of the community of deaconesses and even more important than physical care. Since physical care belonged to the daily routine it was presumably not worth mentioning in too much detail. For, of course, the teachers at the motherhouse knew perfectly well how each step of physical care was to be performed.[37] Therefore the Protestant nurses described each small case study of successful or failed attempts to heal the patient's condition of the soul.

Care of the soul

The narratives about conflicts with patients reveal how the pious nurses proceeded with those who resisted their religious teachings. According to the "Instructionen"[38] the nurses initially offered to read to the patients from the Bible or wholesome writings and to pray the Psalms with them. In addition, singing the hymns together was supposed to strengthen the sufferer's faith. Patients who did not want to be bothered with God or the Protestant faith had to endure the (at times not so) gentle pressure that the deaconesses exerted. Especially with severe cases the deaconesses saw an urgent need for action. They told dying patients about the approaching end and asked them whether they would be able to pass God's judgment.[39]

The deaconesses regarded some patients by default as sinful because of contemporary moralizing concepts of particular diseases. Syphilis patients endured judgmental approaches, as did patients with consumption, who supposedly had led extravagant lives with excessive diets and lax morals. Since the end of the 18th century the state had shown an increased interest in the bodies of its subjects as economic resources. Particularly people from the lower social classes were to be trained in health-conscious behavior. While the state did not explicitly require such training, an improved overall health of its people conformed with its population policies. Consequently an excessive lifestyle with respect to diet took on a moral dimension and the patient himself was held responsible for the loss of his health. Deaconesses reported from impoverished neighborhoods that fathers would drink at the tavern instead of providing their children with healthy food. Observing a lack of faith and immorality, they regarded the sinful, excessive lifestyle as the "germ" for the consumption that was spreading among the poor.[40] The letters by the Kaiserswerth nurses contain many complaints about consumption patients who were perceived as a special challenge with respect to the care of the soul, since they more frequently rejected the religious training.[41]

By contrast, the nurses identified with pious patients and at times lived through crises of faith together with them. For instance, one nurse read "some passages from Job" to a patient in the final stages of uterine cancer. She suggested to the patient and her husband to identify with Job, who had been tried by God with severe suffering. In this way the nurse also overcame her own crisis of faith.[42] This case, which the nurse described very movingly, illustrates that it was the deaconess who was present at the deathbed and thus was able to address questions and crises of faith, instead of the community pastor, who could only visit the patients every so often. Since the deaconess was on site, the patients and families probably did not call for the pastor in such moments of need.

In special cases, the deaconesses also took on the spiritual guidance of dying patients, as can be deduced from another story that Sister Sophie, a Kaiserswerth deaconess, told the motherhouse in one of her letters: An old lady who suffered from "chest disease" and dropsy was approaching the end of her life. The nurse had diagnosed this and the patient herself was very aware that she was dying. However, her daughter and daughter-in-law apparently refused to believe that the lady would soon pass away and tried to raise her hopes. For that reason they did not fulfill her last wish to call for a pastor to pray with her. Proudly the Sister reported how she consoled the dying patient, stood in for a pastor and stayed with the lady during her last moments.[43] While the deaconesses liked to take on the spiritual tasks of the pastors, at times they also openly criticized how the pastors they encountered in the community perceived their professional tasks. Sister Luise, for instance, complained in 1846: "I think the situation would be different if the pastors visited the poor and sick people more frequently but they don't know them. Dear Pastor, people cannot reform themselves if the Lord does not do it but He has his tool also within mankind."[44]

Since the line between care of the soul and spiritual care was blurred, Fliedner and his successors at Kaiserswerth wrote a number of clarifications on this issue. Accordingly, the deaconess was supposed to be the "spiritual caretaker on a small scale," i.e., she was responsible for the "small" issues of faith and thus was supposed do the groundwork for the pastor. In the opinion of the principals of the motherhouses the pastor was in charge for the "perceptions" of spiritual care that "addressed larger issues." In other words, the pastor was ascribed a leading position in the spiritual care at the hospital. However, in reality the pastors were seldom on site to fulfill their spiritual care duties, since they also performed community tasks outside of the hospital. For that reason it was the nurses who assumed a central role in caring for the souls of the patients.[45]

Terminal care

The Christian nurses considered dying consciously as the last opportunity for the severely ill patient to recognize his or her own sinfulness. Turning to the Lord at this last moment would allow them to die blissfully. The deaconesses' obituaries emphasize in particular the dying phase of the various nurses, inscribing these texts into a tradition that had begun a while before.[46] Since the end of the 18th century the Protestant bourgeoisie, in particular pietistic circles, had been describing the last hours of deceased family members in detail. These depictions showed the piousness of a family and also served as a memory of the departed. Part of the ongoing theme of these descriptions was the emphasis on how patiently the deceased had suffered through great pain.[47]

Building on these bourgeois descriptions of dying, the submissive attitude the nurse showed to God as well as pain and suffering was stressed. During their life the pious caregivers interpreted a severe disease that they barely survived as God's biggest award. Indeed, the deaconesses thank God in many letters that He tried them with a severe disease but let them live. Matthias Benad coined the term "piousness of dying" (*Sterbefrömmigkeit*) for these popular depictions and identified them as the center of the deaconesses' religious self-understanding.[48] The nurses wanted to convey the experience of dying as a religious purification and the feeling of being especially close to God with their severely ill and dying patients.

To begin as early as possible with the care of the soul of dying patients, the deaconesses had a keen interest in the terminally ill patients' knowing at the earliest possible stage about their lethal prognosis. However, in the 19th century many physicians rejected the idea of informing severely ill patients about their imminent death. According to contemporary medical thinking, the physicians assumed that the fear of death could cause an "emotional upset" (*Gemütserschütterung*) and subsequently a deterioration of the physical condition, or even a premature death. Towards the end of the 19th century, the notion of the "emotional upset" was no longer valid, but now the doctors were afraid that terminally ill patients would take their own life right after the physician had explained the imminent end to them. For this reason, many doctors took a critical stand towards the care of the soul by clergymen at the deathbed because they were afraid that the pastors would talk too openly and would frighten the terminally ill patients with such conversations. However, physicians did not necessarily have a negative attitude to Christian terminal care – some physicians regarded themselves as the better spiritual caregivers because, in their opinion, the doctor was the symbol of hope while they believed that the patients perceived the clergyman as a messenger of death.[49]

In principle there was a conflict between the physicians' idea of how to deal with dying patients and the deaconesses' Christian convictions. At times the doctors demanded that the deaconesses conceal from the patients that they were dying. In such situations the nurses were in conflict between their professional duty to obey the doctors and the Christian duty to provide their patients with a death in peace. There are very few descriptions of such conflicts in the letters by the nurses, presumably because the deaconesses were only interested in the doctors' orders in the area of physical care. The care of the soul was regarded as the deaconesses' domain. Here they asked the principals of the motherhouse for advice. Many letters by the nurses reveal that the deaconesses initiated the religious terminal care independently and without any reservations. There seem to have been conflicts only when physicians explicitly required them not to talk with the terminally ill patients about their imminent death: pursuant to the guidelines of service, the nurses had to obey doctors' orders. However, when doctors remained silent on the question of informing dying patients about their situation and providing religious aid, the deaconesses acted of their own accord.[50] In one case a deaconess who took care of a terminally ill girl had to obey the doctor's orders to conceal the girl's imminent death from the parents. The parents were still full of hope that their child would get well again and the doctor did nothing to change that belief, which the nurse clearly condemned. In another case, two community nurses even wanted to terminate the care because the doctor had demanded from them that they should lie to their patients who suffered from typhus. Here the situation was resolved when the patients learned the truth through other channels.[51]

In many letters the deaconesses describe the experience of their patients' suffering, dying, and death as an "uplifting feeling" that made the sisters feel "God's almightiness." This handling of death can be seen firstly as a deeply felt religiosity. Yet it also served as a mechanism to cope with this borderline experience during which the deaconesses working in home care were often completely on their own. Caring for dying patients who strictly refused a religious monitoring of death was consequently very hard for them. For example, the deaconesses emphasized in their letters how they went to these sinful terminally ill persons "with a heavy heart which had not changed leaving them."[52] In the nurses' descriptions, the condition of the soul of these godless critically ill people was reflected in the visible mortal agony these "sinners" suffered. At times the pious nurses became so afraid watching this pain that they could only approach the deathbed of these "difficult" patients in the company of a second deaconess.[53] Fear of the "devil incarnate" and a possible contestation of their own faith may well have been reasons why the nurses sometimes, when they were alone, walked away from the deathbed and into the center of the room.[54]

Another good illustration for how uncanny handling death was for young nurses is a letter that describes how the deaconess overcame her "fear of a corpse" during her practical experience, which had haunted her during her time of training in the motherhouse. Together with a woman from the community, she undressed the dead woman. Since she was the only nurse present, she had to overcome her fear.[55]

Conclusion

In the 19th century deaconesses were bound by a strict set of rules, norms and even social control. A praxeological perspective enables the illustration of how practices of Protestant nursing care were integrated into these structures while simultaneously creating them and also shifting their boundaries. The catalogue of self-examining questions is a nice example of the daily or at least regularly ritualized performative creation of the order and the normative ideas set by the motherhouse. A Sister's personal copy of the examining questions reveals, however, the extent to which such a normative framework was reworked and, through that revision, also adopted in real life. This process of revising and adopting also becomes apparent in the many "new editions" of the "House Order and Rules of Service" with which Fliedner responded to the practical experiences of the community of deaconesses.

The order and training of deaconesses already laid out the opportunities for spheres of action within the strictly hierarchically organized work of the nurses: as the case stories presented reveal, the line between spiritual care, which was one of the core competencies of the pastor, and care of the soul, which was the nurses' main area of competence, was blurry. At times the deaconesses consciously adopted the tasks of a clergyman and had many criticisms of how the pastors performed their tasks.

Apparently this activity of the nurses that fell in the pastors' domain was perceived as a problem, so the principals had reasons to clearly define the tasks of nurses and pastors in the area of spiritual care at the hospital.

The relationship between deaconesses and physicians that was also clearly defined in the "House Order and Rules of Service" was also more complex in real life. The deaconesses received some training in the area of small surgery and they were in principle allowed to perform such medical tasks when no surgeon was available. In other words the deaconesses were able to enter the realm of doctor's competency by deciding and performing themselves procedures such as bloodletting, cupping and applying leeches or fontanelles.

Yet the requirement to obey the physician at all times collided with the deaconesses' central task, namely to care for the soul. Fliedner and the nurses regarded the care of the soul as the competency of caregivers and thus placed it at the core of their notion of Protestant nursing care. For that reason the nurses experienced a conflict between their duty for obedience and their commitment to the dying patients' salvation when the doctor demanded to conceal from the patients their imminent death. In general, however, the nurses decided when to initiate their care for the soul of the dying patients without consultation with the doctors.

The care of the soul as the core area of Protestant nursing care points to the significance of female religiosity in the daily practice of nursing care these nurses experienced. Their role as facilitators of the Christian faith that they had adopted within the community of deaconesses enabled them to encounter pastors and physicians alike in a self-confident manner. Hence the religious foundation of the work of Protestant nurses did not only contribute to their humble attitude with respect to male authorities that had so far been the main point of emphasis in the studies of deaconesses. Rather their task to bring the Christian faith to the patients and to take care of their souls also had an empowering effect for the deaconesses. Studying the simultaneity of subordination and empowerment more thoroughly could initiate a change of perspective and thus a reassessment of the history of nursing care in the 19th century.

Notes

1 Translated by Ulrike Nichols.
2 S. Reichhardt, 2007, "Praxeologische Geschichtswissenschaft. Eine Diskussionsanregung." *Sozial. Geschichte*, 3, 22, pp. 43–65.
3 On the "practice turn" see T. Schatzki, K. Knorr-Cetina and E. v. Savigny 2001 (eds.), *The Practice Turn in Contemporary Theory*, Routledge: London; A. Reckwitz, 2003, "Grundelemente einer Theorie sozialer Praktiken. Eine sozialtheoretische Perspektive", *Zeitschrift für Soziologie*, 32, 4, pp. 282–301; Reichardt, Praxeologische Geschichtswissenschaft.
4 P. Bourdieu, 1999, *Sozialer Sinn. Kritik der theoretischen Vernunft*, Suhrkamp: Frankfurt am Main (P. Bourdieu, 1980, *Le sens practique*, Paris).
5 C. Bischoff, 1997, *Frauen in der Krankenpflege. Zur Entwicklung von Frauenrolle und Frauenberufstätigkeit im 19. und 20. Jahrhundert*, Campus: Frankfurt am Main.
6 J. Schmidt, 1998, *Beruf: Schwester. Mutterhausdiakonie im 19. Jahrhundert*, Campus: Frankfurt am Main.

7 S.C. Köser, 2006, *Denn eine Diakonisse darf kein Alltagsmensch sein. Kollektive Identitäten Kaiserswerther Diakonissen 1836–1914*, Leipzig: Evangelische Verlagsanstalt.

8 R. Habermas, 1994, "Weibliche Religiosität – oder: Von der Fragilität bürgerlicher Identitäten," in K. Tenfelde and H.U. Wehler (eds.), *Wege zur Geschichte des Bürgertums*, Vandenhoeck & Ruprecht: Göttingen, pp. 125–148; I. Götz Von Olenhusen, 1995, "Die Feminisierung von Religion und Kirche im 19. und 20. Jahrhundert," in I. Götz von Olenhusen (ed.), *Frauen unter dem Patriarchat der Kirchen*, Kohlhammer: Stuttgart, pp. 9–21; U. Gause, 1998, "Frauen und Frömmigkeit im 19. Jahrhundert: Der Aufbruch in die Öffentlichkeit," *Pietismus und Neuzeit*, 24, pp. 309–327; U. Gause, 2001, "Friederike Fliedner und die 'Feminisierung des Religiösen' im 19. Jahrhundert," in M. Friedrich, N. Friedrich, T. Jähnichen and J.C. Kaiser (eds.), *Sozialer Protestantismus im Vormärz*, LIT-Verlag: Münster, pp. 123–131.

9 Letters, Archive of the Fliedner Cultural Foundation (Archiv der Fliedner Kulturstiftung = AFKSK).

10 For reconstructing the practical and theoretical training in nursing care that the deaconesses received, additional handwritten sources from the archive in Kaiserswerth are enlightening. For instance, the transcripts a nurse on probation took during a "Medical Course" offer insight into the kind of medical training and lessons on physical care the deaconesses received; see: T. Fliedner, Medicinischer Cursus, Heft I–III, AFKSK, Sign.: Rep. II: Fd 1.3. Fliedner's "Instructions for the initial care of the soul" formed the basis of the practice of the so-called care of the soul, i.e. tending to ensure the salvation of the patients; see: Theodor Fliedner, Instruktionen für die erste Seelenpflege bei einem Kranken (Instructions for the initial care for the soul of a patient), AFKSK: Rep. II: Fb.

11 Since the Middle Ages Catholic orders had been dedicated to the care of poor patients. After the Reformation many monasteries were closed. Most of the orders that survived the Reformation were dissolved in the 18th century when, as a result of the Enlightenment, a secularization process began. Around 1830 a new wave of founding Catholic orders for nursing care began, since at this time the State embraced the Catholic care for poor patients as a measure in the fight against poverty; see: R. Meiwes, 2000, *"Arbeiterinnen des Herrn". Katholische Frauenkongregationen im 19. Jahrhundert*, Campus: Frankfurt; R. Meiwes, 2008, "Katholische Frauenkongregationen und die Krankenpflege im 19. Jahrhundert," *L'Homme. Europäische Zeitschrift für Feministische Geschichtswissenschaft*, 19, 1, pp. 39–60.

12 C. Sachße and F. Tennstedt (eds.), 1980, *Geschichte der Armenfürsorge in Deutschland. Vom Spätmittelalter bis zum 1. Weltkrieg*, Kohlhammer: Stuttgart, pp. 222–243.

13 Schmidt, Beruf: Schwester, p. 249; Köser, Denn eine Diakonisse, p. 93.

14 Köser, Denn eine Diakonisse, pp. 91–92.

15 R. Habermas, 2008, "Mission im 19. Jahrhundert. Globale Netzte des Religiösen," *Historische Zeitschrift*, 287, pp. 646–647.

16 K. Nolte, 2009, "Pflege von Leib und Seele – Krankenpflege in Armutsvierteln des 19. Jahrhunderts," in S. Hähner-Rombach (ed.), *Alltag in der Krankenpflege: Geschichte und Gegenwart/Everyday Nursing Life, Past and Present*, Franz Steiner Verlag: Stuttgart, pp. 23–45.

17 Women could only sign contracts including working agreements with their guardian's approval. If they were not married, the closest male relative adopted that role.

18 E. Kleinau and C. Opitz (eds.), 1996, *Geschichte der Mädchen- und Frauenbildung*. Vol. 2: Vom Vormärz bis zur Gegenwart, Campus: Frankfurt am Main, pp. 85–202.

19 Bischoff, *Frauen in der Krankenpflege*, pp. 82–83.

20 Schmidt, Beruf: Schwester, pp. 167–182.

21 Schmidt, Beruf: Schwester; SC Köser, 2001, "'Denn eine Diakonisse darf = kann kein Alltagsmensch sein.' Zur Konstruktion kollektiver Identitäten in der Kaiserswerther Diakonie," in M. Friedrich, N. Friedrich, T. Jähnichen and J.C. Kaiser (eds.), *Sozialer Protestantismus im Vormärz*, LIT-Verlag: Münster, pp. 109–121.

22 One of the first municipal hospitals deaconesses were placed in was the hospital in Saarbrücken. W. Klein, 2002, "'Sie sehen mir alle mit freundlichen Gesichtern entgegen.' Die Beziehung zwischen Patienten und Krankenschwestern im Saarbrücker Bürgerhospital in der Mitte des 19. Jahrhunderts." *Medizin, Gesellschaft und Geschichte*, 21, pp. 63–90.

23 A. Sticker, 1960, *Die Entstehung der neuzeitlichen Krankenpflege. Deutsche Quellenstücke aus der ersten Hälfte des 19. Jahrhunderts*, Kohlhammer: Stuttgart, pp. 37–42; 282–319.

24 T. Fliedner, *Haus-Ordnung und Dienst-Anweisung für die Diakonissenanstalt zu Kaiserswerth* (House order and rules of service for 'Institution for Deaconesses in Kaiserswerth'), 1852, AFKSK, Sign.: Rep II Fc1.

25 Ibid.

26 Köser, Denn eine Diakonisse, pp. 191–251.

27 Fliedner, Haus-Ordnung.

28 E.C. Hummel, 1986, *Krankenpflege im Umbruch. Ein Beitrag zum Problem der Berufsfindung "Krankenpflege"*, Hans Ferdinand Schulz Verlag: Freiburg i.Br., pp. 14–15.

29 R. Felgentreff, 1998, *Das Diakoniewerk Kaiserswerth 1836–1998. Von der Diakonissenanstalt zum Diakoniewerk – ein Überblick*, Heimat- und Bürgerverein Kaiserswerth e.V.: Düsseldorf-Kaiserswerth, pp. 21–24.

30 C.E. Gedike, 1854, *Handbuch der Krankenwartung. Zum Gebrauch für die Krankenwart-Schule der K. Berliner Charité-Heilanstalt sowie zum Selbstunterricht*, August Hirschwald: Berlin; J.F. Dieffenbach, 1832, *Anleitung zur Krankenwartung*, August Hirschwald: Berlin.

31 Bischoff, *Frauen in der Krankenpflege*.

32 Passing on the empirical knowledge from generation to generation, these surgeons learnt their craft from experienced doctors.

33 T. Fliedner, Medicinischer Cursus, Heft I, § 20.

34 T. Fliedner, Medicinischer Cursus, Heft II, § 61.

35 Letters, Kleve Gemeinde (Community of Kleve) 1845–1854, AFKSK, Sign.: 1337.

36 Fliedner, Instruktionen; S Kreutzer and K Nolte, 2010, "Seelsorgerin 'im Kleinen' – Krankenseelsorge durch Diakonissen im 19. und 20. Jahrhundert," *Zeitschrift für medizinische Ethik*, 56, pp. 45–56.

37 From the sources it is impossible to reconstruct whether and to what extent the competent execution of physical care was monitored. The principals may have gained an impression of the physical care during their occasional visits at the locations to which the nurses had been sent. Presumably they could assume that everything was done properly when neither doctors nor patients complained.

38 Fliedner, Instruktionen.

39 Letters, Kleve Gemeinde (Community of Kleve) 1845–1854, AFKSK, Sign.: 1337, Sister Louise Türner and Sister Lisette Steiner: September 24 1847.

40 Letters Gemeinde Elberfeld 1846–1862, AFKSK: Sign.: 1787, Sister Elisabeth Born, June 30 1849.

41 K. Nolte, 2010, "Schwindsucht – Krankheit, Gesundheit und Moral im frühen 19. Jahrhundert," *Medizin, Gesellschaft und Geschichte*, 29, pp. 47–70.

42 Letters, Privatpflege (Private Care) 1888–1893(1894), AFKSK, Sign.: DA 201, Sister Sophie Stock, October 10 1893; K. Nolte, 2010, "Pflege von Sterbenden im 19. Jahrhundert. Eine ethikgeschichtliche Annäherung," in S. Kreutzer (ed.), *Transformationen pflegerischen Handelns. Institutionelle Kontexte und soziale Praxis vom 19. bis zum 21. Jahrhundert*, Vandenhoeck & Rupprecht: Göttingen, pp. 87–108.

43 Letters, Privatpflege, Sister Sophie Stock, January 2 1894.

44 Letters, Kleve Gemeinde, Sister Louise, February 18 1845.

45 Kreutzer/Nolte, Seelsorgerin 'im Kleinen'.

46 Köser, Denn eine Diakonisse, p. 364.

47 U. Gleixner, 2005, *Pietismus und Bürgertum: eine historische Anthropologie der Frömmigkeit. Württemberg 17. – 19. Jahrhundert*, Vandenhoeck & Rupprecht: Göttingen, pp. 195–209.

48 M. Benad, 1996, "Sterbefrömmigkeit im 'Boten von Bethel' 1894–1900," in M. Benad (ed.), *Diakonie der Religionen*, Peter Lang: Frankfurt am Main, pp. 39–48; Köser, Denn eine Diakonisse.

49 K. Nolte, 2010, "Ärztliche Praxis am Sterbebett in der ersten Hälfte des 19. Jahrhunderts," W. Bruchhausen and H.G. Hofer (eds.), *Ärztlicher Ethos im Kontext. Historische, phänomenologische und didaktische Analysen*, V&R press: Göttingen, pp. 39–58.

50 K. Nolte, 2008, "Telling the Painful Truth – Nurses and Physicians in the Nineteenth Century," *Nursing History Review*, 16, pp. 115–134; Heller, A., 1996, "'Da ist die Schwester nicht weggegangen von dem Bett . . .' Berufsgeschichtliche Aspekte der Pflege von Sterbenden im Krankenhaus in der ersten Hälfte des 20. Jahrhunderts," in E. Seidl and H. Steppe (eds.), *Zur Sozialgeschichte der Pflege in Österreich. Krankenschwestern erzählen über die Zeit von 1920 bis 1950*, Maudrich: Vienna, pp. 192–211.

51 K. Nolte, "Telling the painful truth."

52 K. Nolte, 2006, "Vom Umgang mit Tod und Sterben in der klinischen und häuslichen Krankenpflege des 19. Jahrhunderts," in S Braunschweig (ed.), *Pflege – Räume, Macht und Alltag*, Chronos: Zürich, pp. 165–174.

53 Letters, Kleve Gemeinde, Sister Dorothee Haube, February 11 1853.

54 Letters, Wuppertal-Elberfeld, Krankenhaus (Hospital), 1844–1850, AFKSK, Sign.: 1778, Sister Johanne Niendieker, January 1 1862.

55 Letters, Kleve Gemeinde, Sister Dorothee Haube, February 15 1848.

11

AGENTES DE ENLACE

Nursing professionalization and public health in 1940s and 1950s Argentina

Jonathan Hagood

On 26 July 1952, Eva Perón, the wife of the president of Argentina, passed away after a protracted battle with uterine cancer. Perón was affectionately known as "Evita" by the millions of primarily poor and working class people to whom she had been the public face of the Perón administration and of Peronism, its populist political program. Just months before, on May 7, the Argentine Congress had named her the "Spiritual Leader of the Nation," a title no one else would ever hold. Perón was joined in her final days by María Eugenia Álvarez, her personal nurse and the director of the School of Nursing operated by the Fundación Eva Perón (FEP), the charity organization created by Perón to implement social welfare programs that included the distribution of food, clothes, and medicine as well as the construction of homes, schools, and medical facilities.

In 1943, a fifteen-year-old Álvarez had talked her way into the two-year nursing program run by the Sociedad de la Beneficencia de la Capital, the well-heeled and elite-run charity organization that the upstart and populist FEP later superseded. For two years Álvarez worked during the day in the hospital "like a servant" and attended classes at night.[1] Years later, she met Perón when the first lady toured the Hospital Rivadavia where Álvarez worked, and Álvarez subsequently served as the director of the FEP's School of Nursing from 1951 to 1955, when a military coup removed President Perón from power. When later asked about the differences between the FEP's school and the program where she had received her nursing education just a decade before, Álvarez remarked, "Everything was completely different: the Foundation dignified the work of the nurse. It was another time . . . quite different, because [the FEP] had a first class curriculum."[2] With this distinction Álvarez drew attention to the two main ambitions of nursing professionalization that took place in 1940s and 1950s Argentina: greater respect and more rigorous education. Álvarez also drew attention to the FEP's nursing graduates, "who have been heads of nursing at the most important hospitals in the country [while] others are now directors of nursing schools at the highest levels, in reality true professionals."[3] With the phrase "true professionals," Álvarez signaled nursing's principal goal.

This chapter proposes that an examination of the historical development of nursing professionalization will enhance our understanding of the history of health care specialization in particular and the professionalization of occupations in general. The case of nursing professionalization in Argentina illustrates how contingent social, economic, and political factors as well as the interaction of health professions have shaped nursing professionalization.

By the early twentieth century, histories of medicine focused on great doctors or the intellectual history of the *material medica*, touching on histories of professionalization only tangentially, if at all. The initial effects of social history on the study of medicine in the 1930s led to initial histories of a medical "profession," but this approach was limited until sociologists in the 1940s and 1950s developed an interest in medicine as well as professions and occupations.[4] Even for sociologists, the concept of professionalization was implicitly historical because it included the idea that professions moved through a sequential set of stages, a feature that also linked professionalization to contemporary theories of modernization.[5]

For historians working on medical specialization – in general, research on specialization among physicians and not other health professionals – Rosen remains the definitive starting point. He argued that specialization depended on two main causes: social and economic forces (particularly urbanization, immigration, and what twenty-first-century scholars would label "globalization") and "antecedent and contemporary medical factors."[6] Later historians appended the list of socio-economic forces to include the pursuit of status within markets for medical services, and national studies such as those by Stevens viewed specialization as a necessary response to inevitable scientific advances and the growth of medical knowledge.[7]

More recently, Wiesz proposed two phases of specialization among physicians, with the transition between the two taking place roughly at the end of the nineteenth century.[8] One of his central arguments is that physicians collaborated with patients and institutions to divide medical work into categories. A sense among physicians of a united medical profession, medicine's commitment to scientific research, and the continued classification of medical knowledge meant that specialization was initially more about knowledge production and its dissemination rather than particular and differentiated skills or practices.

In the time between the work of Stevens and Weisz, many historical studies focused on medical specialties and histories of the medical profession in national contexts. These histories later became sources for synthetic attempts by sociologists to expand theories of professionalization, which linked it to social structures, interest groups, and the overall social, economic, and political environments in which professionalization took place. For example, Freidson distinguished between "professional dominance," generally achieved in concert with the state, and "consulting status," achieved through the support of the public.[9] Later sociologists explored relationships between professions and the concept of professional "encroachment."[10] Work that includes Larson's concept of an intentional "professional project" and Abbott's "system of professions" largely ignores specialization by recasting it as segmentation within a profession or as a collection of mini- or sub-professions.[11]

More recently, Freidson proposed understanding professionalization as the development of occupational control over work distinct from market or organizational forms of control.[12] Evetts summarizes the contemporary sociological understanding of a profession "as essentially the knowledge-based category of service occupations that usually follow a period of tertiary education and vocational training and experience."[13] Evetts also identifies the emergence of a different interpretation among sociologists of "professionalism as a discourse of occupational change and control."[14]

In summary, the literatures on medical specialization and professionalization agree that the development and maintenance of a self-regulating and externally validated specialty or profession is the product of social, economic, and political factors; relationships with other specialties and professions negotiated in the context of power; and the discourse about a given specialty or profession created by both members and other stakeholders. This last point is particularly relevant to the health care sector with its multiple professions – a "professional ecosystem" – and a clear, hierarchical power structure based on physician control. In this case, both theory and empirical evidence support the idea that the health care professions developed in the context of a discourse about those professions created by members, other health care professions, and patients, among others.

Historians of nursing have not entirely ignored the questions of specialization and professionalization, and research has highlighted historical factors such as the expansion and contraction of the pool of qualified nurses, debates over what constituted "qualified," subordination and competition within a hierarchy of health professions, and changes in employment setting and status – in particular, the move from private-duty home care to hospital work. For example, Schultheiss highlights the role played by gender and class in the professionalization of nursing in nineteenth-century France where, unlike in the US or the UK, men controlled nursing reform.[15] In their study of a training school for nurses in Minnesota, Olson and Walsh argue for balancing the view of nursing professionalization as a series of stages linked to rising standards in education with a recognition of nursing as a collection of manual skills learned through apprenticeship.[16]

Still, many historical studies of nursing professionalization have not taken advantage of the theoretical perspectives available through the literature on medical specialization and professionalization. Studies such as those by Ettinger on nurse-midwifery in the first half of the twentieth century and Ward on the history of nursing in New Jersey are informative and well-written but remain under-theorized.[17] The opportunity available to historians of nursing is to use the literature of medical specialization and professionalization to understand more meaningfully the process by which nurses struggled to become recognized professionals. More importantly, making nursing the object of analysis de-centers the specialization and professionalization of physicians or other health professionals by placing these processes within a broader context that emphasizes intra-professional competition and engages a larger discourse of health, healing, work, and occupation. Using models that view medicine as normative to understand the nursing profession may potentially present problems as medicine – at least in the twentieth century – emphasized biomedicine over holistic healing, curing over caring, and a particular and historically situated relationship with the state. Nevertheless, the history of nursing professionalization clearly reflects the influence of the medical profession as a model both imposed from outside nursing and to which nurses often self-consciously aspired.

Nursing professionalization in Argentina

This chapter makes four basic arguments about the professionalization of nursing in 1940s–1950s Argentina. First, although the perception of nurses' subordinate position did not change, physicians did begin to articulate the need to view nurses as professional members of a health care team. Second, the pace of nursing professionalization quickened through self-organization, improved standards of education, and Peronism's active involvement. Third, nurses became the agents through which the Peronist state incorporated the people (particularly the underserved rural and interior public) into its public health schemes while the nurse also embodied the idealized qualities of the Peronist woman. Finally, understanding the shared vision of Argentine nurses as *agentes de enlace* (liaisons) infuses the traditionally subordinate role of the nurse *vis-à-vis* the physician with a strong claim on linking not only patients to physicians but the greater public to the health care sector itself.

Physicians' perceptions of nurses

In the late 1930s, no one doubted the secondary status of nurses. Writing in the official magazine of the Cruz Roja Argentina (the Red Cross of Argentina), Eduardo A. Méndez stated clearly:"The nurse must collaborate with the physician, rendering unconditionally to him all the moral and professional help of which she is able, given that both merge into a common society whose capital is the effort in the fight against sickness."[18] Nevertheless, at the time physicians had started to consider the need for better education and an elevated understanding of the role nurses could – and did – play because of the increasing complexity of medical care and the growing number of patients filling the hospitals and clinics of a rapidly urbanizing and industrializing Argentina. In the early 1940s, many physicians responded to this need by calling for more training and the formal licensure of nurses and, more importantly, were aware of their responsibility for training nurses in the workplace as well as in nursing schools. For example, one physician wrote in 1947 in *El Médico Práctico*, a journal that circulated widely among physicians in Buenos Aires:"Shaping the mind and spirit of the physician's assistant does not depend solely on the professor in the School of Nursing . . . this task, in large part, belongs to the physician."[19] On one hand, this attitude lends itself to a view of nurses by physicians as "educated allies."[20] On the other hand, "shaping" also implies a tremendous amount of control and power over nurses' professional development.

El Médico Práctico later editorialized about the differences between the ways in which physicians and the public should regard nurses and how they in fact did so. According to the editors, physicians and the public alike needed to dignify the nurse and consider her not, as people had traditionally treated the nurse, as a "mechanical servant or a domestic laborer."[21] The lack of a formal education did not necessarily present a problem, as the editors reminded readers of "untrained" nurses who nevertheless were "efficient and effective collaborators."[22] They remarked that these nurses' "lack of academic qualifications did not prevent their intelligence and feeling from making an accurate observation that was enough for the physician because he cheerfully appreciated the intervention."[23]

Notwithstanding the efforts to raise the professional status of nurses, the Asociación Médica Argentina (AMA) noted in 1956: "it can be argued that the nursing profession is necessarily dependent upon the medical profession on *what* to do, but on *how* to do it nursing will be much more independent the higher its development and maturity as a profession" (emphasis in original).[24] The AMA linked this dependence to two factors: a lag between the entry of recent, well-educated nursing graduates into the workforce and the continuing absence of state regulation. With the former, the AMA had no doubts that new nurses were well-trained and able collaborators, but "most of the time the physician has been in contact with another type of nurse coming from a general educational background without basic professional preparation and therefore much more dependent on the doctor to carry out her work."[25] Indeed, a 1953 government report documented that 62 percent of the approximately 18,000 nurses in Argentina fell under the legal provision that allowed workers with more than ten years' experience to claim the title of *enfermera* despite lacking formal nursing education.[26]

The pace of professionalization

In terms of organization, the 1940s saw the first regional and national conferences on nursing. The First Congreso Panamericano de Enfermería (Pan American Nursing Conference) took place in Santiago, Chile from 14 to 20 December 1942 under the auspices of the Universidad de Chile and the nation's Asociación de Enfermeras. In 1949, the Pan American Health Organization (founded in 1902 as the Pan American Sanitary Bureau and incorporated into the newly formed World Health Organization in 1949) sponsored two regional nursing conferences on general nursing: one in San José, Costa Rica and another in Lima, Peru. The conferences sprang from "the desire to provide nurses the opportunity to discuss their problems amicably and to reach conclusions and recommendations that would benefit the profession."[27] The long-term goals were to foster the development of national associations and international (that is, Pan American) federations of nurses, standardize nursing education, and develop a common nursing lexicon.

The first Congreso Argentino de Enfermería (Argentine Nursing Conference) took place in July 1949 at the Universidad de la La Plata. Delegates proposed recognizing that the title of *enfermera asistencial* should require three years of training with the hope of one day making this a four-year bachelor's degree; the development of a federal law recognizing and regulating nursing as a liberal profession, which in this context placed nursing in the same legal category as professions such as physicians, engineers, and lawyers; and the creation of nursing schools affiliated with universities that would teach the techniques and history of nursing, professional ethics, and public health.[28] Clearly implicit in these recommendations was the perception by conference attendees – including nurses, physicians, and public health officials – that in 1949 nursing education in Argentina did not meet these standards.

Dr Cecilia Grierson, the first female physician in Argentina, had founded the first nursing school in Argentina in 1892. Nursing programs affiliated with the Red Cross opened in 1920. Some physicians and medical researchers also took action; for example, the Instituto de Medicina Experimental, which specialized in cancer treatment, opened a school of nursing in 1924. Director Ángel H. Roffo later recalled: "Except for some very worthy examples, the whole system of nursing that dominated our local and national hospitals consisted of many women – wrongly called nurses – with ambitions of profit, without higher education, without culture, and with even less preparation."[29]

Despite these early efforts at nursing education, in the early 1930s physicians did not consider nursing a true profession – most, as physician Pedro Escudero observed, considered nurses "simply servants dressed in white."[30] The main problems were the demanding length of the workday, the lack of professional regulation or coordinated management of nurses, and the sense that obtaining employment as a nurse depended not on merit but on political and social relationships. Escudero believed that nursing suffered from "a particular and worsening moral state."[31] Describing as "useless" the efforts made to end the practice of nurses receiving a monetary gratuity from patients upon their discharge from the hospital, Escudero argued that its banishment – and, by extension, the professionalization of nursing – could never be achieved while "nurses are recruited from Spanish and Italian peasants and among elements of the political parties," betraying his ethnic and class prejudices.[32]

By the early 1940s, proposals for new and revised nursing programs by hospitals, non-profit institutions, and public universities in Argentina as well as articles published in physicians' trade journals (there were as yet no journals devoted to nursing) made it clear that the three-year program was the ideal for training professional nurses. Questions remained, however, about how much primary and secondary education should be required for entry into these "graduate" programs; who (the Red Cross, universities, or the state in its municipal, provincial, or federal form) should run them; and the extent of specialization in fourth and later years of study. By 1948, nurses common in Argentina included *enfermeras asistenciales* (the unspecialized nurse with a three-year degree) and public health nurses, transfusionists, X-ray nurses, laboratory nurses, obstetrical and gynecological nurses, and nurses expert in the care of tuberculosis patients and of children, all of whom undertook some advanced study.[33]

Also by this time, twenty-six nursing schools of many types operated in Argentina. This variety led to concerns about standards of quality, particularly because nursing remained a profession unregulated by the state. The *Revista de la Cruz Roja Argentina* argued that, although "a good part of these carry out efficient work that has already been widely recognized," those who cared about nursing education recognized "a disparity of programs, conditions, and rules for admission practices that diminish the overall value of this weighty task."[34]

Peronism and nursing

Up to this point, the professionalization and development of nursing in Argentina had taken place organically. However, the election of Juan Perón to the Argentine presidency in 1946 ushered in the era of Peronism, and, like the rest of Argentine society, nursing was not immune to populist attempts at appropriation. Under the direction of Ramón Carrillo, the newly formed Ministerio de Salud Pública (MSP, initially the Secretaría de Salud Pública) oversaw the development of a national health plan and a national sanitary code; the construction of new hospitals and health clinics; and the coordination of municipal, provincial, and federal public health services as a highly visible part of Perón's overall plan for making the state the agent of social justice for the poor and working classes. With the creation of the MSP, Carrillo could leverage the full power of the state to initiate and implement public health reforms and investment in the nation's health care sector. Yet the creation in 1948 of the Fundación Eva Perón (FEP) mitigated the effectiveness of the state's involvement because the FEP's portfolio of social action projects – such as hospital construction, the distribution of medical supplies, and the training and education of nurses – competed directly with the MSP's legislative mandate. In general, historians view the competition between the MSP and the FEP as a typical example of Peronism's "multiple presence," its tendency to pursue a particular policy goal in more than one way; Perón's preference for the type of autocratic and personalist approach that the FEP, as a private organization, but not the MSP, as a government ministry, could provide; or the interpersonal conflicts prevalent within the movement – Carillo and Eva Perón famously avoided being in the same room with one another.[35]

In the area of nursing professionalization, the MSP opened its *Escuela de Enfermeras de Salud Pública* in 1947. The FEP's own School of Nursing, ostensibly founded in 1948, took two years to get off the ground. The FEP claimed that its school differed from other nursing schools run by the Red Cross, universities, municipalities, and the MSP in that it was intentionally created to "constitute a revolution in the idea of a school for nurses under the capitalistic system" – training poor women to be nurses while at the same time training nurses to care for the poor.[36]

Despite this rhetoric, by its formal dedication in 1950 the school closely resembled the common Argentine ideal for nursing education. Its physical plant included classrooms and a formal connection to hospital facilities also built by the FEP. The palpable energy, sense of mission and purpose, and the enhanced public image are undeniable, but at its core the FEP's School of Nursing appears to have followed the same curriculum as other contemporary nursing programs. Three years of education left students as *enfermeras diplomadas* with the opportunity to specialize further during a fourth year of resident study.

In contrast to this curricular similarity, the FEP's nursing students' place of residence distinguished them from students at other schools. The FEP embraced the residential concept, or nurses' home, that had to that point been an aspirational component of nursing education in Argentina. A description of the ideal location for nursing students' housing in relation to the school and hospital written ten years earlier made clear the relationship between a "home" for students and a place to learn and work.[37] The ideal of nursing students living in a controlled environment also went a long way toward ameliorating the common view of the nurse as a woman with loose morals, a girl too easily subject to the otherwise unwelcome advances of men, or a single woman on the prowl for a physician- or patient-husband. Some nursing schools in rural and provincial Argentina followed this model, but the majority of schools – particularly those in urban Buenos Aires and the MSP's nursing school – did not include a residential component, in large part because most nursing students needed to support their educations and, more significantly, their families, by working while in school. In contrast, the FEP zealously embraced the ideal of the nursing-boarding school and the advantages it provided for shaping the character of the women who enrolled, who by all accounts were predominantly from the poor and working classes.

At the same time, the nurse took on the image of the ideal Peronist woman. As a highly visible presidential spouse, Eva Perón made great strides in terms of a view of women as active members of Argentine society, culture, and politics. However, Perón did so within the limits of traditional views of gender, reinforcing the established view of women as first and foremost mothers and housewives. Perón also consistently emphasized the feminine qualities of "kindness, generosity, selflessness, and sacrifice" in her speeches, publications, and conversations with people.[38] Of these characteristics, nurses, other medical professionals, and politicians most commonly used "selflessness" (*abnegación*) when describing the ideal nurse. In this way Perón contributed to a discourse that articulated public roles for women through both the use of generalities that mirrored traditional gender stereotypes and particular programs that positioned women in front of issues such as education, health care, and nutrition. Because of this, women "acted under the idea that there was continuity and not rupture between their daily lives [as women] and political action."[39]

In this context, the FEP and other nursing schools made great efforts to cultivate a positive and more prestigious image of the *enfermera* than had previously existed in Argentine society. This project built on an older attempt by nursing proponents to dignify nurses by identifying their positive and ideal traits. Abraham Abramoff, a physician practicing in Argentina, had earlier proposed: "the focus of nursing is not only a scientific and intellectual discipline but an embodiment of goodness and conscience. Nurses must be a synthesis of scientific knowledge and hands-on practical knowledge."[40] A statement from 1943 about nurses noted that, "to work effectively, the nurse must have good health, initiative, ingenuity, common sense; she should be discreet and adapt to the means that she encounters; it is important that in her relations with the workers she is of strict impartiality, both from the political and religious points of view."[41] Many contemporary descriptions of the ideal nurse emphasized similar themes. For example, a guide to nursing included: "The nurse will also be happy and cheerful and, in a special way, should be courageous in times of crisis or danger in order, first, that her own fear does not cloud her vision of what to do and also so that the patient does not realize any panic in the caregiver."[42]

In a speech given at a graduation ceremony for nurses in Rosario in 1943, Abelardo Irigoyen Freyre, the first Minister of Public Health for the Province of Santa Fe, reminded those in attendance that the older, "pre-professional" nurses, those without formal training, were nevertheless worthy members of the health care sector. However, with the state's rising interest in public health, "the *enfermera de salud pública* appears as a fundamental necessity for the health of the province."[43] Irigoyen Freyre defined many tasks for nurses, but their success, he argued, came from their innate feminine qualities: "she has by natural condition the softness and tact, the tenderness and feeling that a task of this nature demands. She has the necessary patience and perseverance, and she has the insight and consciousness through her own natural and spiritual disposition."[44]

Nurses also understood themselves and their work in gendered terms. Speaking at a "Día de la Nurse" ceremony on June 21, 1940, nursing student María Lina Laporta declared that "the mission of the Nurse is the most sublime that a woman can pursue."[45] Fellow student Clotilde Elia Donadille added that the word "nurse . . . means a woman of generous feelings, mild-mannered, and kind words that in forgetting herself has as her sole aspiration the good of others."[46]

The nurse as public health liaison

Sponsorship of and emphasis on *higienismo* from 1880 to 1930 by the Argentine state meant that the government largely refrained from becoming directly involved in people's lives, preferring instead to focus on improvements to the sanitation infrastructure, medical evaluations of immigrants, and practices drawn from medically and scientifically informed criminology. While the rhetoric of *higienismo* may have been intense, in practice its proponents accomplished very little.[47] As a consequence, serious discussion of the need for state involvement in the health care sector began in earnest in the late 1930s and early 1940s among concerned physicians not allied with *higienismo*. The new debate centered on the "crises" in Argentine medicine caused by rapid industrialization and urbanization: increasing patient loads, diseases caused by overcrowded and unsanitary living conditions, and a crumbling and inadequate medical infrastructure. In general, up through the 1930s the Argentine health care sector effectively restricted consistent and effective medical care to those who could afford to pay for it themselves, and this meant that the health of the vast majority of Argentina's inhabitants, particularly the growing urban population, suffered. By the early 1940s, *higienismo* had clearly lost the debate to social medicine, which called directly for increased state involvement in public health.

Carrillo and the MSP leadership identified the location of public health problems as the underserved interior and rural areas – underserved because physicians generally declined to work there. Carrillo's proposed organization of a public health infrastructure depended on a multi-tiered plan that would extend health care into these areas. At the top, the MSP proposed large urban hospitals of 500 or more beds. At the bottom, Carrillo proposed *centros de salud*, or health clinics, staffed by a nurse and capable only of emergency hospitalization.[48] Carrillo advocated a policy that prioritized improving the top and bottom tiers – particularly the *centros*. The latter were most likely to target underserved areas, had a smaller financial footprint than the largest urban hospitals, and could be up and running relatively quickly; however, Perón's power was based in the rapidly industrializing urban centers to which inhabitants of rural Argentina immigrated daily.

The straightforward way in which this plan imagined the professional and workplace relationship between physicians and nurses highlights the manner in which the MSP saw nurses as critically important links between the Argentine people and the state's public health apparatus – "extend[ing] the action of the physician by visiting distant patients and fulfilling the orders that her boss entrusts to her under his responsibility."[49] As proposed, the base level *centros* functioned with only a nurse in residence who worked under the direction of a physician making the rounds of a number of *centros* (not unlike a circuit judge or minister). The physician's "home clinic" was larger and also staffed by a nurse.

Interestingly, an earlier proposal from 1944 included much larger facilities at the bottom tier of a national public health infrastructure. These *centros* would have provided preventive and curative medical care to the residents through a limited number of beds and a team that included, at a minimum: two physicians, a dentist, a pharmacist, a midwife, a social worker, paramedics, nurses, a cook, and a custodian.[50] The fact that the new, smaller *centros* proposed for the country's interior would be staffed almost entirely by nurses underscored the MSP's retreat from physician-staffed *centros*, doomed by a profound lack of interest among physicians in moving to rural areas.

In principle, the MSP's nursing school would have provided the large number of nurses required to staff the *centros*. These nurses would also have come from the FEP's School of Nursing – if only because of its emphasis on reaching out to the underserved rural interior and recruiting provincial students who would ostensibly return home after graduation. In practice, even if the MSP and FEP had been able to graduate enough nurses to staff all of the MSP's proposed *centros* (few of which were actually constructed), most newly graduated nurses made the same choice as physicians: to remain in Buenos Aires.

These practical realities differed from the rhetorical connections made between nurses and public health. As early as 1940, in her proposal to reorganize and unify all schools of nursing in Argentina, María Elena Ramos Mejía recognized the new and important role for the public health nurse as "the one that links the patient to the hospital."[51] In addition to working in the hospital, the vision of the public health nurse placed her in smaller clinics and dispensaries, in the new factories that industrialization had brought to Buenos Aires, and in the homes of patients and their families. Speaking at a nursing conference in 1942, María Elena Bruno, director of the oldest Catholic school of nursing in Argentina, declared that the nurse could expand her role when working outside of major cities and within the field of public health, no longer "confined to the care of the patient" in the hospital but instead involved in health education and preventive care.[52]

As later shaped by the rhetoric of Peronism and the plans of the MSP and FEP, nursing's growing role in public health drew on the vision of the innately feminine nurse to create the nurse as a link between the physician and the patient: "For patients, the nurse plays the role of the *agente de enlace* (the liaison), being, if it can be said, an extension of the brain and the hand of the physician. She is a conductor . . . The physician gives the nurse the means to heal the sick, and she gives the physician the means to act effectively."[53] This vision combined the nurse's subordinate role, her feminine attributes, and her ability to act effectively as the connection between the patient and the physician.

Conclusion

As proposed above, the literatures of medical specialization and professionalization offer many theoretical frameworks for understanding nursing professionalization as the product of socio-economic factors, relationships with other health professions as negotiated in terms of subordination to power, and the discourse on nursing created by nurses, physicians, and politicians, among others. The case of nursing professionalization in Argentina clearly demonstrates how the social and economic changes unleashed by urbanization and industrialization and the political force of Peronism affected both nurses as individuals and nursing as a profession. The attempts in the 1940s and 50s to professionalize nursing took place in the context of physicians striving to control public health efforts while competing with the populist politics of public figures such as Perón and institutions such as the FEP. As a consequence, nurses inherited a discourse of *dignificación* and *abnegación* from both sides: from the physicians who sought to maintain control of the hospital and from the politicians who sought to maintain control of the public square; but in the process nurses also participated in making new connections between themselves, patients, physicians, and the state.

The desire of physicians to routinize large aspects of public health, differentiate themselves vertically by preferring work in the urban metropolis of Buenos Aires rather than the rural and provincial interior of the country, and delegate primary and preventive care to nurses also shaped nursing professionalization in Argentina in the 1940s and 1950s. The fact that the new, smaller *centros* in the country's interior would be staffed almost entirely by nurses underscored the delegation by physicians of the day-to-day aspects of public health and the resulting development of nursing's claim to the domain of public health.

Throughout the 1930s, physicians in Argentina developed solutions to the health care crises that beset society while excluding both nurses as individuals and nursing as a proto-profession. Relying on the body of academic knowledge that made up social medicine, physicians developed a portfolio of public policies aimed at creating a vast, interconnected public health infrastructure that would bring modern medicine to those members of society for whom health care had always been out of reach. Carrillo's MSP and its public health proposals relied heavily on plans drawn up in the late 1930s and early 1940s by physicians sympathetic to social medicine, and these proposals were therefore consistent with a long-term shift in an increasing number of Argentine physicians' understanding of public health: from individual to social welfare, from voluntary to obligatory coverage, from individual responsibility to a sense of solidarity, and from medical care to social welfare.[54]

When attempting to implement these solutions, however, physicians encountered competition not from nursing or another medical profession but from the political project of Peronism, which proposed alternative though complementary public health solutions. Both physicians and politicians agreed that the collective and individual health of the Argentine people had suffered, but while physicians limited themselves to the domain of medical practice, politicians took to heart the fundamental concept of social medicine that social, cultural, and economic factors influence people's health and made it a useful and highly legible restatement of its central call for social justice. The politicians understood that in order to treat the public health crisis the state needed to improve economic conditions, break down social inequalities, and directly address the non-biological factors that unjustly caused the public health crisis in Argentina, in addition to addressing the working class's need for health care. In words taken from the FEP's description of its nursing school, the Peronist political project understood "that the reason of its existence [was] the . . . reparation of social injustice."[55] From this perspective, women enrolled in the FEP's nursing school not only because of the nursing education that it offered, which was essentially the same as in other schools, but also because the FEP's vision of nursing fused the nursing profession with Peronism's message of social justice, something that physicians' visions of social medicine had never been able to achieve.

In conclusion, neither did nursing in Argentina simply claim public health nor did physicians delegate it to them. Instead, physicians left the day-to-day work of public health open to the nursing profession because physicians' proposed solutions to the nation's health care crises were limited in comparison to the political message of Peronism. In addition, physicians' own preference for urban Buenos Aires at the expense of the rural and provincial interior of Argentina left large figurative and literal spaces within the health care sector that nursing readily filled. Again, nurses in Argentina did not claim public health; rather, nursing benefited from its ability and willingness to carry out the necessary day-to-day work of public health and to act as a link between the public and two groups (physicians and politicians) with rival solutions for the public health crisis. In the end, because physicians and politicians understood nurses as *agentes de enlace*, the nurse became, at least rhetorically, for physicians a vital link between the patient and public health and for politicians a vital link between the people and the state.

Notes

1 Álvarez, M.E. 2010, *La enfermera de Evita*, Instituto Nacional de Investigaciones Históricas Eva Perón, Buenos Aires, p. 23.
2 *Ibid.*, p. 59
3 *Ibid.*
4 See Shafer, H. 1936, *The American Medical Profession, 1783–1850*, Columbia University Press, New York; Shryrock, R. 1937, "The Historian Looks at Medicine," *Bulletin of the History of Medicine*, vol. 5, pp. 887–894; Stern, B. 1945, *American Medical Practices in the*

Perspectives of a Century, The Commonwealth Fund, New York; Straus, R. 1957, "The Nature and Status of Medical Sociology," *American Sociological Review*, vol. 22, pp. 200–204; Parsons, T. 1951, *The Social System*, Free Press, New York; and Hughes, E. 1958, *Men and Their Work*, Free Press, New York.

5 Burnham, J. 1996, "How the Concept of Profession Evolved in the Work of Historians of Medicine," *Bulletin of the History of Medicine*, vol. 70, no. 1, pp. 1–24.

6 Rosen, G. 1944, *The Specialization of Medicine with Particular Reference to Ophthalmology*, Froben Press, New York.

7 Stevens, R. 1966, *Medical Practice in Modern England: The Impact of Specialization and State Medicine*, Yale University Press, New Haven, CT; and Stevens, R. 1971, *American Medicine and the Public Interest*, Yale University Press, New Haven, CT.

8 Weisz, G. 2006, *Divide and Conquer: A Comparative History of Medical Specialization*, Oxford University Press, New York.

9 Freidson, E. 1970, *Profession of Medicine*, Dodd Mead, New York.

10 See Gieryn, T. 1983, "Boundary Work and the Demarcation of Science from Non-Science: Strains and Interests in the Professional Ideologies of Scientists," *American Sociological Review*, vol. 48, no. 6, pp. 781–795; Abbott, A. 1988, *The System of Professions: An Essay on the Division of Expert Labor*, University of Chicago Press, Chicago; and Halpern, S. and Anspach, R. 1993, "The Study of the Medical Institutions: Eliot Freidson's Legacy," *Work and Occupations*, vol. 20, no. 3, pp. 279–295.

11 Larson, M.S. 1977, *The Rise of Professionalism: A Sociological Analysis*, University of California Press, Berkeley and Abbott, *op cit.*

12 Freidson, E. 1994, *Professionalism Reborn: Theory, Prophecy and Policy*, Polity Press, Cambridge, UK; and Freidson, E. 2001, *Professionalism: The Third Logic*, Polity, London.

13 Evetts, J. 2006, "The Sociology of Professional Groups," *Current Sociology*, vol. 54, no. 1, p. 135.

14 *Ibid.*, p. 138.

15 Schultheiss, K. 2001, *Bodies and Souls: Politics and the Professionalization of Nursing in France, 1880–1922*, Harvard Historical Studies, no. 139, Harvard University Press, Cambridge, MA.

16 Olson, T. and Walsh, E. 2004, *Handling the Sick: The Women of St. Luke's and the Nature of Nursing, 1892–1937*, Ohio State University Press, Columbus. See also Ramos, M. 1997, "The Johns Hopkins Training School for Nurses," *Nursing History Review*, vol. 5, pp. 23–48; and Schwirian, P. 1998, *Professionalization of Nursing: Current Issues and Trends*, Lippincott, Philadelphia.

17 Ettinger, L. 2006, *Nurse-Midwifery: The Birth of a New American Profession*, Ohio State University Press, Columbus; and Ward, F. 2009, *On Duty: Power, Politics, and the History of Nursing in New Jersey*, Rutgers University Press, New Brunswick, NJ.

18 Méndez, E.A. 1938, "Ética y orientación profesional de la enfermera," *Revista Oficial de la Cruz Roja Argentina*, vol. 16, no. 185, p. 27.

19 Petrarca, O. 1947, "Los ayudantes del médico, en el hospital," *El Médico Práctico*, vol. 3, no. 27, p. 6.

20 See D'Antonio, P. 1993, "Legacy of Domesticity: Nursing in Early Nineteenth-Century America," *Nursing History Review*, vol. 1, pp. 229–246; and Fairman, J. 2009, *Making Room in the Clinic: Nurse Practitioners and the Evolution of Modern Health Care*, Rutgers University Press, New Brunswick, NJ.

21 "Los Enfermeros Deben ser Considerados como Colaboradores del Médico," Anon. 1953, *El Médico Práctico*, vol. 9, no. 104, pp. 1–2.

22 *Ibid.*

23 *Ibid.*

24 "La Enfermera y su Lugar," Anon. 1956, *Revista de la Asociación Médica Argentina*, vol. 70, no. 831–832, p. 376.

25 *Ibid.*

26 Carrillo, S. 1953, *Organización de Escuelas de Enfermería*, Ministerio de Salud Pública de la Nación, Buenos Aires, p. 13.

27 Pan American Health Organization 1949, *Actas del Primer Congreso Regional de Enfermería y del Segundo Congreso Regional de Enfermería*, World Health Organization, Washington, DC, p. 112.

28 "Votos y recomendaciones del Primer Congreso Argentino de Enfermería," Anon. 1950, *Boletín de la Oficina Sanitaria Panamericana*, vol. 29, no. 3, pp. 323–324.

29 Roffo, A.H. 1941, "Escuela de Nurses del Instituto de Medicina Experimental," *Boletín del Instituto de Medicina Experimental*, vol. 18, no. 2, p. 1189.

30 Escudero, P. 1932, "La enfermera religiosa y la enfermera laica en los hospitals," *El Día Médico*, vol. 5, p. 5.

31 *Ibid.*

32 *Ibid.*

33 Bogliano, R. 1948, "Estado Actual de la Enfermería Argentina," *Revista de la Cruz Roja Argentina*, vol. 25, no. 301–306, p. 45.

34 *Ibid.*

35 See Plotkin, M.B. 2003, *Mañana es San Perón: A Cultural History of Perón's Argentina*, Scholarly Resources, Wilmington, DE; and Ramacciotti, K. 2009, *La política sanitaria del peronismo*, Editorial Biblos, Buenos Aires.

36 Fundación Eva Perón 1953, *Escuela De Enfermeras*, Servicio Internacional de Publicaciones Argentinas, Buenos Aires, p. 14.

37 "Proposiciones relativas a la organización de una Escuela de Enfermeras," Anon. 1940, *Revista de la Cruz Roja Argentina*, vol. 18, no. 206, p. 19.

38 Barry, C. 2009, *Evita Capitana: El Partido Peronista Feminino 1949–1955*, Editorial de la Universidad Nacional de Tres de Febrero, Caseros, Argentina, p. 150.

39 *Ibid.*, p. 153.

40 Abramoff, A. 1939, "Acerca del ejercicio de la profesión de enfermero," *Retoños, Revista Mensual del Hospital Italiano de Santa Fe y Colonias*, vol. 6, no. 72, p. 23.

41 "La enfermera en la industria," Anon. 1943, *Revista de la Cruz Roja Argentina*, vol. 21, no. 235–236, pp. 21–22.

42 Huelin Martaza, R. 1942, *La enfermera: En el hogar y en la clínica*, Editorial Molino, Buenos Aires, p. 7.

43 Irigoyen Freyre, A. 1943, *Problemas de Sanidad y de Asistencia Social*, Universidad Nacional del Litoral, Santa Fe, Argentina, p. 334.

44 *Ibid.*, pp. 337–338.

45 "Día de la Nurse," Anon. 1940, *Revista de Medicina y Cancerología*, vol. 14, no. 11, p. 28.

46 *Ibid.*, p. 30.

47 See Rodriguez, J. 2006, *Civilizing Argentina: Science, Medicine, and the Modern State*, University of North Carolina Press, Chapel Hill.

48 Martone, F.J. 1951, *Administración sanitaria y medicina social*, Ciordia y Rodríguez, Buenos Aires, p. 224.

49 Carreño, D.C. and Yanzon, R. 1946, *Planificación Sanitaria: Distribución de Unidades y Centros de Salud en la Región Cuyana*, C. Carulli, Buenos Aires, p. 8.

50 "Sobre oficialización de la medicina dióse a conocer un informe," Anon. 1944, *Mundo Médico*, vol. 8, no. 103, p. 42.

51 Ramos Mejía, M.E. 1940, *Plan De Unificación De Todas Las Escuelas De Enfermeras*, Buenos Aires, p. 1.

52 Bruno, M.E. 1942, "Escuela de Enfermeras de la Obra de la Conservación de la Fe," in *Primer Congreso Panamericano de Enfermería*, December 1942, Santiago, Chile, p. 11.

53 Dalloni, D. 1946, "Enfermeras y Médicos," *Revista de la Cruz Roja Argentina*, vol. 23, no. 273–274, p. 35.
54 Belmartino, S. 2005, *La atención médica Argentina en el siglo XX: instituciones y procesos*, Siglo Veintiuno Editores, Buenos Aires, p. 97.
55 Fundación Eva Perón, p. 15.

12

A MISSION TO NURSE

The mission hospital's role in the development of nursing in South Africa c.1948–1975

Helen Sweet

This chapter traces the development of nursing in the deprived rural areas of South Africa served by a range of mission hospitals from different denominations, from the beginning of official apartheid in 1948 through to their take-over by the "Bantustan" governments in the mid-1970s. It explores the development of nursing in South Africa, asking what was the role of mission hospital nursing (found primarily in rural areas) within this troubled political history of South Africa during the mid-twentieth century. Mission hospitals were of particular significance to nursing history in this country as, for many years, they constituted the main training centers for black South African nurses and the main providers of biomedical healthcare for black South Africans. This chapter asks: what were the personal, professional and political dilemmas faced by foreign missionary nurses within South African nursing and what were their main roles? Also, how were African nurses able to develop professionally while working under the constraints of the apartheid system during the period 1948–1975? Finally it considers the role of the mission hospital in the history of nurse training and employment during this period.

Background

Among published works on colonial medical history, *Curing Their Ills* by Megan Vaughan[1] focuses on encounters between European medicine and southern African societies in the nineteenth and twentieth centuries, including the role of the missionaries within that encounter. Several PhD theses have also contributed significantly to the understanding of South African nursing and medicine before and during apartheid – in particular, Welcome Siphamandla Zondi's research on medical missions and African demand for Western biomedicine[2] challenged the idea that European medicine was imposed on unwilling black Africans. Simonne Horwitz included some valuable nursing history in her study of Baragwanath provincial hospital[3] – the hospital providing for

Soweto, Johannesburg, whose staff experienced at first hand many of the outcomes of the atrocities of apartheid; and Vanessa Noble's research on the racially segregated training provided by the University of Natal's "non-European" medical school in Durban has also uncovered the daily difficulties facing hospital staff and medical students working, teaching and training under apartheid.

Of the notable works relevant particularly to the history of nursing, only a small number have been written and published in the post-apartheid era, while fewer still relate to the rural mission hospital and its role in primary healthcare provision. One of the first such significant contributors to nursing history has been Shula Marks, and particularly her monograph *Divided Sisterhood*.[4] Marks reveals the racial tensions within the health professions as a direct outcome of apartheid legislation and ideology while exploring the "crisis of identity" from which the profession suffered through the tensions not only between classes and hierarchical structures but also of racial divisions imposed from without and within. Anne Digby[5] has also written widely on the history of medicine in South Africa, including several chapters on, and references to, nursing history. Digby explores the social history of medicine within its political, social and economic context, providing examples of cultural crossover and medical pluralism while documenting the discrimination of race, class and gender within the South African medical and nursing professions, in both community and institutional practice. Other articles by Digby, written in collaboration with Helen Sweet, address aspects of mission and state hospital nursing more directly[6] together with one article recently published looking at South African rural primary healthcare.[7] Digby and Sweet looked more specifically at the impact of these issues within nursing – in particular the role of nurses as culture brokers and student nurses' struggles against colonial and apartheid attitudes and restrictions. Sweet has also written elsewhere on the subject of South African mission nursing and medicine and looking at the place of missionary nursing within colonial nursing more generally.[8]

Earlier work by missionary doctors such as Michael Gelfand,[9] and James McCord with John Douglas,[10] presented somewhat triumphalist and colonialized pictures of missionary medicine, or concentrated on the histories of individual institutions. Nevertheless, the extensive empirical survey of medical missions by Drs Aitken and Gale on which Gelfand's book was based[11] includes valuable statistical information relating to nurse employment. Added to these are a plethora of memoirs and mission hospital histories written by health professionals (mostly doctors) who worked in South Africa's mission hospitals. These include Francis Schimlek's history of St Mary's Mariannhill Hospital,[12] Anthony Barker's views of working at the Charles Johnson Memorial mission hospital[13] and more recently Jens Kargaard's tales from Mangusi Mission Hospital[14] near the border with Mozambique. All give individual views of the clinical experience, cultural obstacles and, to a lesser extent, the role of their hospital's nursing staff, while Ronald Ingle's[15] reflections on the final years of All Saints Mission Hospital in the Transkei reveals the political background to the nationalization of South Africa's mission hospitals.

A substantial amount of work on nursing history by an Afrikaner nurse-leader, Charlotte Searle, was published during the second half of the twentieth century.[16]

Searle's nationalistic leanings are expressed in her historical writing with the result that accounts of black African nurses are grossly devalued; therefore much of the contribution of the mission hospitals to the development of South African nursing goes largely unrecognized by her. American Lutheran missionary nurse June Kjome's[17] memories of her time differ quite noticeably from Searle's outlook. Kjome worked at several of the KwaZulu mission hospitals and her autobiographical sketches throw light on the day-to-day experiences of nursing. These, together with a series of oral histories undertaken by Sweet, including one with Kjome forty years after the latter wrote her book, have been invaluable in understanding the missionary nurse's role and providing a retrospective view of the impact of apartheid on the nursing and medical professions.

In 1995 an African matron, Grace Mashaba, provided a welcome but relatively conservative historical account of the rise of black nurses within the nursing profession in her book *Rising to the Challenge of Change*.[18] In it are surprisingly few words of criticism of the (white) leaders of nursing, many of whom had upheld apartheid within the profession, thereby impeding professional development and representation on racial lines. This was written from Mashaba's personal experience as a pioneering African nurse-leader and academic and therefore fits into the genre of autobiography rather than history. *African Nurse Pioneers*,[19] published nine years later by another African nurse leader, Maso Buthelezi, is very much more outspoken in its critical approach and fiercely condemnatory towards the impact of white colonialism on women generally and on nursing development more specifically. Yet throughout this book, the role of the mission hospital appears to be the exception to her antipathy, since she and many of the nurse pioneers she discusses came from mission backgrounds, perhaps reflecting the significance of these institutions. These final two books by African nurses with contrasting views of their profession's history, yet with notable accord when considering the contribution of the mission hospitals, suggest that a closer study of these hospitals, and the nurses who trained and worked in them, is long overdue.

The institution of apartheid

Although an unofficial form of racial segregation existed before 1948, the much harsher system of official "apartheid" was introduced and often brutally enforced by the National Party which came to power in 1948. The Party claimed that South Africa did not comprise a single nation, but was made up of four distinct racial groups: "white," "black," "coloured," and "Indian," with white people being in the highest social group with most privileges and ("black") Africans constituting the lowest social group (with only basic rights and minimal civil liberties).[20] The Group Areas Act (No. 41) of 1950 and subsequent Acts over the next twenty years then assigned official racial groupings to different residential and business sectors in urban areas, thereby excluding blacks from living in the most developed areas, and led to non-whites being forcibly removed to black "townships" for living in the "wrong" areas. Pass laws required non-whites to carry a pass book in order to enter the "white" regions of their own country, for example to work at a hospital in a "white" area when living in a non-white area. These groups were split further into thirteen nations or racial federations.

Most public services were segregated, including education and medical care, providing black people with services greatly inferior to those of white people. From 1970 black political representation in mainstream politics was abolished and Africans legally became members of one of ten artificially created, ethnically based "homelands" or "Bantustans" (of which KwaZulu was one), rather than citizens of South Africa. In rural areas, where the African population was concentrated in officially designated reserves, there was insufficient land to farm and high hut taxes to pay, so that men were forced to leave their families and work as migrant labor in white-owned mines, industries and farms. Therefore thousands of Africans formed a vast migrant workforce, often living in crowded single-sex hostels near their jobs and separated from their wives – described officially as "superfluous appendages." Sexually transmitted diseases and tuberculosis became commonplace among migrant workers, who also transmitted these diseases to their families on their occasional visits home to the rural "reserves."

In South Africa over 39% of the total (almost 49 million) population is still categorized as "rural."[21] Throughout the period under consideration here, and right up to the end of apartheid, these rural communities were almost entirely black African.[22] As a direct result of official and unofficial apartheid, for much of the twentieth century remote rural areas have therefore been continuously disadvantaged in receiving poor access to biomedical healthcare. A system of official district surgeons served over-large districts with the result that much healthcare had to be provided by nursing and medical missionaries until the mid-1970s, when the state officially nationalized and took over most of the mission hospitals. Pluralistic patient choice in accessing either traditional medicine or biomedicine rested on these alternatives together with the services of a few general practitioners, or, more conveniently, the widely available traditional healers and itinerant unlicensed practitioners.[23]

Clearly indigenous or traditional medicine represented an important enduring alternative to Western biomedicine and was felt to present a threat and challenge to missionary doctors and nurses throughout the apartheid period, both in the acquisition and treatment of patients and in training African nurses brought up within this culture. Whereas missionary medicine by the twentieth century took a largely biomedical rather than spiritual approach to treatment, despite often preaching Christianity within the ward setting, traditional healing took a more multifactorial or holistic approach, in having no distinction between healing and religion. These methods were viewed by most medical missionaries as heathen, based on superstitious or supernatural beliefs, and therefore were perceived as evil.[24] Yet for the African population these were often the first port of call, provided by local people rather than the less familiar practices of white doctors and nurses in uniforms representing officialdom.

Nursing in South Africa: The colonial context (1891–1948)

Looking back in 1963 at the previous fifty years of nursing in South Africa, it was noted that in the first issue of the *South African Nursing Record* in 1913, the editor had written that nursing there was: "not so much a *profession* as a collection of trained nurse units drawn from all the corners of the earth – and one thing was noticeable – it was the rarest possible thing to find a South African-trained nurse in any senior position" (emphasis in original).[25] This was because virtually all senior nurses were at that time "white," and most had been trained in Europe or the USA. This statement reflected a situation in the period immediately following South Africa's Act of Union (1910), in which colonial racial divisions were already firmly entrenched along with a hierarchy of class and gender, permeating the medical and nursing professions. However, the power relationship between state-run colonial medicine and missionary medicine (organized and controlled by religious bodies) based overseas meant that the latter was not necessarily the central instrument of colonialism as was once assumed, but was in fact set "at the very margins of the state, and outside the state altogether – in the education of medical assistants, midwives and nurses, undertaken for the most part by the missions."[26]

Yet ironically South Africa was the first country in the world to have legislation providing for training and registration of nurses and midwives, achieving this through the Cape Colony's Medical and Pharmacy Act of 1891. This ensured that nursing education became legally recognized, state as well as mission-run nursing schools inspected and approved, and statutory curricula and examinations for nurses provided. In theory this was regardless of race, yet it took almost twenty years for the first (black) African nurse, Cecilia Makewane, to train, qualify and be accepted for the Nursing Register as a Registered Nurse at Lovedale (Church of Scotland) Mission Hospital in the Eastern Cape in 1908. The emphasis was clearly on training white women, and the inferior education provided for African children effectively meant that they did not meet the high standards required for admission to state-run training schools. However, mission schools had higher standards of education and it would have been a natural progression for girls to move from the mission school to meet the lower qualification entry standards of the mission hospital. As missions were established in rural areas, with their remit to bring Christianity and "civilization" to the native Africans, the nurses, non-medical staff and patients were almost all Africans. Apart from missionaries, white nurses generally worked in more affluent urban areas demarcated as "white," caring for white patients or supervising black nurses, or as private nurses to white families.

The relationship between black and white nurses was thus a complex and subtly changing one throughout the twentieth century, and perhaps nowhere more so than in the mission hospitals during the apartheid era. Buthelezi claims that the history of African nurses has been neglected because: "White nurses were the core, the fulcrum and the nurse leadership in South Africa. White nurses colonized nursing and African nurses."[27] She claims the lives of black South African women in general, and nurses in particular, have been "neglected, ignored, de-voiced, divorced and devalued" while "struggling against the multiple jeopardy of class, ethnicity, gender and race within the most devastating, horrendous necrophilous regimes."[28] To understand this we need to appreciate the impact "apartheid" had on the nursing profession.

The evolution of nursing under apartheid

In line with apartheid legislation, the Nursing Act (1957) established segregated racial registers for nurses and made it a criminal offense for a white nurse to be put under the supervision of a nurse belonging to a "lower" racial group regardless of educational experience or qualification. In terms of the Act, the South African Nursing Council (SANC) was to maintain separate nursing rolls or registers for the different "racial" groups of Africans and "Coloureds" (mixed race, but in this instance including Indians). The Council was increased from 25 to 33 members, all of whom were to be white. They had the power to prescribe uniforms, badges or other identification signs in respect of the races, as well as differential training. Black nurses were prohibited from holding any official positions within the South African Nursing Association (SANA) and the SANC, and were denied direct representation on their representative bodies, forcing them into racially defined sub-organizations within those bodies referred to as the "Bantu Nurses' Associations." This was also a political move directed at African women generally, to strengthen Pass Laws as: "in order to register with the Nursing Council (compulsory for any practicing nurse) women had to produce their new identity numbers, which meant in turn taking out a pass"[29] and "in the public hospitals matrons often played a key role in insisting that this be done."[30] The Act evoked outrage from a large number of women's groups, from the ANC Women's League to the Anglican Church and Mothers' Union. The Federation of South African Nurses and Midwives was set up in 1957 as a non-racial alternative to SANA.

At large, racially segregated, urban teaching hospitals such as Groote Schuur in Cape Town, King Edward VIII in Durban, or Baragwanath in Soweto, Johannesburg, state-employed nursing staff were perceived as a "moving population" in which "trained nurses [recruited] from overseas, mostly Britain, proved a valuable, if largely temporary, component of the nursing staff."[31] At these hospitals, racial segregation was therefore much more evident than in mission hospitals and African nurses trained and worked in separate parts of the hospitals on "black" wards overseen by senior "white" colleagues. Conversely, the relatively small size of rural mission hospitals' staff, drawn largely from the local inhabitants, not only presented a much more intimate and therefore culturally acceptable face of medicine, but also created a tightly knit community.

Mission hospital development

For the early missions any medical expertise was targeted towards mission staff but gradually expanded to provide care for the rural communities in which they worked, so that eventually "throughout most of Africa, Christian missions . . . provided vastly more care for African communities than did colonial states."[32]

Probably for demographic reasons, the two provinces where the majority of mission hospitals were situated were the Eastern Cape and the province now called KwaZulu Natal, as both had large populations of black Africans with extremely poor access to any public services – as non-governmental bodies, the missions obviously aimed to provide care where government facilities were found most lacking. The hospitals were usually established in very remote rural areas during the inter-war years, although some were founded slightly earlier. They often evolved from hutted mud-thatched clinics run by trained nurses generally working alone or with a native assistant, with their patients sometimes having to travel large distances and cross difficult terrain to reach them.

A central aspect of the history of medical missions that has often been ignored or neglected is the role of the missionary nursing sisters in founding and establishing dispensaries, clinics and even small hospitals, often running them into the 1960s and 1970s without a doctor or with just the sporadic assistance of a visiting (state-appointed) district surgeon. This model seems to have been the rule rather than the exception.[33] As a missionary doctor explained:

> Little money was needed to convert a *rondavel* (round mud hut) into a ward and thus create a hospital. The physic was basic, herbal and available. Sterilization was by a dip in carbolic or a period in the oven after the missionary's wife had finished baking. Tooth-pulling without benefit of analgesia, gave, in exchange for a moment of red agony, ease with no expense at all.[34]

There were occasionally tensions between the medical and nursing missionaries and the colonial doctors – in some cases the local GP or district surgeon would work happily with the mission's nursing staff,[35] but where there was a resident missionary doctor from the outset, there was a greater perceived degree of competition. Many of the trained missionary nurses had come from Scandinavia, Germany or Austria, Britain and the USA, often with the intention to stay for several decades, answering a spiritual call while also wanting to use their nursing training to good effect – perhaps best described as a combined social conscience and spiritual vocation.[36] They came from Catholic and Protestant backgrounds and were not employees of the state but of the Christian missions that supported them. Language initially represented a barrier, as they could not speak the indigenous language and so had to rely on interpreters and had minimal understanding of local customs. Yet most learned basic conversation quite quickly. As American missionary nurse June Kjome explained, "Except for moral support I was not much use in the early days. Until I knew the Zulu language and customs, my nursing contribution was limited."[37] For white nurses establishing the first mission hospitals where traditionally women were subservient, and in competition with a range of traditional healers, the cultural bridges that had to be crossed should not be underestimated.

Language and other cultural issues also represented a problem for mission hospital staff, including trainee nurses.[38] The official rules of the SANC demanded that recruitment and training required all nurses to speak and be examined in either English or Afrikaans, yet they also needed to be able to communicate with hospital staff and patients, which sometimes presented problems both for foreign missionary nurses and for nurses coming from other parts of South Africa. In addition all African nurses from admission to training school onwards were expected to adopt the Western biomedical culture of the hospital and to leave behind their traditional roots. These included beliefs in traditional medicine, and observation of a range of cultural taboos as well as a culture of female subservience. They had to adopt a lifestyle that may have been quite alien and that for many would have included a quite different understanding of health and disease.

For many the role of culture broker between white nursing and medical staff and black patient was a difficult path to tread, and nurses might fervently denounce traditional medicine when working in the clinical field yet express belief in it or even consult a *sangoma* or *inyanga* (traditional healers) when off-duty – a dual practice described as "latent pluralism" which constituted part of the "diplomacy" African nurses had to practice.[39] Nevertheless, the impact of this on healthcare provision for Africans would, for the most part, appear to have been a positive one, providing the reassuring presence of patients' advocates from their own backgrounds among the daunting hospital team of (mostly) white doctors and senior nursing staff. This may have done much to encourage people to attend hospitals and clinics, and to understand their treatment. The alternative view, presented by Marks, was that nurses were trained to become "harbingers of western values" and that "ideas of professionalism and status" created a distance between nurses and their patients.[40] While this may well have been the case in some hospitals, and certainly missionaries were very negative towards what they saw as ignorance and superstition, in the smaller mission hospitals I have studied, arrogance and judgmental disapproval were attitudes that were severely discouraged as being non-Christian by the period of this chapter's study. This fluid historical context is particularly significant as political situations and attitudes changed quite dramatically during this period.

South Africa was one of the most intensive areas of global missionary activity, with numerous different Christian denominations from different countries establishing hospitals and schools attached to their missions. Until amalgamation under the umbrella of the South African Medical Missions in the 1970s "each [denomination] jealously guarded its own [mission hospital's] existence and independence."[41] Growth of missionary medicine in the country meant that by the time the Nationalist Party came to power, in 1948, there were at least 62 mission hospitals in South Africa providing 3000 beds plus extremely busy outpatient departments together with many more mission-run outreach clinics staffed mostly by nurses. By 1970 this number had risen to 110. Consequently, an estimated one in every five hospital beds in the country was in mission hospitals.[42] During the immediate post-war period (1945–1950) many of these hospitals had been expanded, modernized and re-equipped. While this modernization might be perceived as being in line with the state's centralized approach to healthcare, representing a move away from community-based primary care, it more probably reflected improvements delayed by the war but long overdue. As more doctors were recruited by mission societies, hospitals also required facilities such as X-ray, pathology, operating theaters and pharmacies increasing the demand for larger, purpose-built hospitals which in turn increased the need for nursing staff. However, mobile outreach clinics remained a high priority for these hospitals and these were mostly staffed by nurses and occasionally visited by a doctor.

Dr Anthony Barker, Medical Superintendent at the Charles Johnson Memorial Mission Hospital in Nqutu, writing in 1970, felt the major contribution mission hospitals had been able to make to healthcare from his own grassroots viewpoint had been in pediatrics, particularly with kwashiorkor (a childhood form of acute protein deficiency malnutrition) and in preventive medicine, especially polio, diphtheria and tuberculosis. Yet he admitted:

> We were forever aware we were treating the symptoms of an unfair, diseased society, rather than getting at the roots of all this pain. It did not require much insight to recognize that though "our" district had a fairly sophisticated service, those who lived in the next had little or nothing at all . . . Sadly I must own that mission hospitals, even good ones – and many were very good indeed – could never, in their nature, provide the radical answer to a society sick in measure that it was founded on discrimination and injustice.[43]

The final comment typified the strong social consciences of many medical and nursing missionaries as well as the constant struggle throughout this period against an almost overwhelming demand for healthcare but extremely limited resources.

Despite Barker's reservations, the medical missionary system was seen in retrospect as having made major contributions to disease eradication and/or control programs and training of doctors, medical assistants, nurses and midwives and even contributing towards particular medical research projects, while providing: "a comprehensive health care program based on a chain of rural health centers and satellite dispensaries that brought curative and preventative medicine to the whole population within the area covered."[44] Added to this, most mission hospitals' community outreach work increased during this period through mobile and very basic static clinics usually run by nurses, as described later.

Elijah Zulu came to work for Hlabisa hospital in 1953, running the garage, trucks and ambulances, as did carpenter colleague Joel Filela. Together they wrote in *Izibani* of the importance of the hospital to their community as a whole in terms of employment, training and in learning vocational skills as well as providing healthcare. At the end of the article they noted: "so we do not have to leave our families to seek work in the cities" – with migrant labor as one of few options for employment for young men and later also for young women, this was an important point. In fact Mashaba suggested that skills taught by the missions and mission hospitals also improved the marriageable prospects of a lot of women, including a substantial number of nurses: "not just the ones who were nursing, but those who were doing domestic work, doing housekeeping and that sort of thing, that they could say that they'd worked at the Hospital, and that gave them a sort of status." In particular, it was felt that the black nurse had, by the 1960s, become "an influential and prestigious woman in her society."[45]

This was clearly true, as the hospitals represented significant employment for men and women directly and also indirectly within the community through the number of services a hospital requires to function. However, Dr Buhr, a doctor at Emmaus and Hlabisa mission hospitals in the late 1960s, maintained it was still "a drop in the bucket. I mean, how many of our middle and upper grade nurses were married? And we never saw their husbands because their husbands lived in Durban and Johannesburg, and they were just as much a part of the separation and migrant labor thing as everybody else."[46]

Despite this, it certainly represented a valuable "drop in the bucket" for those given training and employment – for example, in 1964 in the twelve Lutheran mission hospitals across the South Eastern region of South Africa there were 215 African student nurses, plus a further 308 trained or semi-trained African nurses and one African doctor, and 505 other African members of staff including clerks, domestics, engineers, electricians, porters, evangelists and pastors. In comparison these hospitals employed a total of 52 American, European or white South African doctors, nurses and "others."[47] Similar statistics could probably be applied to other Anglican and non-conformist mission hospitals.

African nurse training by mission hospitals

Although many became highly competent and experienced practitioners, the majority of African mission hospital nurses trained only to a basic level for which they were awarded a Hospital Certificate, or received a practically based training with minimal theoretical teaching to be admitted to the Roll of Auxiliary Nurses rather than gaining the higher State Registration or Degree level. This was because most of these hospitals failed accreditation status for higher levels of training because they lacked a sufficient combination of facilities, range of experience, numbers of qualified teaching staff, etc. Nevertheless, the four year training taken just to reach Enrollment level typically comprised "classroom lectures combined with practical experience and including anatomy, hygiene and cookery, first aid, medical and surgical nursing, midwifery and bible study"[48] with operating theater and accident department experience being added a few years later. Training to State Registration level could only be achieved by a further "bridging course" involving more theoretical knowledge and further theory and practical examinations, at one of the few training schools accredited to provide this training to black nurses.

One of the exceptions to this was St Mary's Mission Hospital in KwaMagwaza, which graduated to providing for full State Registration by 1944, by which time its inpatient numbers had risen to over 700 annually. Therefore competition from non-Zulu Africans as well as local girls, for probationers' posts, remained fierce throughout the hospital's life as a mission hospital.[49] Yet despite this and an extensive rebuilding project in 1960 it seemed that even this hospital might have to be closed or relocated because it was in an apartheid-designated "white area," and nurse training was consequently suspended from 1962–3. KwaMagwaza was situated in a major sugar-cane growing area demanding a large Zulu workforce and this was a significant factor in the swift overturning of the decision to close the hospital, so that full training was resumed in 1963.

The largest and most significant mission training hospitals were at Lovedale in the Eastern Cape (Transkei) and McCord's Hospital in Durban. Lovedale's pioneering role in nurse training has been described as "hierarchical but caring" and 'liberal paternalism"[50] – a seemingly contradictory concept referring to the reinforcement of views throughout training that African culture was deficient and that biomedical healthcare exemplified a superior (white) civilization. Yet while these nurses were being encouraged to renounce their African culture and to relocate themselves in the hospital hierarchical system that inevitably had white superiors at the top of the ladder, they were simultaneously being encouraged to have higher aspirations and to become useful citizens and missionaries to their own people. Similar challenges faced McCord's Hospital, which was situated in a white area in Durban and was threatened with closure in 1972 but saved by some astute political moves by the American medical management. At both these hospitals and also at several non-mission training institutions such as Baragwanath Hospital, an increasing number of postgraduate courses became available in areas such as management, education, community and public health nursing, all of which enabled nurses to seek promotion. But their horizons, regarding where they could work, would remain limited by apartheid's restrictions for several more decades.

The quarterly journal of Hlabisa mission hospital, *Isibani*, provides numerous examples of the personal cultural divide the African student nurses had to cross during their training, many of them being recruited from other parts of South Africa. These nurses had also to learn the Zulu language in addition to coping with the ordeals of hospital experiences, including living away from home, the terrors of working in an operating theater, encountering birth and death, and nursing male patients. Student Nurse Ndzunga describes a three-day journey back to her home for a week's Christmas holiday and remembers when she first went to Hlabisa "not having any idea of the whereabouts of Zululand to start with" and yet on returning home she felt "almost a Zulu-girl from a Mission Hospital!"[51]; while Probationer Nurse Gcaleka explains that some people had told her "the first thing you do in the hospital is to face a corpse. They told me that this is to prove whether you are afraid of the corpse . . . I was praying that I mustn't be afraid of it!" She also said she came on duty every day, not knowing about "off duty" until someone realized and it was finally explained to her.[52] In particular there were many areas of cultural taboo. Zulu nurse Grace Mashaba recognized that the culture of her community was in a sensitive transitional stage so that, "the black nurse had also to exercise diplomacy in dealing with this issue [of cultural transition] if she were to survive."[53] Student as well as trained nurses often had to exercise this diplomatic role as culture brokers between (white) doctors and sisters and (black) patients.[54] For example, a white doctor might suggest a patient should eat more protein and vitamins, the nurse would appreciate the woman's combined social and cultural circumstances made this impossible so she would try to explain this to the doctor; or the doctor might ask if the patient had consulted with a "witch doctor" and, while realizing the denial she translated for the doctor was baseless, she would actually explain to the patient the dangers of taking two types of medicine at the same time!

Cultural divisions were recognized by some of the more enlightened doctors – for example, George Gale, Medical Superintendent at the Tugella Ferry Church of Scotland Mission Hospital and a strong proponent of social medicine, vividly described the problems of Zulu midwifery practice as he perceived them, recommending that:

The medical man must at all costs avoid the facile short-cut to success in Native medical practice – *experto credo* – by allowing himself to be regarded as a super-magician. This is competing with the *inyanga* (Native doctor) at his own level – that of a mountebank exploiting the credulity and superstitions of simple people. Equally important is it that the doctor should have the active cooperation of his nursing staff. In my own hospital I have had the loyal help of Native nurses from the beginning. The approach to Native patients is, of course, easier for them, both by reason of their knowledge of the vernacular and because of their more ready recognition of Native ideas furtively expressed. It is essential that the nurses should have had a full training, in order that they may be unshaken in their knowledge of and belief in scientific medicine. Incomplete training has obvious dangers . . . Their help is needed, not only in the treatment of disease itself, but also in the task of liberating the Native masses from the ignorance and superstition which shackle them alike in sickness and in health.[55]

Another disparity in the period 1948–1979 was the (relatively) small numbers of fully trained black nurses compared with their white counterparts registering with the SANC. This was despite the fact that the "white" population growth was declining while there was a rapidly growing "black" and "coloured" population. Nevertheless, within the decade 1960–1969 numbers of "coloured" and African nurses had doubled as the numbers of training institutions increased their intakes of students at all levels.[56] However, any increase in numbers of African nurses achieving full registration was not welcomed by many of the white nurse leaders, who wanted the higher qualification to be reserved for white nurses – as Charlotte Searle, Directress of Hospital Services in the Transvaal, in a statement to the Select Committee commented. She was supporting the 1955 Nursing Amendment Bill (which later became enacted by Parliament in 1957) in an attempt to overturn what she regarded as the more liberal and undesirable provisions of the 1944 Nurses Act:

> We enquired whether the provincial authorities really intended training non-European nurses for the full certificate (i.e. as RNs) to any extent because if they did our attitude would have to be quite different . . . if we had known at the time that the policy of the provincial authorities was just the opposite we, and I for one, would certainly not have agreed to the introduction of the Bill . . . We would have fought it to the last ditch. We certainly would not have liked to do something which would ultimately have wrecked the European nursing services in South Africa.[57]

In contrast, Nurse June Kjome writing a few years after the 1957 act had been passed, commented that "apartheid permeates all phases of life: places of residence, education, occupation of land, employment, business rights, buses, other public services and most churches."[58] Many years later she explained how this had affected her for the rest of her life:

> My experience in South Africa made an activist out of me for, you know, against racism and apartheid and all the injustices which you have there. If you

don't look at the root causes of poverty, you're just feeding it . . . And the whole premise of apartheid just, when I realized that the destruction of the Zulu social life also went with the migrant labor system.[59]

One mission doctor also described the unfairness of this racist system that impinged on day-to-day hospital administration:

There were certain . . . policy decisions that the (white) Matron and the Superintendent were making at Emmaus, that we disagreed with, and part of it had to do with our friend . . . who was an [African] nurse there, one of the senior nurses, and she had quite a conflict with the Matron, and we became part of that, and took her side because her position sounded reasonable, and . . . they just weren't willing to make any changes . . . both the Superintendent and the Matron . . . All we know is, we ended up in the middle of some political things, and it did involve blacks versus the white administration staff, and so that's when they [the Lutheran mission] chose to move us to Hlabisa hospital.[60]

This disparity can also be found in the salaries given to nurses of equal rank and qualification but different skin colour, as shown in Table 12.1.

Christian ministries of most denominations were deeply affected by the prevailing ideology of "separate development" and white supremacy and many – though not all – stated their opposition openly. This presented a complex dilemma to nurses from grass-roots level up: while white nurses continued to work and teach within the mission hospitals, they effectively prevented black nurses from reaching a post higher than "sister," yet without the missions providing, financially supporting and running the hospitals, training of black nurses would have been dramatically reduced and rural African healthcare seriously affected. On the other hand, it was part of the principles of the segregationist policy that black patients should be cared for by black nurses, making it inevitable that in hospitals that were labeled "non-European," the white

Table 12.1 Racial discrimination in South African nursing salaries, 1972

Nurse grade	% of 'white' salary (according to respective grade)
"European" Sister	(100%)
"Coloured"/Asian Sister	58
"Black" (African) Sister	47
"European" student nurse	(100%)
"Coloured"/Asian student nurse	65
"Black" (African) student nurse	47

Source: South African Institute of Race Relations (1973), *The African Homelands of South Africa*, p. 166. Johannesburg: SAIRR.

("European") sisters were withdrawn and replaced by black ("Bantu") nurses. In the Orange Free State and Transvaal there were fewer mission hospitals and therefore fewer hospitals where white nurses continued to practice except at the most senior levels of nursing education and management. To carry out their policy to the full, it was therefore the aim of the government to take over all mission hospitals and to remove the influence of overseas white personnel whose liberal Christian ethos conflicted with Nationalist Party policies.

One aspect of apartheid restrictions that has been hitherto overlooked is, rather ironically, the heavy burden of responsibility that fell on the (mostly young white) senior nursing staff running mission hospitals where there was minimal or no medical cover. This is of particular significance when comparing the previous training and working experience many of these nurses would have received in the USA and Europe with that of equally or more experienced, yet racially enforced lower-status, African nurses. Sisters regularly had to move to take charge of wards with which they were less familiar, including theater and maternity, or stand in for the laboratory or X-ray technician if they were away. All trained nurses running outreach clinics in remote areas had to work with a considerable degree of initiative and often outside their recognized role without access to a doctor or telephone.

Endemic diseases prevalent in many of the rural parts of South Africa during this period, and reflective of the poor living conditions associated with the impact of apartheid legislation, included tuberculosis, bilharzia, typhoid, amoebiasis, venereal diseases, malnutrition including pellagra and kwashiorkor, and gastroenteritis. There were also occasional outbreaks of cholera, malaria, polio, measles and chickenpox, which temporarily swamped the hospital's resources. Trauma cases were again regular features of medical and nursing reports – in particular burns and scalds, lacerations, fractures and head injuries from axe, knobkerry and stick fights, and bites and other injuries caused by snakes and wild animals – much of this would have presented a professional and cultural challenge to the young, relatively inexperienced white nurse.

A Methodist missionary nurse running a small Zulu hospital at Maputa, writing about her early experiences in the late 1940s and early 1950s, described routinely having to deal with scabies; malnutrition; a variety of wounds, often from stick fights under the influence of alcohol; toothache; burns; leprosy; VD; and maternal and internal complications.[61] Most of her cases were dealt with as outpatients and the nearest doctor was a district surgeon 60 miles away. The problem continued throughout the period considered here, so that as late as 1981 a law was eventually passed permitting nurses working in remote "black" areas to perform the functions of doctors if there were none "available" – this term was never defined, yet was accepted by all parties.[62]

These were possibly problems familiar to other foreign nurses working in mission hospitals in impoverished rural areas, although this combination of trauma and diseases may have been specific to South Africa. Similarly, in 1965, Canadian nurse Doris Nelson at the small Ununjambeli Mission Hospital mentions having to do a course in plumbing and electrical wiring and comments on "the headache of hospital administration including accounts and book-keeping with P.A.Y.E. income-tax forms, Workmen's Compensation forms and Unemployment Insurance forms."[63] In some cases further training had to be undertaken at Johannesburg or Durban to facilitate South African nurse-registration – for example, June Kjome, writing in 1958, described the maternity departments in South African hospitals as: "quite different than in the USA . . . Our [South African] nurses are trained to give care to the mothers before delivery, then they actually deliver the normal cases themselves here, and give nursing care afterwards to mothers and newborns."[64]

But the dilemma was that mission hospitals were providing the bulk of the training and employment for black nurses, while mission schools until their closure by the government in the early 1950s had produced many of the girls with better levels of education and cultural awareness for recruitment into nursing. With the closure of these schools as part of governmental policy to clamp down on education for blacks, this supply of potential students was soon to be placed under some strain. Despite this, the first black matron in Natal was appointed in 1963 at Edendale Hospital,[65] and at Hlabisa mission hospital the first African sister (Sister Zama Sibeko) was appointed, within just a few years becoming matron of the large Empangeni Provincial Hospital, 40 miles away, and by the mid-1970s the first black (Zulu) matron, Hermina Nxumalo, was in place, making the nursing staff entirely African. She, like all her successors to date, had mission school and mission hospital backgrounds.

End of an era

Much of the white population had shifted away from the free health services provided by the government by the early 1970s while, with the nationalizing of mission hospitals by 1979, almost all non-whites became totally reliant on those services. The report of the National Health Services Commission in 1945, foreshadowing the future, had recognized the value of mission hospitals and recommended subsidies based on bed occupancy.[66] By 1970 the great majority obtained all their funds for capital development and 90% of their running costs from the state. Takeover by the government was seen by many as a *fait accompli*, and it was left largely to the doctors to try to salvage any crumbs of independence for the hospitals with mission hospital boards retaining the right to continue to appoint their own staff, until full nationalization.[67]

With pressure from government for an escalated nationalization program for the mission hospitals, ending independent status for all but a few, the missionaries' position in apartheid South Africa became increasingly untenable, as most refused to become civil servants. It was ever more difficult to find white (American or European) nurses willing to come to supervise nurse training, and white South African nurses did not want to work in these black, deprived rural areas. Anticipating this, the University of Natal working with McCord's Hospital's school of nursing began running Diploma courses for "non-European," i.e. non-white, Sister Tutors from the mid-1960s. By the time the state took over mission hospitals and the missionaries had left, higher promotional avenues had been created and to a certain extent problems relating to career advancement had resolved themselves.

There were a few exceptions to state take-over. For example, McCord Zulu Mission Hospital in Durban, which was state-aided, was never taken over by the state. This was partly because it was originally owned by its missionary founders Dr James and Margaret McCord, who bought the land with donations together with their own money, later donating it to the American Board of Missions in the 1920s. From the 1930s it was governed by a Hospital Board that included many influential local people. Although threatened by closure or removal several times under the Group Areas Act (1950), the hospital was able to survive because of influential contacts especially in local Durban and provincial political circles. Despite several threats to close the hospital because of its location in a "white" residential area, by the late 1970s it was clear that the Durban municipality had a vested interest in keeping the McCord Hospital open in order to treat black workers and domestic servants, therefore the hospital's urban status effectively made all the difference.[68]

Another mission hospital in KwaZulu Natal that has managed to continue its existence as an independently run hospital to the present day is St Mary's Roman Catholic Hospital at Mariannhill, just outside Durban, which retained a large training school for nurses and midwives,[69] but these large hospitals were the exception to the rule and the smaller, more rural mission hospitals were almost all transferred to the state between 1973 and 1976. Although it would appear that some African nurses had resented mission control and favored a more rapid "Africanization" under the apartheid Bantustan "solution," they nevertheless experienced divided loyalties to the mission hospitals where many had trained, and concern for their future. Ominously, the 1978 Nursing amended Act (no. 50) made strike action by nurses a statutory offense with fines of up to 500 rands or one year in jail, or both, suggesting this concern was well founded.

Conclusion

This overview of missionary nursing has considered some significant issues of politics, race and culture, divisions in the professional sisterhoods, the constructs of culture broking, and important rural/urban differences. The crossing of cultures and religions was clearly complex, as white missionary nurses inevitably imposed their values and methods of healthcare, strict discipline, religious beliefs and underlying Western culture on their African staff, trainees and patients. At the same time, these Americans and Europeans were placed in positions of authority within mission hospitals, often being forced to confront situations, diseases and trauma for which they were largely unprepared. Despite this, the mission hospitals were very significant to rural communities, both as healthcare providers and as employers and consumers of a range of services. From the nursing viewpoint in particular, they offered thousands of African women the opportunity to train and to work as professionals. Due to the relatively small size and limited clinical experience of many of these hospitals, training was rarely taken beyond the level of enrolled nurse except at a few hospitals, and because (by definition) they were run by foreign non-governmental agencies, and therefore administered by "white" staff, the missions may be accused of holding back the opportunities for career advancement for "black" Africans – albeit not by intention but because of apartheid legislation.

By 1970 the South African government was providing a large proportion of almost all mission hospitals' funding.[70] So it was virtually a foregone conclusion that by 1975 the state had taken over control and management of most of these hospitals, nationalizing them and placing them under the jurisdiction of the Bantustan authorities. Many missionaries felt they were deserting a sinking ship, leaving their African staff and patients to the mercy of an unmerciful apartheid system.

However, the loss of the missionaries was repeatedly regretted with great sincerity by many hospital workers whom I interviewed, who felt standards and morale fell noticeably following nationalization, as did the sense of "family" that was often mentioned, with individual doctors and nurses who had stayed for more than twenty years still visiting and keeping in touch over forty years later! While the legacy of these rural hospitals and clinics has to be acknowledged, many suffered subsequently from lack of governmental funding during the remainder of the apartheid era. However, despite the passage of time, many have survived into the post-apartheid era and continue to form the focus of primary healthcare throughout this region today, retaining some of their old mission traditions such as morning prayers, and the original hospital graduation traditions.

Looking at the role of the mission hospitals in the education of African women as nurses and hospital staff, this chapter has revealed insights into the development of new and important avenues of work for women in South Africa, as well as offering a different perspective on the controversial subject of the contribution and influence of missions.

Notes

1 Vaughan, M. 1991, *Curing their Ills: Colonial Power and African Illness*. Cambridge: Polity Press.

2 Zondi, Welcome S. 2000, "Medical missions and African demand in Kwazulu-Natal, 1836–1918." Unpublished PhD Thesis, University of Cambridge Modern History Faculty.

3 Horwitz, S. 2006, "A history of Baragwanath Hospital in Soweto." Unpublished DPhil Thesis, Modern History Faculty, University of Oxford.

4 See for example: Marks, S. 1990, *The Nursing Profession and the Making of Apartheid*, paper presented at History Workshop: "Structure and Experience in the Making of Apartheid," University of the Witwatersrand, Johannesburg, 6 – 10 February 1990. Available at (accessed 7 February 2013): http://wiredspace.wits.ac.za/bitstream/handle/10539/7925/HWS-267.pdf?sequence=1; Marks, S. 1994, *Divided Sisterhood: Race, Class and Gender in the South African Nursing Profession*. London: St Martin's Press; Marks, S. 1997, "The legacy of the history of nursing for post-apartheid South Africa" in A.M. Rafferty, J. Robinson and R. Elkan (eds.) *Nursing History and the Politics of Welfare*. London: Routledge; Marks, S. 2002, "'We were men nursing men': Male nursing on the mines in twentieth-century South Africa" in W. Woodward, P. Hayes and G. Minkley (eds.) *Deep hiStories: Gender and Colonialism in Southern Africa*. Amsterdam: Rodopi, pp. 177–205.

5 Digby, Anne 2005, "Making a medical living: The economics of medical practice in the Cape c.1860–1910" in H. Deacon et al. (eds.) *The Cape Doctor in the Nineteenth Century: A Social History*. Amsterdam: Clio Medica 74, pp. 249–280; Digby, A. 2006, *Diversity and Division in Medicine: Health Care in South Africa from the 1800s*. Cambridge: Cambridge University Press; Digby, A. 2007, "'Western' medicine and witchcraft in South Africa: Initiatives at Victoria Hospital, Lovedale" in M. Harrison, M. Jones, and H. Sweet (eds.)

From Western Medicine to Global Medicine. Hyderabad: Orient Blackswan, pp. 221–248; Digby, A. and Phillips, H. with Deacon, H. and Thomson, K. 2008, *At the Heart of Healing: Groote Schuur Hospital 1938–2008.* Cape Town: Jacana; and Digby, A. 2008, "'Vision and vested interests': National health service reform in South Africa and Britain during the 1940s and beyond." *Social History of Medicine* 21(3), pp. 485–502.

6 Digby, A. and Sweet, H. 2001, "Nurses as culture brokers in twentieth-century South Africa" in E. Waltraud (ed.) *Plural Medicine, Tradition and Modernity, 1800–2000,* London: Routledge, pp. 113–129; Sweet, H. and Digby, A. 2004, "Race, identity and the nursing profession in South Africa, c.1850–1958" in S. McCann and B. Mortimer (eds.) *New Directions in the History of Nursing.* London: Routledge, pp. 109–124.

7 Digby, A. and Sweet, H. 2012, "Social medicine and medical pluralism: The Valley Trust and Botha's Hill Health Centre, South Africa, 1940s to 2000s." *Social History of Medicine* 25(2), pp. 425–445.

8 Sweet, H. 2004, "'Wanted: 16 nurses of the better educated type' – Provision of nurses to South Africa in the early C20th." *Nursing Inquiry* 11(3), pp. 176–184; Sweet, H. 2009, "Expectations, encounters and ecclesiastics: Mission medicine in Zululand, South Africa" in M. Harrison, M. Jones, H. Sweet (eds.) *From Western Medicine to Global Medicine: The Hospital Beyond the West.* Hyderabad: Orient Blackswan, pp. 330–359.

9 Gelfand, M. 1984, *Christian Doctor and Nurse: The History of Medical Missions in South Africa from 1799–1976.* Mariannhill: Mariannhill Mission Press.

10 McCord, J.B. and Douglas, J. 1951, *My Patients were Zulus.* New York: Rinehart and Co.

11 Aitken, R.D. and Gale, G. n.d. "The papers on medical missionaries and medical hospital missions in South Africa" 1928–1956. Microfilm. Borthwick Institute for Archives, York University.

12 Schimlek, Francis 1953, *Mariannhill: A Study in Bantu Life & Missionary Effort.* Mariannhill: Mariannhill Mission Press.

13 Barker, A. 1959, *The Man Next to Me: An Adventure in African Medical Practice.* New York: Harper and Brothers; Barker, A. 1970, "Medical Missions – what of the future?" *Seek* (October).

14 Kargaard, Jens 2004, *Out of Africa: A Doctor's Life.* Wansdsbeck: Reach Publishers.

15 Ingle, Ronald 2010, *An Uneasy Story: The Nationalising of South African Mission Hospitals 1960–1976: A Personal Account.* Pretoria: Institute for Missiological and Ecumenical Research.

16 See for example: Searle, C. 1965, *The History of the Development of Nursing in South Africa, 1652–1960: A Socio-historical Survey.* Pretoria: The South African Nursing Association; Searle, C. 1991, *Towards Excellence: The Centenary of State Registration for Nurses and Midwives in South Africa 1891–1991.* Durban: Butterworths.

17 Kjome, June 1963, *Back of Beyond: Bush Nurse in South Africa.* Minneapolis: Augsburg Publishing House.

18 Mashaba, G. 1995, *Rising to the Challenge of Change: A History of Black Nursing in South Africa.* Cape Town: Juta.

19 Buthelezi, M.S.T. MaDlamini 2004, *African Nurse Pioneers in KwaZulu Natal – 1920–2000.* Victoria, Canada: Trafford.

20 The term "Coloured" referred to a heterogeneous or mixed-race ethnic group while "Indian" referred to anyone from an Asian background. "White" only included Afrikaans or other non-Coloured European descendants and "Black" or "Native" referred to black Africans.

21 Data for 2008 according to the World Bank, taking rural as defined by national statistical offices, see: www.tradingeconomics.com/south-africa/rural-population-wb-data.html (accessed 31 July 2011).

22 Cooper et al. stated in 1993 that, "Africans are in the majority at just over 38-million, making up 79.6% of the total population. The white population is estimated at 4.3-million (9.1%), the coloured population at 4.2-million (8.9%) and the Indian/Asian population at just short

of 1.2-million (2.5%)." Cooper, D., Hamilton, R. and Mashaba, H. (1993), *Race Relations Survey 1992/1993*. Johannesburg: South African Institute of Race Relations.

23 Digby, A. 2005, "Making a medical living" pp. 250–251.

24 See Staugard, F. 1985, *Traditional Medicine in Botswana: Traditional Healers*. Gaborone: Ipelegeng; Digby, A. and Sweet, H. 2001, "Nurses as culture brokers in twentieth-century South Africa."

25 Editorial, SANJ, 1963, Vol. XXX (July 7) citing: Editorial SANJ 1913, "New beginnings" *South African Nursing Record* Vol. I.

26 Vaughan, Megan 1994, "'Health and Hegemony': Representations of disease and the creation of the colonial subject in Nyasaland" in D. Engels and S. Marks (eds.) *Contesting Colonial Hegemony. Gramsci and Imperialism*. London: British Academic Press, pp. 173–201.

27 Buthelezi, M.S.T. MaDlamini 2004, *African Nurse Pioneers*, p. 3.

28 Ibid., p. 1.

29 Marks, S. 1990, *The Nursing Profession and the Making of Apartheid*.

30 Marks, S. 1994, *Divided Sisterhood*, p. 161.

31 Digby et al. 2008, *At the Heart of Healing*, p. 159.

32 Vaughan, M. 1991, *Curing their Ills*, p. 56.

33 Sweet, H. 2009, "Expectations, encounters and ecclesiastics", pp. 344, 357–358.

34 Barker, A. 1970, "Medical missions – What of the future?"

35 Such as KwaMagwasa Anglican Mission Hospital, founded in 1912 by a British missionary nurse, Lucy Mallandaine, and Hlabisa Lutheran Mission Hospital, founded in 1915 by Norwegian nurse Petrine Solveik.

36 Sweet, H. 2004, "Wanted: 16 nurses of the better educated type", pp. 176–184.

37 Kjome, June 1963, *Back of Beyond*, p. 60.

38 After 1994 eleven official languages were designated alongside many more unofficial dialects across South Africa.

39 See endnote 50 below; also: Digby, A. and Sweet, H. 2001, "Nurses as culture brokers in twentieth-century South Africa", pp. 124–125. Unfortunately, numbers of traditional healers during this period were not recorded and it was only in the post-apartheid period that the significance of the healers began to be appreciated.

40 Marks, S. 1994, *Divided Sisterhood*, pp. 210–213.

41 Gelfand, M. 1984, *Christian Doctor and Nurse*, p. 289.

42 Ibid., pp. 257–259.

43 Barker, A. 1970, "Medical Missions – what of the future?"

44 Browne, S.G. et al. 1979, "The contribution of medical missionaries to tropical medicine: service – training – research", *Transactions of the Royal Society of Tropical Medicine and Hygiene* 73: 357–360.

45 Mashaba, G. 1995, *Rising to the Challenge of Change*, pp. 58–61.

46 Private oral history collection KZN17, Dr and Mrs Buhr 16/10/2003 (N. Dakota, USA).

47 1964 "Doctors' notes," *Izibani*.

48 Editorial 1959, *Izibani*, pp. 5–6

49 Mashaba, Themba G. 1982, "The contribution made by the Anglican Missions to nursing education in Zululand." Unpublished MA thesis, University of Port Elizabeth, Port Elizabeth.

50 Digby, A. 2007, "Western medicine and witchcraft in South Africa", pp. 223–224.

51 Nurse Ndzunga 1965, *Izibani*, pp. 13–14.

52 Nurse Gcaleka 1965, *Izibani*, pp. 19–20.

53 Mashaba, G. 1995, *Rising to the Challenge of Change*, pp. 60–61.

54 Digby, A. and Sweet, H. 2001, "Nurses as culture brokers", pp.113–129.

55 Gale, G.W. 1936, "The rural hospital as an agent in native health education," *South African Medical Journal* 10 (August 8), pp. 541–543.

56 Searle, C. 1991, *Towards Excellence*, pp. 237–269: Searle presents SANC figures of 17,947 white nurses registering in 1960 increasing to 24,504 in 1969, compared with 6,149 "Coloured and Bantu" nurses in 1960, rising to 13,699 by 1969; while on the SANC Rolls, white nurses rose from 675 to 887 over the same period and "Coloured and Bantu" nurses rose from 2,426 to 7,468.

57 Quoted in Marks, S. 1990, *The Nursing Profession and the Making of Apartheid*.

58 Kjome, June 1963, *Back of Beyond*, p. 234.

59 Private oral history collection KZN16, June Kjome 06 & 07/10/2003 (Wyoming, USA).

60 Private oral history collection KZN17, Dr and Mrs Buhr 16/10/2003 (N. Dakota, USA).

61 Cookson, N. 1956, "Maputa," *South African Nursing Journal* (October), p. 34.

62 Wynchank, Sinclair (1997) "Women medical doctors in South Africa: Transcultural and other influences before, during and after apartheid", *Proceedings of "Women in Multicultural South Africa" December 12–14, 1996 International Seminar*, Université de La Réunion, Special Editor, Dr Claude Féral.

63 Nelson, Doris 1965, *Izibani*, pp. 7–8.

64 Kjome, June 1959, "Midwifery Department", *Izibani*, Vol. I, No. 2 (February), pp. 8–9.

65 Matron Harriet R. Shezi was the first African matron – appointed in 1958 to KwaThema Bantu (Provincial) Hospital, Springs in the Transvaal.

66 Digby, A. 2008, "Vision and vested interests", pp. 485–502.

67 See Ingle, Ronald 2010, *An Uneasy Story*.

68 I am indebted to Drs Julie Parle, Vanessa Noble, and Catherine Burns and Mr Fabio Zoia for this summary of their extensive research of the McCord Hospital.

69 Catholic Health Care Association of Southern Africa 2011, *In the Service of Healing: A History of Catholic Health Care in Southern Africa*. Johannesburg: CATHCA, pp. 117–120.

70 Horwitz, S. 2009, *Health and Health Care under Apartheid*. Johannesburg: Adler Museum of Medicine, University of the Witzwatersrand, p. 4.

13

NURSING AND THE "HEARTS AND MINDS" CAMPAIGN, 1948–1958

The Malayan Emergency

Rosemary Wall and Anne Marie Rafferty

From 1900 to 1955, British Malaya was the most common destination in the world for British colonial nurses (see Figure 13.1). The Malayan territories in South-East Asia were composed of many races including aboriginal communities, Malays who were largely rural, and various Chinese and Indian immigrant populations, in addition to the British and Eurasians.[1] This complex crucible resulted in racial and political tension. Examining nursing during the Malayan Emergency (1948–1960) highlights the role of the profession during a political crisis, and the problems faced by the Colonial Nursing Service in supplying sufficient nurses for the area. How were British nurses persuaded to travel to Malaya and how did methods compromise stringent recruitment standards? How did the Emergency attract international health organizations' attention to nursing? In particular, in what way did nursing become embroiled in the "hearts and minds" campaign to defeat communist insurgents? This chapter argues that the Malayan case illustrates an early emphasis on rural healthcare and the training of nurses within post-World War II international health policy.

For decades, racial and political tensions had been building in British Malaya. The area was a "patchwork quilt of dependencies with different political and administrative traditions" and representative institutions had not developed to the same extent as in India, Burma and Ceylon.[2] While the Straits Settlements, which included Singapore, were a Crown colony, sultans retained sovereignty of the Federated Malay States (FMS) and Unfederated Malay States (UFMS), although the sultans were compelled to follow advice from British administrators.[3] The political life of the Malayan territories was further complicated by the rapid economic development of the region and the influx of immigrant labor. By 1938, Malaya was the world's most successful producer of natural rubber, bringing huge demands for plantation labor, encouraging migration from India. The colony also mined a third of the world's tin before World

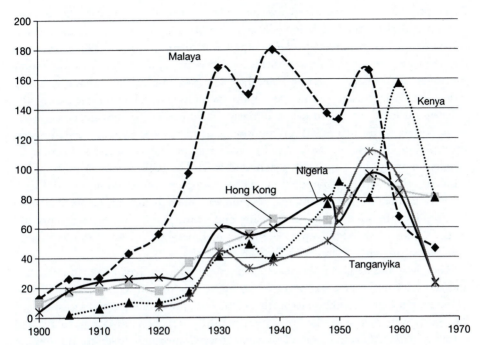

Figure 13.1 Number of British colonial nurses sent to the five most common destinations.

Source: The Bodleian Library of Commonwealth and African Studies at Rhodes House, Oxford, Overseas Nursing Association Collection, Colonial/Overseas Nursing Association, *Annual Reports*, 1897–1966, Brit Emp s400 131.

War II (WWII), an industry that attracted Chinese immigrants.[4] By 1941, although the population of British Malaya was 43 percent Chinese, 41 percent Malay and 14 percent Indian, the Chinese and Indian populations had not been granted political representation. Indeed, conscious of the effect that immigration was having on the population from the 1870s on, the British declared "Malaya for the Malays," developing this ethnic group's political and public sector roles and their education, while operating a *laissez-faire* attitude towards the recent immigrant populations.[5] This resulted in the Malayan sultans' disproportionate influence over the colonial government, which was not in sync with the shifting balance of socio-economic and demographic change.[6]

As part of the Japanese invasion of South-East Asia during WWII, between December 1941 and February 1942, the Japanese gained control of and occupied Malaya and Singapore. British civilians were imprisoned in internment camps. After regaining control in 1945, the British decided to restructure Malaya in order to work toward Malayan self-governance within the Commonwealth. The British government implemented the Malayan Union, excluding Singapore from this new state in order to appease business interests in Malaya who felt threatened by the city's hegemony, and also because the largely Chinese population of Singapore was a concern for Malays. The establishment of the Union involved coercing the sultans to sign over their sovereignty to the British, and opening up citizenship to non-Malays.[7] The

Malay protests regarding the new regime led to the abandonment of the Union, and the British declared the Federation of Malaya in 1948. The Federation gave concessions to Malays, such as making it harder for the Chinese and Indians to gain citizenship, and returning sovereignty to the sultans, with Malaya administered by a high commissioner rather than a governor. Thus, the Federation insulted the Malayan-Chinese who were an important workforce within the colony and had fought against the Japanese during the war.[8] In fact, the Malayan-Chinese communist guerrilla movement developed during WWII, in opposition to Japanese occupation.[9] Additionally, the Malayan Communist Party (MCP) aired grievances about social and economic problems among the Chinese that stemmed from the 1930s. Although many of the Chinese urban and rural populations did not support communism, they did have complaints about the British colonial government which included inadequate medical facilities and the short supply of housing and of food, resulting in high rents and prices.[10] This tension built up to the Malayan Emergency (1948–1960), a violent communist, guerrilla insurgency fought in rural areas.

The Malayan Emergency was one of the most dramatic challenges to British interests and authority in the post-war years, requiring the deployment of some 20 battalions of the British army in addition to nearly 50,000 local police and special constabulary.[11] The stakes were high since the Emergency put the production of Malayan rubber and tin at risk. These Malayan commodities were crucial for earning dollars for the Sterling Area. This bloc was officially formed at the beginning of WWII and included colonies and ex-colonies that fixed their currencies to the British pound, with Britain exchanging sterling for all of the US dollars earned within the Sterling Area. Through this policy, Britain hoped to stimulate markets for its exports and relieve its economic indebtedness to the United States. The insurgency also threatened to open the way for Chinese domination in Malaya at a time when Mao Tse Tung was establishing the People's Republic of China (1949).[12] In January 1950, three months after Mao's victory in China, the British government announced its recognition of the communist government in China, accompanied by Prime Minister Clement Atlee's reassurance that the struggle to stamp out the MCP would continue.[13] If the communists gained control of the Malayan interior, the repercussions would have been far-reaching for the British economy, the control of Singapore, and for relations with the Malayan population and with all Western countries' interests in Asia. Significantly, British policy demonstrated a determination to strengthen British control of the Malayan peninsula, in contrast to the relinquishment of India, Ceylon and Burma.[14] The consequence of this action was that Britain was drawn into a protracted and expensive counterinsurgent campaign.[15]

The "second colonial occupation" is a term used by historians to refer to the post-WWII return of the British in order to re-establish rule over the colonies with a goal to provide the mother country with much-needed raw materials and foodstuffs.[16] This movement supported the increase of British nurses in the colonies. Extra funding from the British Colonial Development and Welfare Fund, and tripartite agreements for Technical Assistance between the World Health Organization (WHO), UNICEF (United Nations International Children's Emergency Fund) and colonial governments led to British government nurses being sent into the Empire in

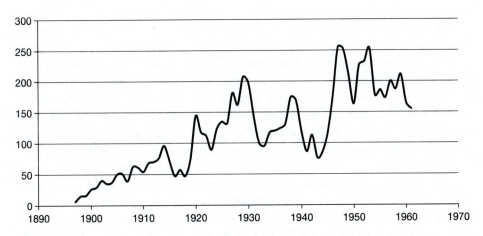

Figure 13.2 Number of Colonial/Overseas Nursing Association nurses sent overseas, 1897–1961.

Source: The Bodleian Library of Commonwealth and African Studies at Rhodes House, Oxford, Overseas Nursing Association Collection, Colonial/Overseas Nursing Association, *Annual Reports*, 1897–1966, Brit Emp s400 131.

unprecedented numbers during the late 1940s, with one of their major roles being to train the local populations in nursing (see Figure 13.2).[17]

Situating post-war Malaya in the historiography of colonial nursing

The nurses who were recruited and employed by the government or its agencies were the largest professional group of female colonial government employees. Between 1922 and 1943, 2,189 nursing sisters were recruited, compared to 83 female teachers and 72 female doctors.[18] Nurses were probably the second largest group of single women in Empire, next to teachers who were employed in Malaya by a wide variety of agencies.[19] Although they initially worked for white populations overseas, the nurses' role in caring for local populations gradually increased, culminating in the training of local nurses.[20] In Britain, colonial nursing was organized by the Colonial Nursing Association (CNA) which was established in 1896, and worked as an agency for the Colonial Office until 1940, when the relationship was formalized with the establishment of the Colonial Nursing Service.[21] In 1918, the organization was renamed the Overseas Nursing Association (ONA), reflecting the work of the nurses in locations outside the official British Empire.[22] From 1896 to 1966, the association recruited 8,450 nurses for work overseas.[23]

The historiography of government nursing in the tropical colonies is slowly building upon the more mature studies of early British nursing in the white dominions.[24] Studies of nurses in British tropical colonies have so far focused on single countries, such as Jhana Gourlay's study of Florence Nightingale's interest in India.[25] West Africa has been a focus for two historians interested in CNA nurses, with Dea Birkett's claim that it was the venue for "by far" the largest number of colonial nurses.[26] However, our research demonstrates that, between 1920 and WWII, South-East Asia became the most common destination for nurses, after which East Africa employed the most.[27] Margaret Jones incorporates colonial nursing into her study of healthcare in Ceylon (present-day Sri Lanka) and in particular reveals the relatively early training of local nurses to higher levels than other colonies.[28] With virtual self-government in Ceylon dating from 1931, this is a rather different case to Malaya, where independence came only in 1957. She also examines the post-colonial incursion of the Rockefeller Foundation following the granting of independence in 1948, and the subsequent involvement of the WHO.[29]

Helen Calloway and Birkett's discussions of colonial nursing in West Africa are incorporated into a substantial body of work on gender and empire. In the 1980s, Calloway's work in this genre established single working British women in empire as a crucial topic. The nurses, lady medical officers and female teachers in empire had perhaps the easiest access to local people.[30] Margaret Strobel and Alison Bashford also briefly acknowledge the role of nurses.[31] Other literature on working white women includes discussions of missionaries with their ideology of religious and cultural superiority (approaches that were not widely successful among Muslims in Malaya), and groups such as teachers with their capacity to connect with local populations.[32] From the perspective of the history of medicine, Lenore Manderson mentions the role of British nurses and health visitors in women and children's health.[33] In many cases this literature reveals that women's roles in Empire enabled close contact with the local communities. As Anne McClintock reminds us, white women were "boundary makers" in Empire.[34]

Although the colonial nurse was subordinate to the male colonial officials and doctors, her lower status and her gender were advantageous for building links with local people, particularly Muslim women. In particular, the local women, whom the British nurses trained and worked with, acted as "cultural brokers," disseminating Western biomedical ideas to the local populations.[35] However, these colonial relationships were complex. The racial and gender hierarchy could be disrupted in situations where white nurses were treated as subordinate to local doctors, as Margaret Jones has illustrated for 1930s Ceylon.[36] Indeed, this was also the case according to one British nurse working in Malaya in the 1920s; Mary Culliton wrote that working with the locally trained doctors in Perak required "tact" as they did not appreciate the training of the British nurses, and offended some sisters by explaining orders in minute detail.[37] WHO male nurse tutor, John Waterer, reported the challenge of male Asian hospital assistants not accepting the authority of the female European sisters and matrons.[38]

The history of nursing in areas of South-East Asia has previously been discussed in terms of the "colonial gaze" of health visitors in Malaya.[39] Nursing auxiliaries volunteering with the St John's Ambulance Brigade in Malaya have been examined within the period during and after the WWII Japanese invasion.[40] Additionally, descriptive accounts of the history of nursing in Singapore have been produced.[41] Catherine Choy's study of Filipino nursing includes a short study of the American nurses who traveled to Asia, but mainly concentrates on the supply of Filipino nurses generated for the American nursing market, and these Filipino nurses' experiences in the USA.[42] Winifred Connerton's extensive exploration of the experiences and influence of American nurses in the Philippines and Puerto Rico depicts the variety of ways in which nurses could travel, whether as missionaries, with the armed forces, or as colonial nurses.[43]

As shown by Figure 13.2, the largest number of nurses in the British Empire operated in the late 1940s and early 1950s. Thus far, this is a neglected period for research on the history of medicine in Malaya as, except for Phua Kai Hong's doctoral thesis on the Malayan health services, the small number of histories of healthcare in Malaya stop before WWII.[44] Yet the challenges of the Emergency and decolonization make this a compelling period for study, with competing political agendas and significant shortages in the healthcare workforce.

The nurse is increasingly a focus for studies of international health organizations. In their studies of the Rockefeller Foundation's International Health Division, John Farley and Barbara Brush have noted the important role nurses played in spreading American schemes of public health around the globe.[45] In addition to Jones' brief account of the WHO incursion into nursing in Sri Lanka, Christine Hallett and Lis Wagner have discussed the role of nurses within the WHO. Focussing on the European Office, they examine the essential role of nurses in the organization's aim to expand primary healthcare which had been articulated in 1978.[46]

Nursing and the "hearts and minds" campaign

The term "hearts and minds" – a strategy of counter-guerrilla warfare – was coined by the High Commissioner for Malaya, Gerald Templer, in 1952. It referred to a "total effort" in political, economic, cultural and social policy and practice in order to gain the support of the Malayan people.[47] Contemporaries usually discussed this strategy in terms of inspiring "confidence" and building or breaking "morale."[48] The nurses who were recruited in order to assist with the hearts and minds campaign in Malaya deliberately reached previously neglected populations as part of the acceleration of "cultural colonialism."[49]

This policy was introduced nearly four years after the declaration of the Emergency as previous propaganda methods had failed in the rural areas of Malaya. Templer arrived in Malaya in 1951, following the death of his predecessor, Henry Gurney, in a guerrilla ambush.[50] Templer's morale-boosting anti-communist campaign was in contrast to Gurney's punitive strategy. Gurney's ruthless program of detention and resettlement to break up guerrilla networks was accompanied by the distribution of millions of leaflets to rural areas, film shows and radio broadcasts, and the rationing of food for the rural communities in order to reduce the supplies reaching the terrorists. His political concessions to the urban elites did not appease the economic and social concerns of the rural Chinese-Malayans.[51]

Templer decided to continue Gurney's plan to resettle Chinese squatters in order to separate them from the guerrillas, hence disrupting the MCP's supply lines. This scheme relocated the rural Chinese population in areas that were often restricted by barbed or electric wire and security guards. In total 500,000 people (10 percent of Malaya's population) were moved into what Templer renamed the "New Villages".[52] The 410 villages had main streets, village committee offices, temples, churches, playing fields, schools, police stations, markets, homes for older people, and in some cases maternity homes, assembly homes and cinemas. These villages housed not only Chinese, but also Malay, Javanese and Indian people. From a healthcare and sanitation perspective, resettlement led to problems such as the lack of adequate supplies of clean water and reliance on voluntary organizations for health clinic services, which Templer was determined to resolve.[53] The prevalence of malaria and water-borne diseases in the villages was particularly challenging for medical officials due to the lack of doctors and nurses.[54]

Most importantly for the history of nursing, the "hearts and minds" campaign included improvements in basic measures such as medical facilities, education and social welfare as part of a "mass exercise in propaganda."[55] Ramakrishna has argued that this was crucial for success in the Malayan Emergency as most Chinese in Malaya were much more concerned about the economic and social problems of their everyday lives than about political reform.[56] Additionally, the campaign included a demonstration of the intention of granting independence, in particular the Malayanization program – enabling Asians, whether Malay, Chinese or Indian, to take senior administrative roles, including those within healthcare.[57]

This type of program, utilizing healthcare to inspire newly independent countries or those on their way to independence to align with capitalist rather than communist countries, became part of international health organizations' policies. This was despite Brock Chisholm, a Canadian and the first Director General of the WHO from 1948 to 1953, being a critic of the Cold War; he hoped to exclude politics from the organization's activities. Yet conflict within the WHO led to many communist states withdrawing, including the USSR and China, because of disagreements regarding WHO administration and policy.[58] John Farley has argued that a "magic bullet" approach of quick solutions to eradicating disease was the route to winning "hearts and minds" within newly independent countries during the Cold War in order to persuade them to align with capitalist rather than communist ideologies. However, Chisholm's influence also inspired an understanding of the importance of social and economic conditions for public health.[59] Additionally, the records of the WHO reveal that there was a commitment to "Technical Health Education" in order to assist training of healthcare practitioners in countries that had been badly affected by WWII.[60]

The Malayan Emergency – a crisis in care

The increase in demand for rubber and tin, stimulated by the Korean War (1950–53), boosted the Malayan government's coffers, enabling increased expenditure on medicine and health.[61] Decisions on healthcare provision changed in 1951 with the introduction of the "member" system to the Malayan Legislative Council. Members of the Council represented commercial and state interests, and were given portfolios, including a Federal Medical Programme under the Member for Health. The Director of Medical Services, in charge of the colonial Malayan Medical Service, became responsible to the Member of Health, advising him on future plans for Malayan healthcare. Prior to 1951, healthcare provision was administered locally and was uneven across the states, particularly in rural areas.[62] In July 1951, Lee Tiang Keng, the Member for Health, requested that medical facilities be established in the New Villages. The aim was not to give the villages any special consideration but to provide them with the same level of service as the rest of the rural population, delivered by male Asian hospital assistants.[63] However, the shortage of staff made this impossible, and existing training schools for hospital assistants were already "fully taxed."[64] Even so, the new measures provided for 32 dispensaries, a further 29 mobile dispensaries, 49 treatment and examination rooms, 25 hospital assistants, 23 hospital attendants, six health inspectors and 156 overseers and labourers for anti-malarial work.[65]

"Hospital assistants" was a term used in Malaya since the late 19th century for male dressers who had been involved in roles including administration, nursing, dispensing, laboratory work, surgery and plastering; the roles also involved serving as clinic assistants, treating minor injuries, storekeeping and radiography, with work not necessarily within hospitals despite their job title. By the 1940s and 1950s these men received the same training as nurses. For 400 villages, 25 hospital assistants were insufficient, so the staff from the existing rural settlements were also stretched over the newly settled areas.[66] Hence, these clinics led to an immediate demand for British nursing staff as a result of the lack of locally trained nurses and assistants.

In 1946, the Malayan medical report presented statistics of its public health staff who conducted much of the rural work. The Director of Medical Services considered that the 28 nursing sisters (usually British nurses in senior positions) and 90 nurses (usually Asian nurses in subordinate roles) for a population of approximately five million was small "by western standards, but it is probably higher than would be found in most of the eastern tropical territories."[67] The rural areas were particularly difficult to cover, considering 47 nursing positions remained vacant within Malaya in 1950.[68]

Despite the demand for nurses, the ONA did not supply enough recruits for rural Malaya. The Emergency deterred nurses from applying to work in the area.[69] Additionally, the deaths of 48 of the British nursing sisters who had served in Malaya during WWII dramatically depleted the post-war nursing workforce in British Malaya. Of colonial nurses working in Malaya and Singapore prior to WWII, four nurses were killed when the Japanese invaded Singapore, 40 were killed while trying to escape on ships, and four more died in the internment camps.[70] As a result of these deaths and the challenges of post-WWII recruitment, the number of British colonial nurses in Malaya and Singapore was only 137 in 1948, whereas it has been 180 in 1939.[71] Although more nurses were required, only nine nurses were appointed to go to Malaya in 1950, and in that year the total number of ONA nurses there decreased to 133.[72] This was at a time of particularly intense terrorist activity, with 4,789 incidents in 1950 and 6,082 in 1951.[73] Guerrilla warfare was nearly under control by 1954, and this led to an increase in nursing recruits. Hence, by 1955 there were 166 British colonial nursing sisters working in Malaya.[74] By March 1953 there was a total of 560 registered nurses in Malaya (including the Asian nurses), but H.M.O. Lester, the Director of Medical Services, believed that the number of nurses should be 2,000 and that a further 2,000 auxiliaries were required.[75]

This nursing shortage in Malaya was exacerbated by the increased global demand for nurses after WWII. British nurses were in high demand for the new British National Health Service and also for the United Nations Relief and Rehabilitation Administration, an organization founded by the Allied nations during WWII in order to provide relief to areas that had been occupied by Axis powers.[76] Additionally, with the second colonial occupation, ever increasing numbers of nurses were going to work across the Empire in the late 1940s (see Figure 13.2).[77]

Recruitment was even more challenging because of the careful assessment of the character of potential colonial nurses in the ONA interview. The word "character" is a chameleon term that covers a code of values, virtues and moral behavior, sometimes explicitly stated but often implicit.[78] In the case of nurses recruited by the ONA it was those behaviors deemed appropriate, combined with the exercise of leadership and authority in the colonial context, which implied a particular type of deportment, demeanor, temperament of self-control, tact, adaptability and resilience, especially important in the tropics, where climate and circumstances could be very trying. Following WWII, the ONA described the type of nurse required: "Character and vision are needed in addition to academic qualifications."[79] The ONA lamented in 1947 that although it had "a greater choice of candidates, there has not been a surplus of good nurses, because heavy demands have come from all Colonies as the Governments build up their staffs after the war and plan developments."[80] The ONA still refused to reduce its required standards of training and character even at this time of political crisis, accompanied by severe nursing shortages. Successful applicants were expected to be dually trained in nursing and midwifery, and have three years' post-qualification experience. Increasingly, particular posts required experience in teaching.[81] In 1950, 298 nurses were interviewed, but only 163 were selected; the ONA argued that "however difficult recruitment may be, it is imperative that there should be no lowering of the standard of the nursing sisters selected, and the Nursing Selection Committee can by no means accept all the nurses who apply and are interviewed."[82] The shortage of ONA nurses resulted in the Malayan government accepting help from the military and calling for assistance from the Red Cross, the St John's Ambulance Brigade and WHO.

A call for help: The military, the Red Cross, St John's Ambulance Brigade, and the World Health Organization

Following the end of the Japanese occupation, the British Military Administration governed Malaya from September 1945 to April 1946.[83] Many army nurses had been working in Malaya during the military administration and some wished to remain. However, in 1946 only seven nurses were released from military service for work in civilian duties and a mere 11 military nurses who had been seconded from elsewhere in Empire to civilian duties in Malaya were allowed to remain for a longer posting.[84] These nurses were required to attend an interview with A.C. Pender, a retired ONA nurse who volunteered to return for this task. Additionally, several other active and retired members of the ONA, who had previously worked in Malaya, volunteered to assist the military nurses in Malaya and Hong Kong, which had also suffered badly from Japanese occupation.[85]

Although such a small number of military nurses could not meet the demand, the recruitment of these nurses was more relaxed than in the African colonies of the British Empire, where military nurses were forbidden to work within the colonial healthcare system due to their lack of midwifery training.[86] The ONA refused to accept the suggestion that military nurses should be recruited for the African colonies, which was made by the Director of Recruitment for the Colonial Service. The association was concerned that a change in standards would cause anger in the colonies as some nurses had specifically undertaken this certificate in order to qualify for colonial service.[87]

In 1950, the Malayan government asked the WHO for help, requesting the assistance of a WHO tutor in public health nursing.[88] Following discussions with the Director of Medical Services and Malaya's Principal Matron, the Member for Health asked for the tutor's contract to be extended and for four more female tutors and a male tutor to be sent by the WHO.[89] In spite of the ONA's difficulty in recruiting from Britain, the WHO decided to try to recruit a male tutor from there in 1952. However, it is not clear in the records from where the candidate, John Waterer, was recruited.[90] The WHO provided further funding in 1953: US$47,000 for a Rural Health Training School at Jitra in Kedah and for four Rural Health Centers. The Western Pacific Secretariat of the WHO claimed that, despite financial challenges, the Organization was attaching "unusual importance" to this project, which was of "very considerable potential value."[91] UNICEF matched this with $47,000 for equipment for maternal and child welfare services.[92] WHO assistance continued, and a further WHO public health tutor arrived in Penang to teach health visitors in 1956.[93]

Although there is no reference to the political challenges of communism in the WHO records in relation to rural health and nursing in Malaya, the concentration on nursing in the colony is revealing. Malaya and the states in North Borneo which were to form unified Malaysia from the 1960s onward, were the only areas of the world to have dedicated WHO nursing programs in the early years of the Organization, between 1948 and 1953, coinciding with the Malayan Emergency. However, WHO nurses took part in many programs across the world, including tuberculosis campaigns and maternal and child health projects.[94]

Assistance from the WHO did not provide an immediate solution as it took time to establish the centers and train staff. With demand for nurses still not met, 370 doctors from the Malayan branch of the British Medical Association (BMA) gathered together in April 1952. They complained about the woeful lack of health services for the New Villages, arguing that where there was a population of over a thousand, a permanent dispensary should be provided. However, the BMA doctors acknowledged that dispensaries would not be easy to provide at a time of staff shortage. It was argued that hospital assistants could run the centers, and doctors would need to volunteer their time.[95]

The colonial Malayan government was fully aware of the inadequate care in the New Villages, and in March 1952 it arranged to pay grants to the British Red Cross Society (BRCS) for supplementary staff. The government hoped that the St John's Ambulance

Brigade (SJAB) would also help to recruit staff. Ninety percent of the charities' costs were paid for by the government, amounting to $1.5 million (Malay dollars).[96] The Red Cross already had a strong presence in Malaya, providing a range of services; for example, maternity and child welfare clinics, welfare work and training in first aid and home nursing.[97] The government also offered aid to church and missionary societies in return for qualified staff.[98] However, except for the China Inland Mission, the missions were reluctant to release their staff for government service.[99]

The BRCS was well advanced in its preparations to send 50 members of staff from Britain by April 1952 – a trained nurse and a welfare worker for each of 25 mobile dispensaries.[100] It had actually anticipated the demand in January and had already written to the County Directors of the BRCS asking them to recruit trained nurses aged 25 to 45.[101] In March 1952, 25 trained nurses were required "at once" with the designation that they should be in excellent health, prepared for "rough conditions" and hopefully able to drive a car. Nursing work was of "great importance in connection with the present Emergency in Malaya, and County Directors are asked to do all they can to make it known as early as possible."[102] In May the age limit was lowered to 21 in order to draw from a "wider choice" of applicants. However, the young applicants had to have "exceptional qualifications" in order to be considered, which were generally undefined but included a "high sense of responsibility."[103] In contrast to the ONA, which produced very few recruitment materials in general, publicity gained for BRCS work in Malaya included Janet Grant speaking on the BBC radio program *Under Twenty Parade* in October 1952.[104] With lower standards, including much less post-qualification experience and without demands for a midwifery qualification, and with much more publicity, the Red Cross was more successful in recruiting nurses for Malaya than the ONA.

With funding provided by the Malayan government, the BRCS built a house for each pair of nurses and welfare workers in the New Villages. Each pair was to look after communities of 10,000 people, half of the population of the New Villages.[105] By August 1953 there were 30 BRCS teams, five from the Australian Red Cross funded by the Colombo Aid Plan for South and South-East Asia, and 25 St John teams. The Red Cross nurses undertook 12-month contracts with the opportunity to extend them for a further year.[106] These organizations covered the traditional Malay villages as well as the New Villages. The BRCS insisted on providing "equal treatment for all races," therefore not just focusing on the Chinese population.[107] Indeed, Templar had promised the sultans that this would be the case as there was religious tension regarding Christian missions in the area.[108]

The Red Cross teams were welcomed with "open arms" and "nothing had been too much trouble" for the Malayan authorities and doctors in helping them to settle in.[109] It was not only the administrative and medical officers who valued their help, but also the "New Villagers" who appreciated their role to such an extent that the guerrillas never attacked their vehicles for fear of angering the Chinese communities and losing potential supporters.[110] Indeed, Mao's directives of 1951 included the cessation of all attacks on Red Cross vehicles.[111] A newspaper report from 1953 claimed that although there had been many communist attempts to "discredit" the Red Cross, the nurses in Malaya had not experienced any violence.[112]

The range of tasks that the nurses and welfare workers were to undertake was enormous; to name a few, they included a daily clinic in their home village, home visits, taking urgent cases to hospital, visiting schools and providing health education, "organizing and promoting" the Junior Red Cross, providing courses on first-aid and home nursing, training "promising girls in the elements of nursing," and advising on health and hygiene.[113] In August 1953, the Member of Health evaluated the work of the Red Cross and SJAB teams and judged that the welfare workers had made a very limited impact and so they would not be replaced. However, the nurses were crucial for rural areas in order to provide "medical treatment facilities."[114] Therefore, the Malayan government negotiated with the BRCS and SJAB for continued provision and replacement of nurses from Britain until 1955. These qualified nurses would train apprentice assistant nurses each time that British welfare workers resigned. The local recruits would receive 12 months' training, followed by further training in hospitals, before returning to work in rural areas. These recruits would also reduce the need for interpreters.[115] This training scheme for rural nurses, coupled with the new training school in Jitra, can be seen as part of the citizenship program described by historian Timothy Harper; community development was introduced into rural areas, including education and reading rooms. This included Malay women being encouraged to take a role in social welfare where they could work and socialize with expatriate British staff employed in this area.[116]

Another tactic used in the Emergency was an earnest incentive of independence to inspire the Malayans to fight communism.[117] Part of this program was the "Malayanization" of public services – the transfer of roles from the British to the Asians, whether they were Malays, Chinese or Indian. The training and promotion of Asian nurses in Malaya had been limited by a belief in the superiority of British nurses, and by the complicated racial mix in Malaya. Muslim Malays were largely reluctant to train as it was unusual for women to work outside of the home, and they lacked formal education.[118] Following WWII, A.G.H. Smart, Medical Adviser to the Secretary of State for the Colonies, visited Malaya and complained that the British were suppressing the career progression of Asian nurses who had clearly proved their capabilities when the British were interned during the war.[119]

In 1949, 66 nurses completed their training at the Penang School and 28 Asian nurses were given posts as health or nursing sisters: positions that were previously held by Europeans.[120] By 1952, nurse-training at the Penang School was awarded reciprocity with the General Nursing Council in the United Kingdom.[121] The emphasis was on training men as nurses rather than hospital assistants from 1951, exemplified by the request for a male tutor from the WHO. Despite the long history of hospital assistants in the country, it was difficult to change their title to nurse as these men thought this meant a loss of prestige, even though the intention was to give them a professional status. Waterer noted with interest that in one state the Asians did not realize that the European sisters were nurses. This change in status was made even more challenging as the colonial government had declared a policy that the number of hospital assistants would be reduced. Despite male hospital assistants outnumbering female nurses before the war, the post-war policy was to aim for only 10 percent of the nursing workforce to be male nurses. A recruitment drive had been aimed specifically at women, marginalizing these men who believed their livelihood was at stake.[122]

In 1955, the process of the Malayanization of the public services was accelerated.[123] The official policy was that British nurses would cease to be recruited from the mid-1950s. Sisters were only to be appointed from the local nursing service from 1955 on. This program accentuated the shortage of senior nurses in Malaya, and by 1956 there were plans to carry on recruitment from other overseas areas, including India.[124] In 1962, the Malayan government invited the WHO back in order to provide technical assistance as teaching staff were urgently needed in order to train staff for the hospitals and public health services. However, this project only required one WHO nurse, and mainly funded fellowships for study overseas.[125]

Although 21 percent of the New Villages still did not receive medical services by 1958, the number of static dispensaries in rural settlements increased from 32 in 1951 to 172 by the end of 1954.[126] In 1954, a mission of the International Bank for Reconstruction and Development reported that health in the colony was "one of the world's outstanding achievements of public health and medicine, a tribute to the British administrators and their medical and public health officers."[127] Randall Packard, a historian of medicine, has noted that healthcare facilities and campaigns increased following WWII, partly influenced by the anti-communist campaign to win hearts and minds. He has argued that except for occasional rural campaigns, these strategies focussed on techno-centric eradication campaigns for diseases such as malaria and smallpox and that until the 1970s, primary healthcare facilities continued to be located around areas of economic activity, which were usually urban.[128] Yet rural health centers were established in the British colony of the Gold Coast in West Africa (present-day Ghana) in the early 1950s, with 23 completed by 1960, so perhaps facilities such as these were not as unusual as has been portrayed.[129] The Malayan Emergency had inspired rural public health provision on a scale that was apparently unique in the British Empire, particularly with provision of such a large nursing workforce, with around 250 British Red Cross or colonial nurses in the area by the mid-1950s.

Discussion

Historian Timothy Harper argues that the Malayan Emergency was the "most major metropolitan commitment to empire in the mid-twentieth century, in terms of the people and resources absorbed"; its goal was the transfer of power to safe hands through a much quicker "civilizing mission" than previously intended, constructing a "pro-western, capitalist and clean" government.[130] The Emergency was associated with the "second colonial occupation" and demonstrates the deployment of nursing as part of a wider strategic effort that, officials perceived, could be effective in counteracting the spread of communism on the ground. One of the features of this "second colonial occupation" was the pouring in of experts with different technical backgrounds into the region to protect trade and commercial interests as well as stimulate the economy, including the health economy. Thus Malaya became a melting pot for interventions from a range of governmental and non-governmental organizations and philanthropies. The nurse was used as a totem and tool in the propaganda war of the British government to demonstrate that it cared about the welfare of villagers. She was an important conduit into the local population and ideally placed to win their trust and confidence, thereby presenting a benevolent image of the British government.

The experiences of nursing in Malaya also reveal an awareness of the need to balance gender considerations with pragmatics in the recruitment of men and skilling and scaling up of training for indigenous workers. The mobilization of sufficient numbers of nurses at the appropriate speed meant that the government could no longer rely on its usual sources. Recruits were sought from a wider range of organizations, and it was this pluralistic world that would increasingly characterize the post-war health regime.

Nursing has much to add to the political history of Malaya. Not only has the detailed history of 1940s and 1950s health services been largely neglected by historians, but the nurse was crucial to the hearts and minds campaign. The Malayan case demonstrates the significant political role that nurses played as proponents of a particular set of values in providing "outreach" to communities on the ground. Before accelerated decolonization, the Emergency brought a second wave of colonization with publicly funded facilities extended to rural areas, and federal and state governments growing in size, assisted by specialists working on civilian projects.[131]

The history of nursing in post-WWII Malaya also has much to add to the history of colonial nursing, demonstrating why it is essential to study the post-war years in order to understand the political and practical role of the colonial nurse, especially considering that this was the period when most colonial nurses were employed. The Emergency also highlights the elitism of the ONA, with its insistence on quintessential good character and experience, and how this resulted in the colonial governments diversifying in their use of agencies for recruitment of nurses.

The use of nurses as part of a wider political strategy was not new.[132] Yet before the Malayan case, nurses had not been recruited with such an explicit recolonizing campaign in mind. Nursing was also drawn into the process of Malayanization, and this dual role during the second colonial occupation and the seriousness of the stakes for the British government put nursing at the center not only of colonial history but of the socio-political history of the region.

Notes

1 B.W. Andaya and L.Y. Andaya, *A History of Malaysia*, Basingstoke: Palgrave, 2001, pp. 3–4.

2 J. Darwin, *Britain and Decolonisation: The Retreat from Empire in the Post-War Period*, Basingstoke: Macmillan, 1988, pp. 105–7.

3 Ibid., pp. 105–6.

4 Ibid., pp. 106–7; K. Ramakrishna, *Emergency and Propaganda: The Winning of Malayan Hearts and Minds, 1948–1958*, Richmond, UK: Curzon, 2002, p. 6.

5 Darwin, *Britain and Decolonisation*, p. 107; Ramakrishna, *Emergency and Propaganda*, p. 7.

6 Darwin, *Britain and Decolonisation*, p. 107.

7 Andaya and Andaya, *A History of Malaysia*, pp. 256–68.

8   R. Stubbs, *Hearts and Minds in Guerrilla Warfare: The Malayan Emergency 1948–1960*, Oxford: Oxford University Press, 1989, pp. 25–37; Ramakrishna, *Emergency and Propaganda*, pp. 9 and 85; Andaya and Andaya, *History of Malaysia*, p. 268.

9   Darwin, *Britain and Decolonisation*, p. 56.

10 Stubbs, *Hearts and Minds*, p. 51.

11 Darwin, *Britain and Decolonisation*, pp. 155–6.

12 Ibid.; N.J. White, *Decolonisation: The British Experience since 1945*, London: Longman, 1999, p. 7.

13 Ramakrishna, *Emergency and Propaganda*, p. 85.

14 Darwin, *Britain and Decolonisation*, pp. 106 and 156.

15 Ibid., p. 106.

16 J. Darwin, *The End of the British Empire: The Historical Debate*, Oxford: Blackwell, 1988, pp. 89–94.

17 Phua Kai Hong, "The development of health services in Malaya and Singapore, 1867–1960," unpublished thesis, London School of Economics, p. 260; S. Clarke, "A technocratic imperial state? The Colonial Office and scientific research, 1940–1960," *Twentieth Century British History* 18, 2007, pp. 463–4; J. Farley, *Brock Chisholm, the World Health Organization, and the Cold War*, Vancouver: University of British Colombia Press, 2008, pp. 128–9; The Bodleian Library of Commonwealth and African Studies at Rhodes House, Oxford, Overseas Nursing Association Collection (hereafter ONA), Annual Report, 1949, MSS Brit Emp s400 131, p. 6.

18 H. Calloway, *Gender, Culture and Empire: European Women in Colonial Nigeria*, Urbana: University of Illinois Press, 1987, p. 14.

19 *The Census of British Malaya, 1921* (London: Waterlow and Sons, 1922), pp. 266–70; J.N. Brownfoot, "Sisters under the skin: imperialism and the emancipation of women in Malaya, c. 1891–1941," in J.A. Mangan (ed.) *Making Imperial Mentalities: Socialisation and British Imperialism*, Manchester: Manchester University Press, 1990, pp. 51 and 57.

20 ONA, Annual Report, 1938.

21 A.M. Rafferty and D. Solano, "The rise and demise of the Colonial Nursing Service: British nurses in the colonies, 1896–1966," *Nursing History Review* 15, 2007, p. 147.

22 H.P. Dickson, *The Badge of Britannia: the History and Reminiscences of the Queen Elizabeth's Overseas Nursing Service, 1886–1966*, Edinburgh: Pentland Press, 1990, p. 14; ONA, Annual Report, 1918.

23 ONA, Annual Report, 1966.

24 For example, S. Marks, *Divided Sisterhood: Race, Class and Gender in the South African Nursing Profession*, Basingstoke: Macmillan, 1994; complemented by more detail on white government nurses in H. Sweet, "'Wanted: 16 nurses of the better educated type': provision of nurses to South Africa in the late nineteenth and early twentieth centuries," *Nursing Inquiry* 11, 2004, pp.176–84; J. Godden and C. Helmstadter, "Women's mission and professional knowledge: Nightingale nursing in colonial Australia and Canada," *Social History of Medicine* 17, 2004, pp. 157–74; J. Godden, *Lucy Osburn, a Lady Displaced. Florence Nightingale's Envoy to Australia*, Sydney: Sydney University Press, 2006.

25 J. Gourlay, *Florence Nightingale and the Health of the Raj*, Aldershot: Ashgate, 2003, pp. 66–73.

26 D. Birkett, "The 'White Woman's Burden' in the 'White Man's Grave': the introduction of British nurses in colonial West Africa," in N. Chaudhuri and M. Strobel (eds), *Western Women and Imperialism: Complicity and Resistance*, Bloomington: Indiana University Press, 1992, p. 177; Calloway, *Gender, Culture and Empire*.

27 CNA and ONA, Annual Reports, 1900–66.

28 M. Jones, *The Hospital System and Healthcare: Sri Lanka, 1815–1960*, Hyderabad: Orient BlackSwan, 2009, pp. 227–61.

29 Ibid., pp. 347–89.

30 Calloway, *Gender, Culture and Empire*; Birkett, "The 'White Woman's Burden."

31 M. Strobel, *European Women and the Second British Empire*, Bloomington and Indianapolis: Indiana University Press, 1991, pp. 29–30; A. Bashford, "Gender, Medicine and Empire," in Philippa Levine (ed.), *Gender and Empire: The Oxford History of the British Empire*, Oxford: Oxford University Press, 2004, pp. 113–33.

32 Strobel, *European Women*; K. Jayawardena, *The White Woman's Other Burden: Western Women and South Asia during British Colonial Rule*, New York: Routledge, 1995; See Wan Faizah binti Wan Yusoff, "Malay responses to the promotion of western medicine, with particular reference to women and child healthcare in the Federated Malay States, 1920–1939," unpublished thesis, University of London, 2010, pp. 16–17 and 103, on Muslims and missionaries; Brownfoot, "Sisters under the skin."

33 L. Manderson, *Sickness and the State: Health and Illness in Colonial Malaya, 1870–1940*, Cambridge: Cambridge University Press, 1996, pp. 210–28.

34 A. McClintock, *Imperial Leather: Race, Gender and Sexuality in the Colonial Contest*, London: Routledge, 1995, pp. 24–5.

35 Manderson, *Sickness and the State*, p. 232.

36 Jones, *The Hospital System*, p. 239; ONA, Mary Culliton to Miss Adams, 21 Nov. 1927, MSS Brit Emp s400 140/4.

37 Mary Culliton to Miss Adams, 21 November 1927.

38 A tutor is the role that was assigned to teachers who worked in the classrooms of British nurse training schools, a position for which university Diplomas of Nursing were required, the first being awarded by the University of London. The World Health Organization Archives (hereafter WHO Archives), John Waterer, WHO Male Nurse Tutor, to I.C. Fang, Final Report of Activities, 22 April 1953 to 20 March 1957.

39 Manderson, *Sickness and the State*, pp. 201 and 211–15.

40 K. K. Liew, "St John's Ambulance Brigade and the gendering of 'passive defence' in British Malaya, 1937–42," *Gender and History* 23, 2011, pp. 367–81.

41 Accounts of nursing in Singapore are provided within Y.K. Lee, "Nursing and the beginnings of specialised nursing in early Singapore," *Singapore Medical Journal* 46, 2005, pp. 600–9; Y.K. Lee, "The origins of nursing in Singapore," *Singapore Medical Journal* 26, 1985, pp. 53–60.

42 C.C. Choy, *Empire of Care: Nursing and Migration in Filipino American History*, Durham: Duke University Press, 2003.

43 W. Connerton, "Have cap, will travel: U.S. nurses abroad 1898–1917," unpublished thesis, University of Pennsylvania, 2010.

44 Phua, "The development of health services"; Manderson, *Sickness and the State*; K.K. Liew, "Specifying fevers: positioning Malaya's health lobbies (1867–1941)," unpublished thesis, University College London, 2007; Wan Faizah, "Malay responses"; J.N. Palmer, "Health and health services in British Malaya in the 1920s," *Modern Asian Studies* 23, 1989, pp. 49–71.

45 J. Farley, *To Cast Out Disease: A History of the International Health Division of Rockefeller Foundation, 1913–51*, Oxford: Oxford University Press, 2003; B.L. Brush, "The Rockefeller Agenda for American/Philippines nursing relations" in Anne Marie Rafferty, Jane Robinson and Ruth Elkan (eds), *Nursing History and the Politics of Welfare*, London: Routledge, pp. 45–63.

46 Jones, *The Hospital System*, pp. 386–9; C. Hallett and L. Wagner, "Promoting the health of Europeans in a rapidly changing world: a historical study of the implementation of World Health Organisation policies by the Nursing and Midwifery Unit, European Regional Office, 1970–2003," *Nursing Inquiry* 18, 2011, p. 364.

47 Stubbs, *Hearts and Minds*, pp. 1 and 169.

48 Ramakrishna, *Emergency and Propaganda*, p. 12.

49 For the use of this term see Manderson, *Sickness and the State*, p. 242; Wan Faizah, "Malay responses" p. 49; Mark Harrison, *Public Health in British India: Anglo-Indian Preventive Medicine, 1859–1914* (Cambridge: Cambridge University Press, 1994), pp. 60–98.

50 Stubbs, *Hearts and Minds*, pp. 1 and 6.
51 Ramakrishna, pp. 54, 57, 72–5 and 103.
52 Stubbs, *Hearts and Minds*, pp. 1, 74, 96, 101–2 and 126–7; Phua, "The development of health services," p. 272.
53 Phua, "The development of health services," p. 282; Stubbs, *Hearts and minds*, p. 105.
54 Stubbs, *Hearts and Minds*, p. 103.
55 Quote from Ramakrishna, *Emergency and Propaganda*, p. 128. See also K. Hack, "'Iron Claws on Malaya': The historiography of the Malayan Emergency," *Journal of Southeast Asian Studies* 30, 1999, p. 115.
56 Ramakrishna, *Emergency and Propaganda*, pp. 2 and 16.
57 Ibid., pp. 66–7; Karl Hack, "Iron Claws on Malaya," p. 115.
58 Farley, *Brock Chisholm*, pp. 2, 6 and 188–90.
59 Ibid., pp. 3, 18 and 122.
60 WHO Archives, Technical Health Education, 4 February 1948, 615/1/5.
61 Stubbs, *Hearts and Minds*, pp. 110–13, 172 and 178.
62 Phua, "The development of health services," pp. 211 and 257–8.
63 The National Archives, London (hereafter, TNA), Extract from Federal Legislative Council Paper 33 of 1952, CO 1022/31.
64 Ibid.
65 Ibid.
66 Ibid.; WHO Archives, Malaya Nursing Education Plan of Operations, Annex 1, 1951, Malaya 1; Elizabeth Hill, Nursing Adviser, WHO, to I.C. Fang, Report – Field Visit to Malaya, May 20 to 26 1952, Malaya 1; John Waterer, Final Report of Activities.
67 Malayan Union, *Annual Report of the Medical Department for the Year 1946*, p. 3.
68 Federation of Malaya, *Annual Report of the Medical Department for the Year 1950*, p. 103.
69 ONA, Annual Report, 1954, p. 10.
70 Dickson, *The Badge of Britannia*, pp. 21–2 and 100–7.
71 ONA, Annual Reports, 1939 and 1948.
72 ONA, Annual Reports, 1950 and 1954.
73 J. Coates, *Suppressing Insurgency: An Analysis of the Malayan Emergency, 1948–1954*, Boulder: Westview Press, 1992, p. 61.
74 ONA, Annual Report, 1955.
75 WHO Archives, Elizabeth Hill to I.C. Fang, Report – Field Visit to Malaya, 20 February to 3 March 1953, Malaya 1.
76 ONA, Executive Council Minutes, 9 April 1946 and 15 October 1946, MSS Brit Emp s400.
77 ONA, Executive Council Minutes, 4 November 1947.
78 Sheryl Nestel, "(Ad)ministering angels: Colonial nursing and the extension of Empire in Africa," *Journal of Medical Humanities* 19, 1998, pp. 257–77.
79 ONA, Annual Report, 1947.
80 ONA, Annual Report, 1947, p. 11
81 ONA, Annual Report, 1948, 1949, 1951 and 1953.
82 ONA, Annual Report, 1950.
83 Stubbs, *Hearts and Minds*, pp. 11–13.
84 Phua, "The development of health services," p. 174; TNA, I.C. Fang, Regional Director, Western Pacific, to the Member for Health, Penang, 2 September 1952; UNICEF Recommendation of the Executive Director for an Apportionment to Malaya for the Expansion of Material and Child Welfare Services and Training, 25 August 1953; I.C. Fang, to the Member for Health, Penang, 9 January 1953, CO 859/415.
85 ONA, Executive Council Minutes, 31 July 1945.
86 ONA, Executive Council Minutes, 2 October 1945.
87 Ibid.

88 Malayan Union, *Annual Report of the Medical Department for the Year 1946*, p. 21.

89 WHO Archives, Lee Tiang Keng to I.C. Fang, 7 May 1951, Malaya 1.

90 WHO Archives, Elizabeth Hill, Nursing Adviser, WHO, to I.C. Fang, Report – Field Visit to Malaya, May 20 to 26 1952, Malaya 1; Elizabeth Hill to I.C. Fang, Report – Field Visit to Malaya, 20 February to 3 March 1953, Malaya 1.

91 TNA, I.C. Fang, Regional Director, Western Pacific, to the Member for Health, Penang, 2 September 1952; UNICEF Recommendation of the Executive Director for an Apportionment to Malaya for the Expansion of Material and Child Welfare Services and Training, 25 August 1953; I.C. Fang, to the Member for Health, Penang, 9 January 1953, CO 859/415.

92 TNA, UNICEF . . . Apportionment to Malaya for . . . Child Welfare Services and Training, 25 August 1953, CO 859/415.

93 Federation of Malaya, *Annual Report of the Medical Department for the Year 1956*, p. 31.

94 World Health Organization Library, Approved and Proposed WHO–UNICEF-assisted Projects, 1949–1953, MH/1951, vol. 5.

95 TNA, Newspaper cutting (unattributed), 3 April 1952, CO 1022/31.

96 TNA, Note beginning, "To supplement the Government staff," 27 March 1952; Memorandum by the Member of Health, Plans for the continuation of the work of the BRCS and SJAB teams in the rural areas after the overseas workers have left the Federation, August 1953, CO 1022/31.

97 The British Red Cross Society Museum and Archive, London (hereafter BRCS), Work the Red Cross Branches are already doing, 1952, 76/31 (1).

98 TNA, Note beginning "To supplement the Government staff," 27 March 1952, CO 1022/31; Phua, "The development of health services," p. 278.

99 TNA, R.J. Minnitt to Dr Pridie, 15 May 1952, CO 1022/31.

100 TNA, Extract from Federation of Malaya Monthly Newsletter No. 39 for the period 16th March to 15th April 1952, CO 1022/31.

101 BRCS, F.H.D. Pritchard, Secretary-General to County Directors, 25 January 1952, Branch Circulars, 1952.

102 BRCS, F.H.D. Pritchard to County Directors, 18 March 1952, Branch Circulars, 1952.

103 BRCS, F.H.D. Pritchard to County Directors, 2 May 1952, Branch Circulars, 1952.

104 ONA, Executive Council Minutes, 15 October 1946; BRCS, F.H.D. Pritchard to County Directors, 9 October 1952, Branch Circulars, 1952.

105 TNA, Federal Government Press Statement, "Spotlight on the Emergency," 17 May 1952, CO 1022/31; BRCS Archives, Annual Report of the Federation of Malaya Branch, 76/31 (1), pp. 1–2.

106 TNA, Memorandum by the Member of Health, Plans for continuation, CO 1022/31; Phua, "The development of health services," p. 278.

107 BRCS, BRCS Federation of Malaya Branch Director's Report, 8 September 1952, p. 1, 76/31 (1).

108 T.N. Harper, *The End of Empire and the Making of Malaya*, Cambridge, Cambridge University Press, 1999, pp. 184–5.

109 Ibid.

110 Ramakrishna's interview with Datin Marshall, *Emergency and Propaganda*, p. 130.

111 Coates, *Suppressing Insurgency*, p. 66.

112 TNA, "Red Cross in Malaya," cutting from *Glasgow Herald*, 15 January 1953, CO 1022/31.

113 TNA, Federal Government Press Statement, CO 1022/31.

114 TNA, Memorandum by the Member for Health: Plans for the continuation of the work of the BRCS and SJAB teams in the rural areas after the overseas workers have left the Federation, 17 September 1953, CO 1022/31.

115 Ibid.; BRCS, British Red Cross Society Federation of Malaya Branch Director's Report, 1952, p. 1, 76/31 (1).
116 Harper, *End of Empire*, pp. 312–14.
117 Stubbs, *Hearts and Minds*, p. 137.
118 Manderson, *Sickness and the State*, pp. 208–10; Andaya and Andaya, *History of Malaysia*, p. 178.
119 TNA, A.G.H. Smart, Report on some aspects of medical planning for Malaya, CO 273/679.
120 Federation of Malaya, *Annual Report of the Medical Department for the Year 1949*, pp. 25 and 103.
121 Federation of Malaya, *Annual Report of the Medical Department for the Year 1952*, p. 21.
122 WHO Archives, John Waterer, Final Report of Activities.
123 Harper, *End of Empire*, p. 197.
124 Federation of Malay, *Annual Report of the Medical Department for the Year 1955*, p. 28; Federation of Malaya, *Annual Report of the Medical Department for the Year 1956*, p. 30.
125 WHO Archives, Plan of Operation for a Nursing Education Project in the Federation of Malaya, 1962, Malaya 32.
126 Stubbs, *Hearts and Minds*, pp. 110–13, 172 and 178.
127 Cited in Phua, "Development of health services," p. 9.
128 R. Packard, "Visions of postwar health and development and their impact on public health interventions in the developing world" in F. Cooper and R. Packard (eds), *International Development and the Social Sciences: Essays on the History and Politics of Knowledge*, Berkeley: University of California Press, 1997, pp. 93–115; R. Packard, "Post-colonial medicine" in Roger Cooter and John Pickstone (eds), *Companion to Medicine in the Twentieth Century*, London: Routledge, 2003, pp. 97–112.
129 S. Addae, *The Evolution of Modern Medicine in a Developing Country: Ghana 1880–1960*, Edinburgh: Durham Academic Press, 1997, p. 86; M. Worboys, "Colonial medicine" in Cooter and Pickstone (eds), *Companion to Medicine*, p. 78.
130 Harper, *End of Empire*, p. 362.
131 Ibid., pp. 195–6.
132 Farley, *To Cast Out Disease*, pp. 239–59; A.M. Rafferty, "Internationalising nursing education during the interwar period" in P. Weindling, *International Health Organisations and Movements, 1918–1939*, Cambridge: Cambridge University Press, 1995, pp. 266–82.

14

COMMUNITY MENTAL HEALTH POST-1950

Reconsidering nurses' and consumers' identity[1]

Geertje Boschma, PhD, RN

. . . but we did have a consumer on the [founding] Board of Directors [of the Riverview Hospital Volunteer Association].

(Registered Psychiatric Nurse, Colleen Dewar)[2]

Well, we had to train the staff [of Pioneer House] because no-one, nobody had done that kind of work before . . .

(Consumer and Mental Health Advocate, David Beamish)[3]

Colleen Dewar, a 1969 graduate from the British Columbia (BC) School of Psychiatric Nursing at Riverview Hospital (RH), the large provincial mental hospital in BC, and David Beamish, consumer and former (or ex-) patient,[4] from this same hospital were intimately involved with the process of deinstitutionalization in BC, Canada.[5] In the early 1980s, they engaged with the newly founded Riverview Hospital Volunteer Association (RHVA),[6] and helped establish Pioneer House, one of the first non-profit small-scale residential care facilities in the area. The mission of the RVHA was to enact a new rehabilitative model of care aimed at providing patients discharged from RH with support *and* control during their transitions into the community.[7] Rather uniquely, Pioneer House was operated by psychiatric nurses, volunteers, and consumers who had joined forces as the RHVA, forming an unusual alliance of professionals and patients working in parallel pursuit of appropriate community services. Sharing ties to RH, they drew on their institutional experiences as resources from which they renegotiated their work, identities, and places in community mental health. The development of Pioneer House was part of a larger social process of deinstitutional-ization that characterized mental health care in the second half of the 20th century.[8] Using the establishment of this 30-bed residential facility as a case-example, drawn from an oral history project I recently conducted with Margaret Gorrie in the

Canadian context,[9] we can gain a nuanced understanding of the complex transformation of place and identity the shift from large mental hospitals towards community-based care entailed and the challenges it reproduced from the viewpoint of nurses and consumers.[10]

From the 1950s onwards, Canadian mental hospitals, like those in other western societies, began the deliberate processes of patient depopulation. Increasing numbers of discharged patients had to find their ways in a convoluted and uncharted domain of community mental health.[11] Somewhat different from its US counterpart, this was a long-term process in Canada, lasting for several decades, and in BC continuing into the 21st century.[12] Post-WWII economic prosperity and entitlement to health as a right enhanced the establishment of public funding for health care in Canada, while confidence in new professional and therapeutic insights and the availability of new psychotropic medication stimulated the idea that people hospitalized because of mental illness could benefit from returning to their home communities. Confidence in science and research reinforced this trend.[13] As mental hospitals engaged with a process of reform and renewal, new social, medical, and therapeutic environments had to be created, not only inside but also outside the confinement of a custodial institutional structure, based on new 20th century managerial, professional, and scientific foundations.[14] Not unlike institutional contexts of large mental hospitals, newly established community services were challenged to find a balance between rehabilitative, supportive care and bureaucratic control in what became a new matrix or network of community services in which patients and professionals forged new understandings of place, work, and identity.[15]

Despite the enormous changes experienced by nurses and consumers, who were intimately involved with the construction of new community services, we have little historical examination of deinstitutionalization from their perspectives. Psychiatric mental health nursing historiography does not focus extensively on the period of deinstitutionalization, nor does it often incorporate a patient-perspective. Narrative analysis of the ways nurses and consumers engaged with the establishment and work of rehabilitative community services provides an opportunity to further develop the existing framework of writing the history of psychiatric and community mental health nursing.[16] By means of the Pioneer House case example and an analysis of existing international historiography on mental health care and psychiatric nursing, in this chapter I contend the following points: First, although psychiatric nursing historiography has mainly focused on professional development, I argue that we also require analysis of the ways nurses and patients experienced and contributed to the transformation of mental hospitals. In envisioning new ways of supporting community living that would empower former patients, both groups drew on their institutional experiences to enact it. Nurses engaged with new roles in the mental hospitals and in community work, whereas consumers renegotiated their "patient" identities and established a prominent presence parallel to other professional workers. Additionally, volunteers became drawn into social movement organizations and were purposefully recruited into institutions as of the 1950s to work closely with nurses and patients to lessen isolation and stigmatization. When patient activists, often ex-patients, began in the 1970s to engage with the renewal of mental health services in the community, they radicalized and politicized volunteer activities and patient advocacy, also within the institution. Finally, emphasizing these close connections between institutions and new community services, institutional environments, I argue, did not "end" with the move to a matrix of community-based services. These services, enacted by the people who "built" them, expanded and "loosened up" institutional places, but also recreated their dilemmas in new contexts. In doing so, the various parties involved had to accommodate, differing in their views around the parameters of care and rehabilitation, the inevitable compliance with bureaucratic control, and ultimately about the balance between the two—very much like their predecessors in the institution had done previously.

Mental health historiography through the lens of nurses and patients

Mental health historiography that has emerged since the 1980s has largely focused on the rise of the 19th century asylum or mental hospital.[17] Analysis of the work of attendants and nurses in the asylum—and I speak here to the Anglo-American literature —appeared in studies centering on the inner workings of the asylum.[18] These studies contested an earlier, sweeping critique of the mental hospital as a place of great confinement,[19] of expanding medicalization and social control,[20] or as a "total institution"—an oppressive, totalitarian organization, appearing in the wake of a broader counter-cultural and civil rights movement.[21] In mental health care, counter-cultural activism generated anti-psychiatric protest against the poor circumstances in large mental hospitals and lack of patient rights, in some countries as early as the 1950s, but spreading throughout the western world in the 1960s and 1970s.[22] Psychiatry and the alleged hegemony of the medical model became the target of vivid public debate and activism of patients, families, and professionals in the 1970s. The social critique was deeply anti-medical, in that medicalization was explained as a mechanism of social control rather than a humanitarian effort striving towards the greater good.

In the 1980s, social and medical historians argued that a careful analysis of asylum dynamics as negotiated realities of multiple groups, such as patients, families, and physicians, but also of attendants, nurses, and other staff would nuance the revisionist conclusions.[23] The analysis of mental health nursing as a new field of paid and professional work has been written into this history. Nursing scholars emphasized nursing's place within the asylum hierarchy,[24] using categories of class and gender to explore the asylum's inner workings and complex power dynamics that determined an often precarious balance between care and control, while other scholars began to study the experience of patients.[25] At the turn of the 20th century asylum, attendants and nurses held little power in the system, encompassing the lowest groups in the asylum hierarchy, just above patients. In a way, the analysis of the power dynamics and realities of day-to-day care through the lens of nurses' (and patients') work belied the idea of the asylum as either a fully medicalized or a "total" institution.

In an analysis of the Friends Asylum in Philadelphia, D'Antonio focused explicitly on the lay model of care that had pre-dated the medicalization of the asylum, depicting it as a large family household rather than a medicalized institution.[26] Also using a social historical framework, I analyzed nurses' day-to-day work and the power dynamics shaping the professional development of psychiatric nurses in Dutch asylums.[27] At the turn of the 20th century, most asylums had become medical institutions headed by medical superintendents. Presumably to improve the attendants' alleged lack of morality and skill, psychiatrists implemented a training model for personnel drawn from the powerful, deeply gendered model of nurse training that had just begun to emerge in general hospitals. Their goal was to instill personnel with a morality of civic respect and humanity (itself a very class-based and gendered idea) and to provide the new nurses with basic nursing skills to assist them in new somatic treatments. Likewise, the model proved an effective staffing system and raised the psychiatrists' own professional profile. Most mental hospitals in western countries adapted to this model.

My study was among several that appeared during the 1990s and early 21st century analyzing the history of mental hospital-based psychiatric nursing using social history approaches with a continued focus on institutional care and professional development.[28] A new, critical, social historiography on nursing in general sparked these studies.[29] Furthermore, a desire to provide psychiatric nurses with voice and professional identity also influenced this work.[30]

Two themes dominated this historiography. First, analyses of professional development and (authoritative) power addressed psychiatric nurses' desire for jurisdictional control over education and practice and for improvement of working conditions. Several authors emphasized that psychiatric nurses' ambivalent alliance with science and higher education stemmed not only from their entanglement in a gendered power relation with medicine, but also from an ambivalent relationship with general nursing. Church, for example, perceived American psychiatric nurses' integration within general (hospital and public health) nursing education as a great step forward.[31] Others, such as Dingwall et al., applying a social control framework, noted that an impression of steady improvement of mental nurses' status and effectiveness based on a professionalization framework might be misleading. They felt mental nursing was best depicted in its relationship to the average patient experience in the "average" institution, which even post-1950s in the British National Health Service was still one of continued social control, medicalization, marginalization, custodial habits, and lack of funding.[32]

Neither the professionalization thesis nor the social control frameworks, however, sufficiently concede that such conclusions also reflect national differences with regard to nursing's link with science and higher education. In the United States (US), to which context Church referred, the passage of the 1946 National Mental Health Act and the subsequent establishment of a National Institute for Mental Health led to the availability of funding for academic, university (graduate) education in psychiatric nursing—a trend virtually unheard of in most other countries at that time.[33] The rise of psychiatric nursing as an advanced nursing specialty in the US resulted in part from the early academization of US nursing, which coincided with the mental hygiene movement emerging in the 1920s and 1930s.[34] On the other hand, we have little knowledge of what happened to the extensive nursing workforce in North American mental hospitals once they closed.

Many analyses address the way psychiatric nursing became caught up in power struggles within the fields of medicine (as psychiatrists sought acknowledgement for their own profession within the larger medical arena) and between medicine and general hospital nursing.[35] Battles over psychiatric nursing registration in the UK, but also in Canada, arose between professional organizations of psychiatry and general nursing—with psychiatric nursing caught in the middle.[36] In Canada, this battle enforced regional East–West differentiation, with Eastern provinces following North American patterns of early integration of psychiatric nurses into the registry of general nurses. In Western Canadian provinces, general nursing organizations excluded psychiatric nurses from their registries, leading psychiatrists to establish diplomas for psychiatric nurses under the wings of the provincial mental health services branches in the 1930s. Eventually, psychiatric nurses organized themselves into their own professional associations in these Western provinces in the 1950s, while general hospital schools also incorporated training in psychiatric nursing in their programs, including two- or three-month "affiliation" experiences in the mental hospitals. As a result, in Western provinces two separate licensing bodies continue to exist: one for registered nurses and one for registered psychiatric nurses.[37] In Quebec, patterns were slightly different, in that it had large institutions but also early strategic interaction between institutional staff and families.[38]

Several studies of psychiatric nursing in Western Canada also explored the intertwined influence of region, union connections, and gender on professional identity.[39] Prebble has observed similar influences in psychiatric nursing in New Zealand, while Braunschweig studied Swiss psychiatric nursing using these categories.[40] Regional differences importantly shaped nurses' work and education and need more analysis to also explore the way nurses' work outside of the asylum evolved.

A second theme, addressed in several of these studies, is the day-to-day reality of nurses' work and interaction with patients, albeit mostly in an institutional context. I argued that a performative perspective forms a useful analytic lens, not only to "see" nurses' work but also to explore family and patient interaction with mental health service.[41] Within the latter view, power is perceived from a discursive perspective, asking how nurses enact, negotiate, and accommodate their work in the everyday interaction with patients and in the broader relational network of which they are part. Similarly, the way patients and families accommodated to the pressures placed on them in dealing with mental illness and negotiating care and control have been examined.[42]

Perhaps because of the preoccupation with professionalization and workforce dynamics in institutions, little attention has been given to the fact that nurses in mental hospitals, very similar to their counterparts in general hospitals, obtained a negotiable skill and knowledge base that many—particularly women—used upon graduation to find employment in more independent roles in the community.[43] In my study of turn of the 20th century Dutch asylums, I found evidence of graduates from the mental hospital schools establishing homes for "nervous" patients, providing rest, support in convalescence, and daily management of care. Others went to work in private duty, or in a boarding program of family care, sometimes tied to the institution.[44] Hähner-Rombach described similar strategies of family care for female patients of the Zwiefalten asylum in Germany.[45] Such work extended a long tradition of lay models of care beyond the confinements of the institution. A powerful model in this regard is the family care model established in Geel, Belgium, which dates back to the Middle Ages and has often been pondered and studied for its potential to offer an alternative to institutional care.[46]

Another domain of work and prevention "beyond the walls of the institution" arose within the mental hygiene movement during the 1920s and 1930s. Starting in North America, this movement spread internationally in response to concerns about the mental health of the population in relation to immigration-, class-, and race-based fears of degeneration, uncivilized behavior, and alleged "digressing" morality.[47] With strong roots in eugenic ideas, this work has only to a limited degree been analyzed from the perspective of psychiatric nurses.[48] Clifford Beers, a former patient, had an essential role in the establishment of a national committee for mental hygiene in the United States in 1909.[49] Several countries followed this example, and an international federation was formed in 1924.[50] Psychiatrists and nurses engaged with outpatient and public mental health programs in response to initiatives of these national committees, while improvement of mental hospitals also was a central concern. In the Netherlands, for example, social psychiatry expanded in the mental hygiene era, generating new roles for nurses in after-care for discharged patients and preventive mental hygiene programs. In this context, postgraduate education in social psychiatric nursing evolved.[51] In a new study, Aan de Stegge also examines this program and the social value of its qualifications.[52] In Canada, as another example, public health nurses took on roles in mental hygiene in schools, outpatient clinics, and the juvenile court.[53] While it was difficult to engage with such work because of nurses' firm tie to the institutions, they did so nevertheless, influencing the incorporation of preventive work in nursing thought and practice.

Recent analysis of nurses' and attendants' work with families and patients in psychiatry underscores how the boundaries between institutions and families have always been permeable.[54] Long before "the rise of the asylum" in the 19th century, care-taking of people with mental illness occurred in small private or public enterprises or in a religious context with religious orders involving themselves with charitable work, a model that spread around the globe with colonial expansion and evangelical zeal.[55] Boarding patients with families for pay was a common poor relief strategy.[56] Moreover, a beginning analysis on the roles of volunteers and family members in enacting fluid connections between institutions and community is emerging.[57] More study of the interactive dynamics between nurses' work, patient experiences, and volunteer contributions, I argue, provides a promising framework for nuancing the understanding of the post-1950s shift to community care. In my beginning work on the rise of community mental health, I noticed how these groups in particular were of crucial importance in negotiating new connections not only in the community, but also between mental hospitals and community. Examining these groups highlighted that the shift to community care did not mean that institutions ceased to exist. Rather, that they are better depicted as places of negotiation maintained in fluid connections with the individuals, families, and communities using them.[58] Further analysis is needed of the way in which the meaning of institutional care was renegotiated in the community.

New historiography on community mental health

In understanding how psychiatric nurses engaged with new community-based services in the post-WWII period, I argue, the professionalization theme is only partially relevant, as it does not sufficiently engage with an analysis of nurses' work and their interaction with patients and communities. While this aspect might be difficult to analyze for the earlier period, as nurses left little evidence of their work behind, for recent periods oral history can be used to examine how nurses interacted with patients and renegotiated their work as institutions transformed and with the shift to community care.[59] Recent studies have begun to examine nurses' work in the transition to community care post-1950s.[60] Nolan broke new ground with a nuanced portrayal of post-1950s mental health nursing in the UK, addressing the professional battles, but also outlining how nurses' work was shaped by the day-to-day interaction with patients in often chaotic circumstances with few resources available.[61] The UK was one of the first European countries to embrace a deinstitutionalization policy in the 1950s and its new emphasis on community care became a leading example internationally.[62] Community psychiatric nurses were an essential component of new community services, but the "insertion" of their professional experience and nursing knowledge obtained within the institutional context into the rising community system was rarely planned and, if it was, it was most often implemented as an afterthought.[63] In the face of a growing number of short-term admissions, which continued to raise the demand for nursing personnel in mental hospitals, and new departments of general hospital psychiatry, envisioning nursing roles in the community was difficult.[64] It took time to realize that rehabilitation of people with long-term mental illness through new modes of rehabilitative and "active treatment"—turning mental hospitals into alleged new "therapeutic communities"—not only was relevant to a neglected group of largely ignored patients on back-wards of mental hospitals, but would also have to become an ongoing component of psychiatric care in new community services.[65] At first, the organization of community services emerged with little planning. Few leaders in policy considered the experience of psychiatric nurses developed in the mental hospital during a process of renewal from the 1950s through the 1970s a potential resource outside the hospital for such services as medication management, facilitating groups, and rehabilitative support.[66] An exception to this trend is the early emergence of a community psychiatric nursing program in Saskatchewan in the post-1950s era.[67]

Keeping the lens closely on the realities of nurses' work, Sheridan examined new therapeutic roles and rehabilitative practices of nurses in the new domain of rehabilitative community psychiatric nursing in Ireland.[68] She found that the formation of the European Union prompted changes in psychiatric nursing during the 1970s. It generated new directives on professional and academic education, and stimulated a new view on rehabilitation and community care, which was implemented in the nursing curriculum in the 1980s. Similarly, Prebble found that community mental health care in New Zealand shifted the context of nursing education and work; it was no longer tied to its traditional origin in the mental hospital.[69] The psychiatric hospital she studied dissolved administratively into a general hospital board in 1972 and the psychiatric nursing educational program moved into a comprehensive generic nursing program in the polytechnic educational system.

Harrington conducted a detailed analysis of the way nurses, social workers, and other professions constructed community mental health work in Manchester and Salford in the UK from the 1960s onwards, primarily relying on oral history.[70] Harrington provides an important framework for interpreting the process of resettlement of long-term mentally ill people into new community facilities, describing this process as "radicalism in a backwater."[71] In a second wave of anti-psychiatric protest in the late 1970s in the UK, she noted, a group of activist-minded mental health professionals, guided by Wolfensberger's normalization theory and life history approaches, empowered long-neglected patients in the back-wards of an underprivileged mental hospital to reestablish their lives in the community.[72] Turning away from the focus of nurses' work in particular, the construction of community mental health work is also examined in new studies in health geography through the lens of place and community.[73] Based on this work it can be argued that institutional care was part of a longer continuum of place "inside and outside the walls of the asylum."[74] Further studies begin to reveal how many facilities and support services, such as housing, sheltered work, employment, volunteer work, drop-in support, and "technologies" of rehabilitation and medication management had to be renegotiated and reinvented as the framework of community services took shape.[75]

A focus on the multiple groups involved—nurses, consumers, volunteers, other professional groups, and newly evolving experts such as mental health workers and peer support workers with new professional identities—will help to better understand the way new domains of caring work were negotiated within the transformation to community care. Such an analysis is interconnected with multiple areas of historical and interdisciplinary scholarship.[76] In keeping the lens on changes in day-to-day mental health care, it appears that neither nurses nor patients were passively determined by the (professional) scripts placed on them, but related and responded to their circumstances and helped shape them.[77] Gender, professional identity, region, place, and work (not referring to unionism alone but also to nurses' craft, occupational, and expert knowledge) are important analytic categories to examine and deepen our understanding of the transition to community care.[78] A changing therapeutic climate and focus on rehabilitation within and "outside" mental hospitals changed the work and professional identity of nurses. And, as I argue in my case example, consumers (or ex-patients) participated in this process as well, renegotiating their own conceptualizations of identity and work in tandem with nurses and other mental health professionals.

Patient engagement with community mental health work

Patient engagement in activism for patient rights as well as immersion in volunteer and paid mental health work to improve care post-1950s has reframed the way we think about mental health and mental illness. In considering the *work* of nurses and patients as a parallel and performative process, we can nuance the history of patient involvement in transforming mental health care, particularly as of the 1970s, recognizing that both groups simultaneously renegotiated their respective identities in mental health care.

An articulate voice of patients was not a new phenomenon in the 1970s. Although a historiography on patients is a relatively recent phenomenon, an autobiographical literature existed since the beginning of the century, and even before.[79] Notably, Beers' biography had been at the heart of the mental hygiene movement.[80] Whether it was on their experiences of illness or health care, or a critique of the system, patients have used both autobiography and fiction to make their views known.[81] Political engagement, cultural critique, and advocacy for change shaped an emerging historiography, including oral history and (auto)biographical studies on the place of the patient in psychiatry post-1950s.[82] Media and film added to the popularization of the patient experience, with one of the most influential and lasting examples being the 1962 novel and 1975 film, *One Flew Over the Cuckoo's Nest*.[83]

Patients became a new voice in the context of community-based care and had an essential role in its construction, especially after the 1970s. In many places throughout Europe and North America, new collectives of counter-cultural activism resulted in new alternatives of community living.[84] To emphasize their political stance and connection to the "mad or liberation movement," patients resisted their identification with the medical model and many no longer identified as "patient." Instead, being a "user of services" constituted one as a "consumer of services," and having been subjected to services perceived as harmful constituted one as a "survivor."[85] Hence, new identities of ex-patient, survivor, and consumer emerged.[86] By the late 1980s, in North America and abroad, advocates were well integrated into many legal professional policy bodies and advisory councils, able to join a broader effort in health care to articulate patient rights of (consumer) choice and influence policy making.[87] Using patient oral histories to challenge the post-1950s history of mental illness, Davies explored key narrative frames, such as loss, survival stories, and self as patient, in which patients "have made their experience meaningful to themselves and others."[88] She makes a compelling argument about the way in which these stories should be listened to. But she overlooks, I believe, a fourth narrative frame of central importance to patient experiences: narratives of patients as workers. Reaume has analyzed the essential role of patient work in maintaining the asylum economy.[89] In post-1950s anti-psychiatric activism, patient work took on new meaning and obtained new organized forms.[90] Work figured importantly in the stories of consumers in the New Westminster oral history project.[91] From the 1970s onwards, (ex)patients or consumers, at points supported by nurses and other professionals,[92] obtained powerful identities in mental health work as "experiential experts" or "prosumers."[93] That is, they became teachers, mental health workers, and advocates, sharing a parallel presence with nurses, other professionals, and volunteers in many new services and, as I will argue in this chapter, in new and "unusual alliances." The story of the establishment of Pioneer House illustrates the point.

Pioneer House

Opened in New Westminster, British Columbia, in 1982, Pioneer House initially provided housing for about 22 "deinstitutionalized" people as a new experiment in community living.[94] While different iterations of community care already had emerged in British Columbia, such as boarding homes, general hospital wards, smaller "trans"-institutions and free-standing community mental health centers, Pioneer House was a new experiment in community living.[95] A grassroots initiative, based on a consumer-driven self-help philosophy, it was established by an unusual alliance of professionals and patients, both political activists and pragmatists, who, as the Riverview Hospital Volunteer Association (RHVA), drew from their institutional experiences to work together for ex-patient empowerment and control in community transitions. In the development and operation of Pioneer House, professionals and patients simultaneously renegotiated their identities amid the ongoing processes of deinstitutionalization. Ultimately, as a case-example, Pioneer House highlights the fluid connections, or the permeable membrane, between the institution and the community.

In 1982, the RHVA rented an abandoned old-age home, with the idea of constructing a new "model of community living" for ex-mental patients.[96] Approaching the project from a "grassroots" position, rather than simply enacting top-down institutional or governmental policy, staff, volunteers, and residents sought to move away from older hierarchical models, such as the BC Boarding Home Programme (BHP). Started by the BC government in the 1960s to facilitate community placement of long-term hospitalized RH patients deemed no longer suitable for treatment, boarding homes built upon older poor relief patterns and focused on placement, with little anticipation of ongoing support, nor a taking into account of the perspectives of front line workers or persons using the services.[97] Because of regulations governing their licensing, boarding homes could easily (d)evolve into staff-driven, highly regulated structures that constrained rather than enabled a self-directed way of living. Carol Ann Russell, a psychiatric nurse who joined Dewar in the management of Pioneer House a year after it opened, recalled: "[Clients] were leaving RH, they were coming into the community and they were . . . sitting in some living room in a [boarding] house somewhere. They . . . had a more integrated community life at Riverview where there was the store and the movies and the bowling . . . When they came to the community, which was supposedly a better deal for them, there was no infrastructure in place to help integrate these people into the community; [they] were less active than they had been at Riverview."[98] Joining forces to place Pioneer House on a new footing, the RHVA tried to move away from such models.

Instead, Pioneer House aimed for a different ideal, one that asserted ex-patient control rather than professional authority, and promoted meaningful involvement in activities and work.[99] Rather than remaining idle or being told what to do, Pioneer House residents participated in daily household activities—cleaning, cooking, or grocery shopping, for example—or were encouraged to engage in work or education. "Nobody is too ill not to be able to wipe a table," Dewar pointed out. Promoting consumer control and empowerment, house decisions were made via the democratic process of group meetings run by residents themselves: "We . . . used to have a resident's meeting every week, I organized that," Beamish recalled. "Staff could sit in on it but they couldn't participate really." A philosophy of self-help was enacted at Pioneer House by developing work and volunteer projects for residents, helping them to decide and plan for themselves what they wanted to do, or, if necessary, set limits—strategies that supported independence, rehabilitation, and recovery. Russell, referring to previous staff-driven programs, noted "nobody is going to come to their door when they move with a bingo game under their arm saying 'Ok I'm here to activate you.'"

Within the RVHA the ideal of promoting consumer control and empowerment brought together the political influence of one of the first patient activist groups in BC, the Mental Patient Association of Vancouver (MPA), which during the 1970s had also asserted its influence at RH, and the earlier institutional initiatives to "open up" the mental hospital by opening wards and enhancing patient activity through volunteer and "reactivation" activity.[100] Russell remembered Beamish's institutional experience as profoundly influencing the new way of operating at Pioneer House: Beamish was "someone who . . . had been in the system, [and] this [patient-run structure] is what he felt was needed . . . A lot of [what we did] was based on his personal experiences of being a mental patient in the system in those days—and where he saw the gaps." Beamish's institutional experience in turn was shaped by both his experience as a patient and his engagement with the MPA. He became one of the MPA leaders and advocates who negotiated ex-patient representation and a new MPA niche within the RH Volunteer Department.[101] Additionally, although less explicitly, Dewar and Russell brought the skills they originally learned inside the institution to establishing and managing Pioneer House.

When Dewar and Russell started nursing school at RH, in 1967 and 1969 respectively, the coordination of recreational and daily living activities rested with the nursing staff.[102] By then, psychiatric nursing education incorporated an emphasis on interpersonal relations, use of therapeutic milieu, rehabilitation methods, and team nursing in intensive treatment areas; in continued treatment areas, students developed skills in group-work methods.[103] At RH, Dewar and Russell learned to physically care for people living with mental illness—attending to somatic therapies and managing medications—but they also learned ward organization, and facilitation of daily living and rehabilitative activities. At Pioneer House, Dewar and Russell inserted their institutionally learned skills into the community themselves, as there was little forward planning or governmental/official infrastructure in place to do so. They used these familiar strategies to counter the problem that Russell had laid out so well: that there was more community available in the mental hospital then there was outside, in the actual community.

An alliance of political activists and pragmatists

Although nurses and patients working together in new power structures was arguably novel in community care (such a thing wasn't happening in boarding homes, for example), the RHVA alliance had its roots inside the institution. Connections between nurses and patients were built upon these older traditions of hospital renewal and volunteer work initiated at RH in the 1950s by the Canadian Mental Health Association, which had grown into a well-established volunteer department attracting over 300 volunteers by 1973.[104]

Patient activism was a new influence on institutional services at RH in the mid-1970s that soon merged with the existing volunteer structures. In the early 1970s, in a politically charged move, ex-patients themselves began to "volunteer" on Riverview grounds, visiting their peers.[105] These volunteers were members of the Mental Patient Association (MPA)—an ex-patient collective founded in Vancouver in 1971 by consumers who had experienced a lack of community resources and decided to develop services for themselves.[106] With a patient-rights, anti-psychiatry focus, the group operated homes and a drop-in center for discharged patients, aiming to "rehabilitate" the social structure—rather than individual people—and reverse power.[107] Despite the political upheaval, the RH administration soon welcomed their presence and the MPA, spearheaded by Beamish, triggered a new patient-led council, and obtained a permanent MPA office in the existing Volunteer Department.[108] Finding themselves (unusual) allies, the pragmatic, nurse-driven RH Volunteer Department and the politically conscious consumer volunteers formed the RHVA in 1980.[109] Beamish became the ex-patient representative on the board. The result of this alliance was a push to broaden RH volunteer work into a new *outward* and more politicized direction. Bringing together nursing experience, volunteer initiative, and patient activism, forging new relationships on the institutional grounds, RHVA became a new platform for bridging community connections in new ways with Pioneer House as its first experiment.

The Pioneer House effort did not emerge in isolation from larger social changes and was not immune to bureaucratic pressures. Examining this particular initiative in more detail provides the opportunity to understand the way patients and nurses reworked existing institutional pressures and negotiated their place and identity in the community within existing bureaucratic constraints. The MPA influence transmitted into the new RVHA initiative and, at first, the group resisted the so-called medical model or any formal therapy, which to them represented the mental health bureaucracy while friendship and community drove their work.[110] However, in order to have the home approved as a licensed care home in BC, under the Community Care Facilities Act, the association had to hire a professional with appropriate credentials to direct the home.[111] The RHVA board hired well-known-to-them Fran Phillips, a politically minded registered nurse who held a degree and "a wealth of community experience," as the Facility Administrator.[112] Phillips, who had started her career in nursing at the RH School of Psychiatric Nursing, had already worked closely with MPA since the early 1970s as their residence coordinator in Vancouver.[113] Dave Beamish immediately became a senior worker and Colleen Dewar was hired in 1982 to set up the home.[114]

While Phillips and Beamish clearly brought their activist MPA experience to Pioneer House, other staff members, such as nurses Dewar and Carol Russell, who started in 1982 and 1983 respectively, appeared to join for more pragmatic reasons such as the hours and increased flexibility the work allowed, which permitted them to combine their position with their family responsibilities. They further appreciated the relative independence community work provided and were attracted to the non-profit model because of the greater independence it gave them. Russell noted:

> I feel working in a non-profit organization, you can institute changes . . . modify programs . . . without the bureaucracy, and although . . . we were being paid considerably less than what the hospital were paying their nurses . . . [which made it a hard decision], I'm a single parent . . . but I was able to get the flexibility I needed . . . with the satisfaction I was getting from the work . . . I just decided to stay here.[115]

Perhaps because of her more pragmatic lens, Dewar was able to navigate Pioneer House through many bureaucratic obstacles. For example, Dewar introduced the first community self-medication program, skillfully negotiating the bureaucratic regulations:

> We started the first self-medication program. I had to write to Victoria (the BC capital) to receive permission for that. So we started that and we have a module and now in every program we have, we have a graduated self-medication program.[116]

At the time of the interview Dewar was the facilities' executive director.

The unusual alliance sometimes created tension, as different viewpoints had to be negotiated. For example, in the mid-1980s conflicts arose over the sustainability of the model of care that the group—as a collective—sought to maintain and over program funding. Up until the mid-1980s staff had been able to independently decide who would live at Pioneer House. But during that time the provincial government began to assert more control over residential services, in terms of both funding and placement policies, through its local mental health centers and had appointed a placement coordinator at the New Westminister Mental Health Centre (MHC).[117] Pioneer House was part of that jurisdiction. Phillips and Beamish deeply resented such control, preferring to decide who could live in the house for themselves, and were unwilling to accept MHC input.[118] For them, the MHC resembled governmental bureaucracy and seemed only an exponent of medical and bureaucratic control. Disagreement was exacerbated when the regional health authority requested they use a third of the beds in their facility to establish a Community Residential Emergency Short Stay Treatment (CRESST) Program.[119] Phillips and the RHVA Board did not agree on this point, and Phillips resigned. Russell explained it this way:

> There really wasn't any sort of connection with the MHC at New Westminster. So [when] gradually . . . [the MHC] started to [direct placement and] oversee residential programs [we had no liaison . . .] and that wasn't working. We really, really needed to change the relationship that we had with the [MHC in New Westminster] because let's face it, they were contracting our service.[120]

To her and the larger RHVA board it seemed reasonable to accept the proposed change to avoid risking the funding. Pragmatically perhaps, the Board accepted the bureaucratic constraints and new stipulations and established the CRESST program while maintaining the residential component of its program. It did not see this as a way of overruling a democratic, consumer-driven ideal of rehabilitative services, but rather as a strategic response to sustain and protect it in the face of shifting pressures of bureaucratic control and funding. As the RHVA had to renegotiate the power relationships within the group, under the pressure of a certain level of bureaucratic control, it in fact rebalanced accommodation and resistance to such control in order to sustain the model of community living that was the larger interest of the RHVA. In a sense, the conflict let the RHVA confirm its place in the community and also clarified its purpose. In order to maintain a focus on rehabilitative support the question was not about independent care or bureaucratic control, but rather about negotiating the right balance between them. Building community connections as a grassroots development and asserting Pioneer House's place in the new "matrix" of services continued to be a complex and sometimes challenging process—as this case example well illustrates—requiring continued accommodation to larger bureaucratic dynamics not unlike what their predecessors within the institutions also had faced.

Conclusion

Although the nurses who joined the RHVA project had been exposed to ideas and practices of rehabilitation (because the whole RH institution was transformed based on these premises between the 1950s and 1980s), they had not had a chance to take up rehabilitation in the particular politicized way the MPA group understood it. In addition, the new community setting provided them a context to assert their independence as nurses in community mental health. As an organization, RHVA established and renewed its commitment to enhance community living for people with mental illness. Its joined forces strengthened it in renegotiating a new model of support. Rather than "caring for," as Russell put it, the new alliance pushed staff toward a more participatory model that reflected the change of times, a new nurse–consumer relationship, as well as a different professional identity. But disagreement arose as well within the Board and among the staff over the way the balance between care and control should be maintained. In the shift to a matrix of community-based services, patients, consumers, peer support workers, "experiential experts," mental health workers, or "prosumers" established a prominent presence parallel to other workers in the system, such as nurses and other professionals. In the particular case example of this chapter, both groups had experienced the institution and both envisioned and enacted new ways of supporting community living that would empower former patients. However, in doing so, some of the dilemmas of bureaucratic control were also reproduced in the community, for example in the way residential placement became coordinated via the MHC, establishing regional control over a locally initiated organization, thus constraining consumer influence. While Pioneer House represented a reworking of the meaning of a supportive community, new tensions also arose over the way rehabilitation and bureaucratic control should be balanced and negotiated. In this process, nurses and consumers negotiated new identities as community mental health workers. Further analysis of these complex reworkings and realignments of work, place, and identity that formed the new matrix of community-based mental health services will set an important new agenda of community mental health history.

Notes

1 I acknowledge financial support from the BC Medical Services Research Fund, the Social Science and Humanities Research Council of Canada, and the Canadian Institutes of Health Research for this research. I am most grateful for the generous comments and constructive feedback of Catherine Haney, Margaret Gorrie, Patricia D'Antonio, Julie Fairman, and Jean Whelan on earlier drafts of this chapter. I also acknowledge the support of the Open Doors/After the Asylum project team. Most importantly, I thank all the people who participated in this research by sharing their experience, knowledge, and memory through oral history. Without their insights on the development of community living for people living with mental illness I would not have been able to write this chapter.

2 Interview with Dewar, C. by M. Gorrie and author, New Westminster, February 2009. This research is part of a larger project which explores the development of mental health services in New Westminster, BC: 1960–2000 from professional and consumer points of view, funded by the BC Medical Services Research Fund, Vancouver Foundation (G. Boschma, principal investigator, M. Gorrie co-investigator, and C. Haney, research assistant at the time we wrote this chapter). Thirty-five oral interviews were conducted by the investigators and N. Bonifacio, also a research assistant, a subset of which is included in this chapter. Institutional ethical approval from the Behavioral Research Ethics Board of the University of British Columbia and the Fraser Health Research Ethics Board was obtained as well as interviewees' consent. Interviewees who consented to reveal their names are addressed as such; those who did not want to have their names used are referred to by pseudonym. The oral histories are with the author.

3 Interview with Beamish, D. by author, Vancouver, August 2011.

4 Since the emergence of a patient rights movement in mental health in the 1960s, participants have identified with a variety of terms, including ex-patient, survivor, consumer, or people living with mental illness. Terminology also was a political statement to distance themselves from the medical term "patient." While there is still debate over terminology, I have tried to use the terms according to context and time, and to the way people tended to use them themselves to frame their identity, which could be (ex-) patient, survivor, client, or consumer. I will use the terms "patient," former or ex-patient, and "consumer" interchangeably in this chapter. For further discussion see also Tomes, N. 2011, "From outsiders to insiders: the consumer-survivor movement and its impact on US mental health policy," in B. Hoffman, N. Tomes, R. Grob, and M. Schlesinger (eds), *Patients as policy actors: a century of changing markets and missions*, Rutgers, New Brunswick, NJ, pp. 111–31, especially notes 1 and 2, and Shimrat, I. 1997, *Call me crazy: stories from the mad movement*, Press Gang Publishers, Vancouver.

5 The extent to which downsizing occurred in Canada and the timing of it varied from province to province because of its provincially based health care system. Tellingly, RH in BC only permanently closed its doors in 2012, whereas its patient population had peaked at about 4600 patients in 1950—60 years earlier. See Boschma, G. 2011, "Deinstitutionalization reconsidered: geographic and demographic changes in mental health care in British Columbia and Alberta, 1950–1980," *Histoire Sociale/Social History*, vol. 44, no. 88, p. 234.

6 Certificate of Incorporation under the Province of British Columbia Society Act S-15918, Canada, issued on 6 October 1980, certifying the incorporation of the Riverview Hospital Volunteer Association under the act, with Constitution attached, filed and registered. Copy obtained from Colleen Dewar, Pioneer Community Living Association, New Westminster, BC.

7 Interview with Dewar; Interview with Beamish, 2011.

8 Dyck, E. 2011, "Dismantling the asylum and charting new pathways into the community: mental health care in twentieth century Canada," *Histoire Sociale/Social History*, vol. 44, no. 88, pp. 181–96.

9 See note 1 for project details.

10 Boschma, G. 2012, "Community mental health nursing in Alberta, Canada: an oral history," *Nursing History Review*, vol. 20, pp. 103–35; Elliot, J., Toman, C., and Stuart, M. (eds) (2008) *Place and Practice in Canadian Nursing History*, Vancouver: UBC Press.

11 Fingard, J. and Rutherford, J. 2005, "The politics of mental health care in Nova Scotia: the case of the Halifax County Hospital, 1940–1976," *Acadiensis*, vol. 35, no. 1, pp. 24–49; Fingard, J. and Rutherford, J. 2008, *Protect, befriend, respect: Nova Scotia's mental health movement, 1908–2008*, Fernwood Publishing, Halifax; Grob, G. 1994, *The mad among us: a history of the care of America's mentally ill*, The Free Press, New York; Gijswijt-Hofstra, M., Oosterhuis, H., Vijselaar, J., and Freeman, H. (eds) 2005, *Psychiatric cultures compared: psychiatry and mental health care in the twentieth century*, Amsterdam University Press.

12 Boschma, "Deinstitutionalization reconsidered," pp. 223–56; Davis, S. 2006, *Community mental health in Canada: theory, policy, and practice*, UBC Press, Vancouver; Macfarlane, D., Fortin, P., Fox, J., Gundry, S., Oshry, J., and Warren, E. 1997, "Clinical and human resource planning for the downsizing of psychiatric hospitals: the British Columbia experience," *Psychiatric Quarterly*, vol. 68, no. 1, pp. 25–42; Marchildon, G.P. 2011, "A house divided: deinstitutionalization, Medicare, and the Canadian Mental Health Association in Saskatchewan, 1944–1964," *Histoire Social/Social History*, vol. 44, no. 88, pp. 305–29; Menzies R. and Palys, T. 2006 "Turbulent spirits: aboriginal patients in the British Columbia psychiatric system," in Moran J.E. and Wright D. (eds) *Mental health and Canadian society: historical perspectives*, McGill-Queen's University Press, Montreal; Sealy, P. and Whitehead, P.C. 2004, "Forty years of deinstitutionalization of psychiatric services in Canada: an empirical assessment," *Canadian Journal of Psychiatry*, vol. 49, pp. 249–57.

13 Dyck, "Dismantling the asylum"; Marchildon, "A house divided"; Shorter, E. 1997, *A history of psychiatry: from the era of the asylum to the age of Prozac*, Wiley, New York.

14 Boschma, "Deinstitutionalization reconsidered"; Davies, M.J. 2003, *Into the house of old: a history of residential care in British Columbia*, McGill-Queen's University Press, Montreal; Dickinson, H.D. 1989, *The two psychiatries: the transformation of psychiatric work in Saskatchewan, 1905–1984*, Canadian Plains Research Centre, University of Regina, Regina; Hector, I. 2001, "Changing funding patterns and the effect on mental health care in Canada," in Q. Rae-Grant (ed.), *Psychiatry in Canada: 50 years, 1951–2001*, Canadian Psychiatric Association, Ottawa; Ostry, A. 2009, "The foundations of national public hospital insurance," *Canadian Bulletin of Medical History*, vol. 26, no. 2, pp. 261–82.

15 Boschma, "Community mental health nursing"; Dyck, "Dismantling the asylum"; Knowles, C. 2000, *Bedlam on the streets*, Routledge, London.

16 Boschma, G., Scaia, M., Bonifacio, M., and Roberts, E. 2008, "Oral history research," in S.B. Lewenson and E. Krohn-Herrmann (eds), *Capturing nursing history: a guide to historical methods in research*, Springer, New York.

17 Boschma, G. 2003, *The rise of mental health nursing: a history of psychiatric care in Dutch asylums, 1890–1920*, Amsterdam University Press, Amsterdam; Gijswijt-Hofstra et al., *Psychiatric cultures compared*; Moran, J. 2000, *Committed to the state asylum: insanity and society in nineteenth-century Quebec and Ontario*, McGill-Queen's University Press, Montreal; Moran

and Wright, *Mental health and Canadian society*; Thifault, M. 2009, "Au-delà d'un role de protection à l'égard des aliénés: initiation à l'art du nursing à l'Hôpital Saint-Jean-de-Dieu, 1912–1915," in S. Yaya (ed.), *Pouvoir médical et santé totalitaire: conséquences socio-anthropologiques et éthiques*, PUL, Ville de Québec.

18 Digby, A. 1985, *Madness, morality and medicine: a study of the York Retreat, 1796–1914*, Cambridge University Press, Cambridge; Dwyer, E. 1992, "Stories of epilepsy, 1880–1930," in C.E. Rosenberg and J. Golden (eds), *Framing disease: studies in cultural history*, Rutgers University Press, New Brunswick, NJ; Tomes, N. 1984, *Generous confidence: Thomas Story Kirkbride and the art of asylum keeping, 1840–1883*, Cambridge University Press, Cambridge.

19 Foucault, M. 1965, *Madness and civilization*, Pantheon, New York.

20 Scull, A. 1979, *Museums of madness: the social organization of insanity in nineteenth-century England*, Allen Lane, London; Szasz, T. 1974 (1961), *The myth of mental illness: foundations of a theory of personal conduct*, Harper Collins, New York.

21 Goffman, E. 1961, *Asylums: essays on the condition of the social situation of mental patients and other inmates*, Doubleday, New York.

22 Chamberlain, J. 1978, *On our own: patient-controlled alternatives to the mental health system*, Hawthorn Books, New York; Crossley, M.L. 2006, *Contesting psychiatry: social movements in mental health*, Routledge, New York; Hunsche, P. 2008, *De strijdbare patient: van Gekkenbeweging to Cliënten Bewustzijn—Portretten 1970–2000 [The fighting spirited patient: from mad-movement to client (or consumer) consciousness—portraits 1970–2000]*, Uitgeverij Candide, Amsterdam.

23 Digby, *Madness, morality and medicine*; Grob, *The mad among us*; Porter, R. 1987, *A social history of madness*, Weidenfeld & Nicolson, London; Tomes, *Generous confidence*.

24 Boschma, *The rise of mental health nursing*; Nolan, P. 1993, *A history of mental health nursing*, Chapman & Hall, London.

25 Porter, *A social history of madness;* Reaume, G. 2000, *Remembrance of patients past: patient life at the Toronto Hospital for the Insane, 1870–1940*, Oxford University Press, Ontario.

26 D'Antonio, P. 2006, *Founding friends: family, staff, and patients at the Friends Asylum in early nineteenth century Philadelphia*, Lehigh University Press, Bethlehem, PA.

27 Boschma, *The rise of mental health nursing*.

28 Chatterton, C. 2004, "Caught in the middle? Mental health nurse training in England, 1919–51," *Journal of Psychiatric Mental Health Nursing*, vol. 11, no. 1, pp. 30–5; Dooley, C. 1998, "When love and skill work together: work, skill and the occupational culture of mental nurses at the Brandon Hospital for Mental Diseases, 1919–1946," MA thesis, University of Manitoba; Hicks, B. 2008, "From barnyards to bedsides to books and beyond: the evolution and professionalization of registered psychiatric nursing in Manitoba, 1955–1980," PhD dissertation, University of Manitoba; Hicks, B. 2011, "Gender, politics, and regionalism: factors in the evolution of registered psychiatric nursing in Manitoba, 1920–1960," *Nursing History Review*, vol. 19, pp. 103–26; Nolan, *A history of mental health nursing*; Prebble, C. 2007, "Ordinary men and uncommon women: a history of psychiatric nursing in New Zealand public mental hospitals, 1939–1972," PhD dissertation, University of Auckland; Stegge, Aan de, C. 2005, "Changing attitudes towards 'non-restraint' in Dutch psychiatric nursing, 1897–1994," in Gijswijt-Hofstra et al., *Psychiatric cultures compared*; Svedberg, G. 2000, "Narratives on prolonged baths from psychiatric care in Sweden during the first half of the twentieth century," *International History of Nursing Journal*, vol. 5, no. 2, pp. 28–35; Thifault, "Au-delà d'un role de protection"; Tipliski, V. 2002, "Parting at the crossroads: the development of education for psychiatric nursing in three Canadian provinces, 1909–1955," PhD dissertation, University of Manitoba.

29 Dingwall, R., Rafferty, A.M., and Webster, C. 1988, "Mental disorder and mental handicap," in authors (eds), *An introduction to the social history of nursing*, London: Routledge, pp. 142–4; McPherson, K. 1996, *Bedside matters: the transformation of Canadian nursing,*

1900–1990, Oxford University Press, Toronto; Melosh, B. 1982, *The physician's hand*, Temple University Press, Philadelphia; Reverby, S.M. 1987, *Ordered to care: the dilemma of American nursing, 1850–1945*, Cambridge University Press, Cambridge.

30 Church, O.M. 1985, "Emergence of training programs for asylum nurses at the turn of the century," *Advances in Nursing Science*, vol. 7, no. 2, pp. 35–46; Church, O.M. 1987, "From custody to community in psychiatric nursing," *Nursing Research*, vol. 36, no. 1, pp. 48–55; Nolan, *A history of mental health nursing*.

31 Church, "Emergence of training programs"; Church, "From custody to community." According to Prebble, "Ordinary men and uncommon women," Church saw the legacy of the asylum as a hindrance.

32 Dingwall et al., "Mental disorder and mental handicap".

33 Church, "From custody to community"; Worley, N.K. (ed.) 1997, *Mental health nursing in the community*, Mosby, St Louis.

34 Taylor, E.J. 1926, "What progress are we making in mental hygiene and mental nursing," *ICN Bulletin*, vol. 1, no. 2, pp. 81–95; Taylor, E.J. 1935, "The next step forward – psychiatric nursing in Department of Nursing Education," *The American Journal of Nursing*, vol. 35, no. 1, pp. 57–66.

35 Boschma, *The rise of mental health nursing*; Nolan, *A history of mental health nursing*; Tipliski, "Parting at the crossroads."

36 Chatterton, "Caught in the middle?"; Dingwall et al., "Mental disorder and mental handicap"; Hicks, "From barnyards to bedsides to books"; Nolan, *A history of mental health nursing*; Tipliski, "Parting at the crossroads."

37 Boschma, G., Yonge, O., and Mychajlunow, L. 2005, "Gender and professional identity in psychiatric nursing practice in Alberta, Canada, 1930–1975," *Nursing Inquiry*, vol. 12, no. 4, pp. 243–55; Dooley, "When love and skill work together"; Hicks, "Gender, politics, and regionalism"; Martin, A. 2003, "Determinants of destiny: the professional development of psychiatric nurses in Saskatchewan," MA thesis, University of Regina; Nolan, *A history of mental health nursing*; Tipliski, "Parting at the crossroads."

38 Thifault, M.C. 2011, "Hell in the family: married women and madness before institutionalization at the St-Jean-de-Dieu Asylum, 1890–1921," *Nursing History Review*, vol. 19, no. 1, pp. 15–28.

39 Boschma et al., "Gender and professional identity"; Hicks, "From barnyards to bedsides to books"; Martin, "Determinants of destiny"; Tipliski, "Parting at the crossroads"; Wood, S.T. 1998, "Changing times: a historical review of psychiatric nursing education in the province of Saskatchewan," MA thesis, University of Regina.

40 Prebble, "Ordinary men and uncommon women"; Braunschweig, S. 2004, "Die Entwicklung der Krankenpflege und der Psychiatrie-Pflege in der Schweiz," in I. Walter, E. Seidl, and V. Kozon (eds), *Wieder die Geschichtslosigkeit der Pflege*, ÖGVP Verlag, Wien.

41 Boschma et al., "Gender and professional identity"; Boschma G. 2007, "Dominance and resistance in cultural discourse on psychiatric mental health: Oral history accounts of family members," *Nursing Inquiry*, vol. 14, no. 4, pp. 266–78.

42 Boschma, "Dominance and resistance"; Boschma, G. 2008, "A family point of view: negotiating asylum care in Alberta, 1905–1930," *Canadian Bulletin of Medical History*, vol. 25, no. 2, pp. 367–89; Thifault, "Hell in the family"; Thifault, M. and Perreault, I. 2012, "The social integration of the mentally ill in Quebec prior to the Bédard Report of 1962," *Canadian Bulletin of Medical History*, vol. 29, no. 1, pp. 125–50.

43 See McPherson, *Bedside matters*, and D'Antonio, P. 2010, *American nursing: a history of knowledge, authority and the meaning of work*, Johns Hopkins University Press, Baltimore; McPherson, *Bedside matters* for a discussion of this theme in general (hospital) nursing.

44 Boschma, *The rise of mental health nursing*.

45 Hähner-Rombach, S. 1995, *Arm, Weiblich—Wahnsinnig? Patientinnen der Königlichen Heilanstalt Zwiefalten im Spiegel der Einweisungsgutachten von 1812–1871 [Poor, female—insane? Female patients of the Royal Asylum Zwiefalten from the perspective of admission, 1812–71]*, Verlag Psychiatry und Geschichte, Zwiefalten.

46 Goldstein, J.L. and Godemont, M.L. 2003, "The legend and lessons of Geel, Belgium: a 1500-year-old legend, a 21st-century model," *Community Mental Health Journal*, vol. 39, no. 5, pp. 441–58.

47 MacLennan, D. 1987, "Beyond the asylum: professionalization and the mental hygiene movement in Canada, 1914–1928," *Canadian Bulletin of Medical History*, vol. 4, pp. 7–23; Pols, H. 2010 "Beyond the clinical frontiers: the American mental hygiene movement, 1910–1945," in V. Roelcke, P.J. Weindling, and L. Westwood (eds), *International relations in psychiatry: Britain, Germany and the United States to World War II*, University of Rochester Press, Rochester.

48 Braunschweig, S. 2006, "Krankenpfleger, Spitalarchivar und Stammbaumforscher Heinrich Rellstab im Kampf Gegen Erbkrankheiten [Male nurse, hospital archivist and geneologist Heinrich Rellstab in his battle against hereditary diseases]," in author (ed.), *Pflege—Räume, Macht und Alltag. Beitrage zur Geschichte der Pflege [Nursing—space, power and everyday praxis. Contributions to the history of nursing]*, Chronon Verlag, Zurich; Foth, T. 2011, "Analyzing nursing as a dispositif: healing and devastation in the name of biopower: a historical, biopolitical analysis of psychiatric care under the Nazi regime, 1933–1945," PhD dissertation, University of Ottawa; Mansell, D. and Hibberd, J. 1998, "'We picked the wrong one to sterilise': the role of nursing in the eugenics movement in Alberta, 1920–40," *International History of Nursing Journal*, vol. 3, pp. 4–11.

49 Beers, C. 1908, *A mind that found itself*, University of Pittsburgh Press, Pittsburgh.

50 Roland, C.G. 1990, *Clarence Hincks: mental health crusader*, Dundurn Press, Toronto; Thomson, M. 1995, "Mental hygiene as an international movement", in P. Weindling (ed.), *International health organizations and movements, 1918–1939*, Cambridge University Press, Cambridge.

51 Brouns, G. 2010, "Social-psychiatrische verpleegkunde: de ontwikkeling van een verpleegkundig specialisme in het domein van de Nederlandse sociale psychiatrie [Social-psychiatric nursing: the development of a nursing specialty in the domain of Dutch social psychiatry]," PhD dissertation, Universiteit Maastricht; Oosterhuis, H. 2005, "Outpatient psychiatry and mental health care in the twentieth century," in Gijswijt-Hofstra et al., *Psychiatric cultures compared*.

52 Stegge, Aan de, C. 2012, *Gekkenwerk: De Ontwikkeling van het Beroep Psychiatrische Verpleegkunde in Nederland, 1830–1980 [Crazy work: the development of the profession "psychiatric nurse" in the Netherlands, 1830–1980]*, Maastricht University Press, Maastricht.

53 Sillars, D. 1983, "The development of community mental health nursing in Toronto from 1917–1947," MSc thesis, University of Toronto.

54 Thifault, "Hell in the family."

55 Jones, C. 1989, *The charitable imperative: hospitals and nursing in ancien régime and revolutionary France*, Routledge, London; Leiby, J.S. 1992, "San Hipólito's treatment of the mentally ill in Mexico City, 1589–1650," *Historian*, vol. 54, no. 3, pp. 491–8.

56 Boschma, *The rise of mental health nursing*; Shorter, *A history of psychiatry*.

57 Mooney, G. and Reinarz, J. 2009, *Permeable walls: historical perspectives on hospital and asylum visiting*, Rodopi, New York; Whyte, J. 2011, "Visiting the mentally ill: volunteer visitors at Saskatchewan Hospital, Weyburn 1950–1965," *Histoire Sociale/Social History*, vol. 44, no. 88, pp. 289–304.

58 Boschma, "A family point of view"; Cellard, A. and Thifault, M.C. 2006, "The uses of asylums: resistance, asylum propaganda, and institutionalization strategies in turn-of-the-century Quebec," in J. Moran and D. Wright (eds), *Mental health and Canadian society: historical perspectives*, McGill-Queen's University Press, Montreal; Lanzoni, S. 2005, "The

asylum in context: an essay review," *Journal of the History of Medicine and Allied Sciences*, vol. 60, no. 4, pp. 499–505; Moran, *Committed to the state asylum*; Moran and Wright, *Mental health and Canadian society*.

59 Boschma et al., "Oral history research."

60 Harrington, V. 2008, "Voices beyond the asylum: a post-war history of mental health services in Manchester and Salford," PhD dissertation, University of Manchester.

61 Nolan, *A history of mental health nursing*, was one of the first to examine this more recent time period using oral history.

62 Freeman, H. 2005, "Psychiatry and the state in Britain," in Gijswijt-Hofstra et al., *Psychiatric cultures compared*; Oosterhuis, "Outpatient psychiatry."

63 Nolan, *A history of mental health nursing*; for Canada see Martin, "Determinants of destiny."

64 Boschma, "Deinstitutionalization reconsidered."

65 Wilkinson, G. 1994, "Douglas Bennett: in conversation with Greg Wilkinson," *Psychiatric Bulletin*, vol. 18, pp. 622–6; Harrington, "Voices beyond the asylum."

66 Boschma et al., "Gender and professional identity"; Martin, "Determinants of destiny"; Nolan, *A history of mental health nursing*.

67 Martin, "Determinants of destiny."

68 Sheridan, A. 2000, "Analysis of the activities of psychiatric nurses practicing in Ireland, 1950–2000," PhD dissertation, University of Birmingham; Sheridan, A. 2006, "The impact of political transition on psychiatric nursing – a case study of twentieth-century Ireland," *Nursing Inquiry*, vol. 13, no. 4, pp. 289–9.

69 Prebble, "Ordinary men and uncommon women."

70 Harrington, "Voices beyond the asylum."

71 Ibid., pp. 196–258.

72 Ibid. See Wolfensberger, W. 1972, *Normalization: the principle of normalization in human services*, National Institute on Mental Retardation, Toronto.

73 Dyck, E. and Fletcher, C. (eds) 2011, *Locating health: historical and anthropological investigations of place and health*, Pickering and Chatto, London; Elliot, J., Toman, C., and Stuart, M. (eds) 2008, *Place and practice in Canadian nursing history*, UBC Press, Vancouver; Parr, H. 2008, *Mental health and social space: towards inclusionary geographies?*, Wiley-Blackwell, Edinburgh.

74 Bartlett, P. and Wright, D. (eds) 1999, *Outside the walls of the asylum: the history of care in the community, 1750–2000*, Athlone Press, London; Dyck and Fletcher, *Locating health*; Moran and Wright, *Mental health and Canadian society*; Parr, *Mental health and social space*.

75 Boschma, "Community mental health nursing"; Fingard and Rutherford, *Protect, befriend, respect*.

76 D'Antonio, *American nursing*; Dyck, "Dismantling the asylum."

77 Boschma, "Community mental health nursing"; Boschma, G., Haney, C., and Gorrie, M. 2012 "Gender, work, and identity: consumer perspectives on rehabilitation and recovery in mental health care," *Bulletin of the UK Association for the History of Nursing*, vol. 1, no. 1, pp. 8–19.

78 Boschma et al., "Gender and professional identity"; Boschma et al., "Gender, work, and identity"; Elliot et al., *Place and practice*; Hicks, "Gender, politics, and regionalism"; Nolan, *A history of mental health nursing*; Prebble, "Ordinary men and uncommon women."

79 Davies, K. 2001, "'Silent and censured travelers?' Patients' narratives and patients' voices: perspectives on the history of mental illness since 1948," *Social History of Medicine*, vol. 14, no. 2, pp. 267–92; Porter, *A social history of madness*; Reaume, *Remembrance of patients past*.

80 Beers, *A mind that found itself*.

81 Beamish, D. 2003, *King of the world, poems and prose* (chapbook), Vancouver, t.p. verso; Chamberlain, *On our own*; Davies, "Silent and censured travelers?"; Ingram, R. 2005, "Troubled being and being troubled: subjectivity in the light of problems of the mind," PhD dissertation, University of British Columbia; Kaysen, S. 1993, *Girl, interrupted*,

Turtle Bay Books, New York; Plath, S. 1963, *The bell jar*, Faber, London; Shimrat, *Call me crazy*.

82 Baur, N. 2011, "On site: oral testimonies in mental health history," *Social History of Medicine*, vol. 24, no. 2, pp. 484–7; Ingram, "Troubled being and being troubled"; Kerr, D. 2003, "'We know what the problem is': using oral history to develop a collaborative analysis of homelessness from the bottom up," *Oral History Review*, vol. 30, no. 1, pp. 27–45.

83 Kesey, K. 1962, *One flew over the cuckoo's nest*, Viking Press, New York; Hirshbein, L. & Sarvananda, S. 2008, "History, power, and electricity: American popular magazine accounts of electroconvulsive therapy, 1940–2005," *Journal of the History of the Behavioral Sciences*, vol. 44, no. 1, pp. 1–18.

84 Burstow, B. & Weitz, D. (eds) 1988, *Shrink resistant: the struggle against psychiatry in Canada*, New Star Books, Vancouver; Chamberlain, *On our own*; Crossley, *Contesting psychiatry*; Harrington, "Voices beyond the asylum"; "Documentary *Mental Patients' Association* DVD-R 0177005" 1977, directed by R. Patton, produced by S. Blejic and P. Jones, National Film Board of Canada; Morrison, L. 2005, *Talking back to psychiatry: the consumer/survivor/ex-patient movement*, Routledge, London; Tonkens, E. and Weijers, I. 1999, "Autonomy, care and self-realization. Policy views of Dutch service providers," *Mental Retardation: The Journal of the American Association of Mental Retardation*, vol. 37, no. 6, pp. 468–76.

85 Crossley, *Contesting psychiatry*; Shimrat, *Call me crazy*.

86 Tomes, N. 2006, "The patient as a policy factor: a historical case study of the consumer/survivor movement in mental health," *Health Affairs*, vol. 25, pp. 720–9; Tomes, "From outsiders to insiders."

87 Everett, B. 2000, *A fragile revolution: consumers and psychiatric survivors confront the power of the mental health system*, Wilfred Laurier University Press, Waterloo; Hoffman, B., Tomes, N., Grob, R., and Schlesinger, M. (eds) 2011, *Patients as policy actors*, Rutgers, New Brunswick, NJ; Hunsche, P. 2008 *De strijdbare patient: Van gekkenbeweging tot cliëntenbewustzijn—Portretten 1970–2000 [The patient fighter: From mad-movement to client consciousness—Portraits 1970–2000]*, Uitgeverij Candide, Amsterdam; Kneeland, T.W. and Warren, C.A.B. 2002, *Pushbutton psychiatry: a history of electroshock in America*, Praeger, Westport, CT.

88 Davies, "Silent and censured travelers?", p. 273.

89 Reaume, G. 2006, "Patients at work: insane asylum inmates' labour in Ontario, 1841–1900," in J. Moran and D. Wright (eds), *Mental health and Canadian society: historical perspectives*, McGill-Queen's University Press, Montreal.

90 Shimrat, *Call me crazy*.

91 Boschma et al., "Gender, work, and identity."

92 Harrington, "Voices beyond the asylum."

93 Boevink, W. 2000, "Ervaring, Ervaringskennis, Ervaringsdeskundigheid [Experience, Experience-Based Knowledge, Experiential Expertise]," *Deviant*, vol. 26, pp. 4–9; Borkes, K. 2008, "My recovery: a long and winding road," *Peace of Mind—Bi-Annual Newsletter of the Canadian Mental Health Association, Simon Fraser Branch*, vol. 7, p. 11; Interview with Borkes, K. by author and M. Gorrie, New Westminster, April 2009 (Borkes used the notion of prosumer); Tsai, A. 2002, "The experiences of a 'prosumer,'" *Psychiatric Rehabilitation Journal*, vol. 26, no. 2, pp. 206–7.

94 "Pioneer House to open soon under Riverview volunteers" 1982, *Insight, Riverview Hospital Newsletter*, vol. 1, no. 8, p. 1; Interview with Dewar; Interview with Beamish, 2011.

95 Thompson, R.H. 1972, *A summary of the growth and development of mental health facilities in British Columbia, 1850–1970*, Mental Health Branch, BC Government, BC; Tucker, F.G. 1971, "Mental health services in British Columbia," *Canada's Mental Health*, vol. 19, no. 6, pp. 7–12; Riverview Hospital Volunteer Association (RHVA) 1981, "Proposal for the use of Pioneer House," unpublished document.

96 RHVA, "Proposal for the use of Pioneer House."

97 Booth, B. 1961, "Family care homes for mental patients," MSW thesis, University of British Columbia; Boschma, "Deinstitutionalization reconsidered"; Crum, M. and Jamieson, J. 1972, "An analysis of the British Columbia regional boarding home programme," Master's Thesis, University of British Columbia; Fingard and Rutherford, *Protect, befriend, respect.*

98 Interview with Russell, C.A. by N. Bonifacio, New Westminster, August 2009.

99 Certificate of Incorporation (Note 4).

100 Mental Health Services Branch of British Columbia (MHSB) *Annual Reports* (AR), 1951–74, Victoria BC, Deposited in the Woodward Library of the University of British Columbia. Hereafter cited as MHSB, AR, and year: MHSB, AR, 1956, pp. Q63; MHSB, AR 1955, M99; MHSB 1961, pp. H57–8; Baird, S. 1974, "Riverview's volunteer activities—1973," *Newsletter, Mental Health Branch, Department of Health Services and Hospital Insurance*, March 1974, pp. 11–12; Mental Patients' Association 1983, *Head on: into the eighties*, Carolina Publications, Vancouver; Beamish, D. 1976, "MPA Riverview extension program," *In a Nutshell, The MPA Newsletter*, vol. 4, no. 4, p. 5.

101 Beamish, "MPA Riverview extension program."

102 MHSB, AR 1967, pp. G57–8.

103 Ibid., pp. G47–8; Coppard, A.E. 1963, *Rehabilitation programme* (staff publication), Riverview Hospital, British Columbia; Jones, M. 1953, *The therapeutic community: a new treatment method in psychiatry*, Basic Books, New York.

104 CMHA (Canadian Mental Health Association) 1960, *Milestones in mental health: a record of achievements . . . the Canadian Mental Health Association 1918–1958*, CMHA, Toronto; Baird, "Riverview's volunteer activities."

105 Beamish, D. 1973, "Hospital visiting," *In a Nutshell, The MPA Newsletter*, vol. 2, no. 1, p. 5; Strickland, N. 1973, "Way out of a blind alley," *The Province* (Thursday September 27, 1973), p. 42.

106 Mental Patients' Association, *Head on.*

107 Mental Patients' Association, *Head on;* Strickland, "Way out."

108 Beamish, "MPA Riverview extension program"; Interview Beamish, 2011; Interview with Tremere, A. by author and C. Haney, New Westminster, December 2011.

109 Certificate of Incorporation.

110 Interview with Beamish, D. by M. Davies, Vancouver, June 2010 (Obtained from M. Davies, Open Doors/After the Asylum Project); Interview with Beamish, 2011.

111 Crum and Jamieson, "An analysis of the British Columbia regional boarding home programme."

112 Phillips, F. 1976, "MPA residence program: in memoriam," *In a Nutshell, The MPA Newsletter*, vol. 4, no. 2, p. 12; "Pioneer House to open." The sources were unclear about the nature of Phillips' degree, but it met the licensing requirement.

113 Interview with Beamish, 2011; Phillips, "MPA residence program."

114 Interview with Dewar.

115 Interview with Russell.

116 Interview with Dewar.

117 Mental Health Services, BC Ministry of Health, *Annual Report* 1981, Victoria, BC, pp. 90–1.

118 Interview with Beamish, 2011.

119 Interview with Dewar.

120 Interview with Russell.

INDEX

Page numbers in *italics* denotes an illustration

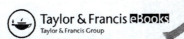